Recent Progress in Urology Research

Recent Progress in Urology Research

Edited by Timothy Lawson

hayle medical
New York

Hayle Medical,
750 Third Avenue, 9th Floor,
New York, NY 10017, USA

Visit us on the World Wide Web at:
www.haylemedical.com

ISBN: 978-1-63241-777-0

Cataloging-in-Publication Data

Recent progress in urology research / edited by Timothy Lawson.
    p. cm.
Includes bibliographical references and index.
ISBN 978-1-63241-777-0
1. Urology. 2. Urology--Research. 3. Genitourinary organs--Diseases. I. Lawson, Timothy.
RC871 .R43 2019
616.6--dc23

Contents

Preface   IX

Chapter 1

**Urinary incontinence, mental health and loneliness among community-dwelling
older adults**   1
Andrew Stickley, Ziggi Ivan Santini and Ai Koyanagi

Chapter 2

**Management of large renal stones: laparoscopic pyelolithotomy versus percutaneous
nephrolithotomy**   10
Yunjin Bai, Yin Tang, Lan Deng, Xiaoming Wang, Yubo Yang, Jia Wang and Ping Han

Chapter 3

Assessing health-related quality of life in urology – a survey of 4500 German urologists   19
A. Schmick, M. Juergensen, V. Rohde, A. Katalinic and A. Waldmann

Chapter 4

**Symptom clusters and related factors in bladder cancer patients three months after
radical cystectomy**   30
Hongyan Ren, Ping Tang, Qinghua Zhao and Guosheng Ren

Chapter 5

**A gonadotropin-releasing hormone antagonist reduces serum adrenal androgen
levels in prostate cancer patients**   37
*Yoshiyuki Miyazawa, Yoshitaka Sekine, Takahiro Syuto, Masashi Nomura, Hidekazu Koike,
Hiroshi Matsui, Yasuhiro Shibata, Kazuto Ito and Kazuhiro Suzuki*

Chapter 6

**Anti-proliferative potential of Glucosamine in renal cancer cells via inducing cell cycle
arrest at G0/G1 phase**   43
*Long-sheng Wang, Shao-jun Chen, Jun-feng Zhang, Meng-nan Liu, Jun-hua Zheng and
Xu-dong Yao*

Chapter 7

**Assembling and validating data from multiple sources to study care for Veterans with
bladder cancer**   51
Florian R. Schroeck, Brenda Sirovich, John D. Seigne, Douglas J. Robertson and Philip P. Goodney

Chapter 8

**Alpha$_{1A}$-adrenoceptor antagonist improves underactive bladder associated with
diabetic cystopathy via bladder blood flow in rats**   58
Saori Yonekubo, Satoshi Tatemichi, Kazuyasu Maruyama and Mamoru Kobayashi

Chapter 9

A low psoas muscle volume correlates with a longer hospitalization after radical cystectomy   66
Yoko Saitoh-Maeda, Takashi Kawahara, Yasuhide Miyoshi, Sohgo Tsutsumi, Daiji Takamoto, Kota Shimokihara, Yuutaro Hayashi, Taku Mochizuki, Mari Ohtaka, Manami Nakamura, Yusuke Hattori, Jun-ichi Teranishi, Yasushi Yumura, Kimito Osaka, Hiroki Ito, Kazuhide Makiyama, Noboru Nakaigawa, Masahiro Yao and Hiroji Uemura

Chapter 10

The neutrophil-to-lymphocyte ratio (NLR) predicts adrenocortical carcinoma and is correlated with the prognosis   71
Taku Mochizuki, Takashi Kawahara, Daiji Takamoto, Kazuhide Makiyama, Yusuke Hattori, Jun-ichi Teranishi, Yasuhide Miyoshi, Yasushi Yumura, Masahiro Yao and Hiroji Uemura

Chapter 11

Real life persistence rate with antimuscarinic treatment in patients with idiopathic or neurogenic overactive bladder: a prospective cohort study with solifenacin   75
Marloes J. Tijnagel, Jeroen R. Scheepe and Bertil F. M. Blok

Chapter 12

Ureteral reconstruction using a tapered non-vascularized bladder graft   79
Lujia Zou, Shanhua Mao, Shenghua Liu, Limin Zhang, Tian Yang, Yun Hu, Qiang Ding and Haowen Jiang

Chapter 13

Heterogeneity in high-risk prostate cancer treated with high-dose radiation therapy and androgen deprivation therapy   85
Daniel N. Cagney, Mary Dunne, Carmel O'Shea, Marie Finn, Emma Noone, Martina Sheehan, Lesley McDonagh, Lydia O'Sullivan, Pierre Thirion and John Armstrong

Chapter 14

The usefulness of flexible cystoscopy for preventing double-J stent malposition after laparoscopic ureterolithotomy   93
Jae-Yoon Kim, Seok-Ho Kang, Jun Cheon, Jeong-Gu Lee, Je-Jong Kim and Sung-Gu Kang

Chapter 15

Presence of transient hydronephrosis immediately after surgery has a limited influence on renal function 1 year after ileal neobladder construction   99
Takuma Narita, Shingo Hatakeyama, Takuya Koie, Shogo Hosogoe, Teppei Matsumoto, Osamu Soma, Hayato Yamamoto, Tohru Yoneyama, Yuki Tobisawa, Takahiro Yoneyama, Yasuhiro Hashimoto and Chikara Ohyama

Chapter 16

Toileting behaviors and overactive bladder in patients with type 2 diabetes   107
Dongjuan Xu, Ran Cheng, Aixia Ma, Meng Zhao and Kefang Wang

Chapter 17

Suprapubic tube versus urethral catheter drainage after robot-assisted radical prostatectomy   114
Zhongyu Jian, Shijian Feng, Yuntian Chen, Xin Wei, Deyi Luo, Hong Li and Kunjie Wang

Chapter 18

Penile cancer in Maranhão, Northeast Brazil: the highest incidence globally?   121
Ronald Wagner Pereira Coelho, Jaqueline Diniz Pinho, Janise Silva Moreno,
Dimitrius Vidal e Oliveira Garbis, Athiene Maniva Teixeira do Nascimento,
Joyce Santos Larges, José Ribamar Rodrigues Calixto, Leandra Naira Zambelli Ramalho,
Antônio Augusto Moura da Silva, Leudivan Ribeiro Nogueira,
Laisson de Moura Feitoza and Gyl Eanes Barros Silva

Chapter 19

Unilateral pedal lymphangiography plus computed tomography angiography for location of persistent idiopathic chyle leakage not detectable by ordinary contrast computed tomography   128
Dingyi Liu, Boke Liu, Weimu Xia, Qi Tang, Haidong Wang, Jian Wang, Yanfeng Zhou,
Jiashun Yu, Wenmin Li, Mingwei Wang, Wenlong Zhou, Sang Hu and Yuan Shao

Chapter 20

Cost implications of PSA screening differ by age   133
Karthik Rao, Stella Liang, Michael Cardamone, Corinne E. Joshu, Kyle Marmen,
Nrupen Bhavsar, William G. Nelson, H. Ballentine Carter, Michael C. Albert,
Elizabeth A. Platz and Craig E. Pollack

Chapter 21

Obesity impairs male fertility through long-term effects on spermatogenesis   141
Yan-Fei Jia, Qian Feng, Zheng-Yan Ge, Ying Guo, Fang Zhou, Kai-Shu Zhang,
Xiao-Wei Wang, Wen-Hong Lu, Xiao-Wei Liang and Yi-Qun Gu

Chapter 22

Antihypertensive drugs use and the risk of prostate cancer   149
Liang Cao, Sha Zhang, Cheng-ming Jia, Wei He, Lei-tao Wu, Ying-qi Li, Wen Wang,
Zhe Li and Jing Ma

Chapter 23

Prognostic significance of epidermal growth factor receptor (EGFR) over expression in urothelial carcinoma of urinary bladder   163
Atif Ali hashmi, Zubaida Fida Hussain, Muhammad Irfan, Erum Yousuf Khan,
Naveen Faridi, Hanna Naqvi, Amir Khan and Muhammad Muzzammil Edhi

Chapter 24

Efficacy analysis of self-help position therapy after holmium laser lithotripsy via flexible ureteroscopy   169
Jie Yang, Rong-zhen Tao, Pei Lu, Meng-xing Chen, Xin-kun Huang, Ke-liang Chen,
Ying-heng Huang, Xiao-rong He, Li-di Wan, Jing Wang, Xin Tang and Wei Zhang

Chapter 25

The effect of mirabegron, used for overactive bladder treatment, on female
sexual function: a prospective controlled study   176
*A. Zachariou, C. Mamoulakis, M. Filiponi, F. Dimitriadis, J. Giannakis, S. Skouros,
P. Tsounapi, A. Takenaka and N. Sofikitis*

Chapter 26

Surgical management of urolithiasis – a systematic analysis of available guidelines   184
*Valentin Zumstein, Patrick Betschart, Dominik Abt, Hans-Peter Schmid,
Cedric Michael Panje and Paul Martin Putora*

Chapter 27

Scrotal hemorrhage after testicular sperm aspiration may be associated with
phosphodiesterase-5 inhibitor administration   192
Yong-tong Zhu, Rui Hua, Song Quan, Wan-long Tan, Qing-jun Chu and Chun-yan Wang

Chapter 28

Fibroblast growth factor receptor 3 (FGFR3) aberrations in muscle-invasive
urothelial carcinoma   196
Young Saing Kim, Kyung Kim, Ghee-Young Kwon, Su Jin Lee and Se Hoon Park

Chapter 29

Prognostic significance of the combination of preoperative hemoglobin and
albumin levels and lymphocyte and platelet counts (HALP) in patients with renal
cell carcinoma after nephrectomy   203
*Ding Peng, Cui-jian Zhang, Qi Tang, Lei Zhang, Kai-wei Yang, Xiao-teng Yu, Yanqing Gong,
Xue-song Li, Zhi-song He and Li-qun Zhou*

Chapter 30

Perineural invasion as an independent predictor of biochemical recurrence in
prostate cancer following radical prostatectomy or radiotherapy
Li-jin Zhang, Bin Wu, Zhen-lei Zha, Wei Qu, Hu Zhao, Jun Yuan and Ye-jun Feng   211

Chapter 31

Decolonization potential of 0.02% polyhexanide irrigation solution in urethral
catheters under practice-like in vitro conditions   221
*Florian H. H. Brill, Henrik Gabriel, Holger Brill, Jan-Hendrik Klock,
Joerg Steinmann and Andreas Arndt*

Permissions

Contributors

Index

Preface

In my initial years as a student, I used to run to the library at every possible instance to grab a book and learn something new. Books were my primary source of knowledge and I would not have come such a long way without all that I learnt from them. Thus, when I was approached to edit this book; I became understandably nostalgic. It was an absolute honor to be considered worthy of guiding the current generation as well as those to come. I put all my knowledge and hard work into making this book most beneficial for its readers.

The area of study related to the diseases of the male and female urinary-tract system and the male reproductive organs is known as urology. The kidneys, urinary bladder, adrenal glands, testes, prostate, seminal vesicles and penis are some of the organs studied under the branch of urology. Both the urinary tract and the reproductive tract are closely associated with each other. Therefore, the diseases of one usually affect the other. Examples of urological disorders include urinary-tract infections, prostate cancer, traumatic injury, kidney stones, congenital abnormalities, etc. Minimally invasive robotic surgery and laparoscopic surgery are two common ways to treat urological disorders. This book elucidates the concepts and innovative models around prospective developments with respect to urology. It strives to provide a fair idea about this discipline and to help develop a better understanding of the latest advances within this field. The extensive content of this book provides the readers with a thorough understanding of the subject.

I wish to thank my publisher for supporting me at every step. I would also like to thank all the authors who have contributed their researches in this book. I hope this book will be a valuable contribution to the progress of the field.

Editor

Urinary incontinence, mental health and loneliness among community-dwelling older adults

Andrew Stickley[1]*, Ziggi Ivan Santini [2] and Ai Koyanagi[3]

Abstract

Background: Urinary incontinence (UI) is associated with worse health among older adults. Little is known however, about its relation with loneliness or the role of mental health in this association. This study examined these factors among older adults in Ireland.

Methods: Data were analyzed from 6903 community-dwelling adults aged ≥ 50 collected in the first wave of The Irish Longitudinal Study on Ageing (TILDA) in 2009–11. Information was obtained on the self-reported occurrence (yes/no) and severity (frequency/activity limitations) of UI in the past 12 months. Loneliness was measured using the UCLA Loneliness Scale short form. Information was also obtained on depression (CES-D), anxiety (HADS-A) and other sociodemographic variables. Logistic regression analysis was used to examine the association between variables.

Results: In a model adjusted for all potential confounders except mental disorders, compared to no UI, any UI was associated with significantly higher odds for loneliness (odds ratio: 1.51). When depression was included in the analysis, the association was attenuated and became non-significant while the inclusion of anxiety had a much smaller effect. Similarly, although frequency of UI and activity limitations due to UI were both significantly associated with loneliness prior to adjustment for mental disorders, neither association remained significant after adjustment for both depression and anxiety.

Conclusion: UI is associated with higher odds for loneliness among older community-dwelling adults but this association is largely explained by comorbid mental health problems, in particular, depression.

Keywords: Urinary incontinence, Lonely, Anxiety, Depression

Background

Urinary incontinence (UI), which is defined as the involuntary leakage of urine [1] is highly prevalent in the general population and can severely affect many aspects of daily life [2, 3]. Although this condition can exist in adults of all ages [3], a large body of research has shown that the prevalence of UI increases with age [4, 5] and that the elderly are especially vulnerable to this condition [6] particularly in a severe form [7, 8]. While previously reported prevalence figures vary due to the different operational definitions of UI employed (type,

severity etc.), an earlier review article presented figures which showed that the prevalence of UI ranges between 9 and 59% in those aged 50 and above [9].

Studies have indicated that UI can have a significant negative effect on the lives of older people [10]. For example, it has been associated with troublesome symptoms such as aches, pain, weakness, and shortness of breath [11], as well as with an increased risk for outcomes such as falls and fractures [12, 13]. The avoidance of physical activity in an attempt to manage/control the condition may also have an effect on overall health by increasing the risk of conditions such as hypertension [14, 15]. In addition, UI is also associated with poorer mental health among older persons including anxiety disorders [16] and depression [16, 17].

* Correspondence: amstick66@gmail.com
[1]The Stockholm Center for Health and Social Change (SCOHOST), Södertörn University, Huddinge 141 89, Sweden
Full list of author information is available at the end of the article

Despite the large number of studies on UI and its associated adverse health outcomes, one condition which has been little studied to date in relation to UI is loneliness. This is an important research gap given that: (a) incontinent individuals can experience feelings of frustration, embarrassment and shame [18, 19] as a result of their condition and will sometimes reduce/avoid social contacts and activities in order to control UI and its effects [18], which may lead to increased social isolation and feelings of loneliness; and (b) loneliness has itself been linked to an increased risk for morbidity and mortality among older persons [20, 21]. To the best of our knowledge, to date, there have been only three studies which have investigated this association. Specifically, two recent studies have shown that older adults (≥57 years old) with UI in Canada and the United States have an increased risk of feeling lonely compared to those who are continent [22] or who have no/less severe UI symptoms (no/weekly/monthly/yearly vs. daily) [23], respectively. An earlier study from the United States also found similar results where UI and UI severity (measured by the quantity of urine loss) were both associated with loneliness among middle-aged and older adults (≥ 40 years old) [24].

Although these studies have advanced understanding of the psychological consequences of UI, there are aspects of the association between UI and loneliness among older adults that are yet to be elucidated. In particular, there has been an absence of research on the role of common mental disorders (CMDs) in this association. This is an important gap in the research as not only are anxiety and depression linked to UI in older persons [16, 17], but other research has highlighted their close link with loneliness in older adults [25–27] and that in middle-aged and older adults, depressive symptoms and loneliness may be reciprocally related [28]. Therefore, there is a need to assess the extent to which CMDs explain the association between UI and loneliness. In addition, until now, there has been no research on whether the specific consequences of UI, such as activity limitations, are important for loneliness in older adults.

Thus, using data from a nationally representative sample of community-dwelling older adults (aged 50 and above) in Ireland, the current study had three aims: (1) to determine if UI is associated with an increased risk of feeling lonely; (2) to examine if the severity of UI, as measured by the frequency of urine loss and activity limitations, is associated with loneliness; and (3) to assess the role of CMDs in the association between UI, UI severity and loneliness.

Methods
Study design and sample
The data used in this study came from the first wave of The Irish Longitudinal Study on Ageing (TILDA) which was conducted by Trinity College Dublin between October 2009 and February 2011. Details of the survey and its sampling procedure have been published previously [29, 30]. In brief, TILDA was a nationally representative survey of community-based adults aged 50 and above living in Ireland. The target sample included every household resident meeting this age criterion. Clustered random sampling was used to obtain a nationally representative sample. Individuals who were institutionalized and those who had doctor-diagnosed dementia were excluded. If severe cognitive impairment (judged at the interviewer's discretion) prevented individuals from providing written informed consent to participate in the survey, they were also excluded [31]. The data was collected by trained interviewers using computer-assisted personal interviewing (CAPI), and with the use of self-completion questionnaires (SCQs). All individuals that underwent a CAPI interview were also asked to complete the SCQ. The overall response rate was 62%, while 84% of those who participated in the survey returned the SCQ [29, 30].

In total, 8504 people aged ≥50 years (n = 8175) and their spouses or partners younger than 50 years (n = 329) comprised the survey sample. In the current study, the analysis was restricted to participants aged 50 years and above and those who completed the SCQ. These conditions were necessary as information on certain variables (e.g., loneliness, anxiety etc.) was obtained from the SCQ. Following these restrictions, the analytic sample comprised 6903 individuals. The Faculty of Health Sciences Ethics Committee of Trinity College Dublin provided ethical approval for TILDA, with written informed consent being obtained from all participants.

Measures
Loneliness (Dependent variable)
The short form of the University of California, Los Angeles (UCLA) Loneliness Scale was used to assess feelings of loneliness [32, 33]. The short form UCLA Loneliness Scale, which assesses subjective feelings of social isolation, is a commonly used measure in loneliness research. The dominant factor underlying the UCLA Loneliness scale is 'perceived social isolation' [34, 35]. The UCLA three-item scale is comprised of three negatively-worded questions relating to feelings of isolation, feeling left out and companionship. The three response options are coded as 1 (hardly ever), 2 (some of the time), and 3 (often). Scores are summed to create a total score that runs from 3 to 9, with higher scores indicating a greater degree of loneliness (Cronbach's alpha = 0.81). Previous research has indicated that this scale has an acceptable degree of reliability and has both concurrent and discriminant validity [33]. As the distribution of the loneliness variable was right-skewed, in this study we used a dichotomous loneliness variable for the regression

analyses. Specifically, in accordance with a recent study, a score of 4–9 was categorized as feeling lonely while a score of 3 (i.e., replying 'hardly ever' to all of the questions) was classified as not feeling lonely [22].

Urinary incontinence (UI) (Independent variable)

Any UI was assessed by the question 'During the last 12 months, have you lost any amount of urine beyond your control?' with the answer options 'yes' or 'no'. For those who responded affirmatively to this question, follow-up questions on the frequency of UI and limitations in activity due to UI were asked. Frequency was assessed by the question 'Did this happen more than once during a 1 month period?' and activity limitations were examined by the question 'Do you ever limit your activities, for example, what you do or where you go, because of UI?' Both of these questions had 'yes' or 'no' as answer options.

Depression

Depressive symptoms were measured with the 20-item Center for Epidemiologic Studies Depression (CES-D) scale [36], which assesses symptoms experienced in the preceding week. Its 20 items are scored on a scale from 0 (rarely or none of the time, less than one day in the week) to 3 (most or all of the time, five to seven days in the week). In order to avoid an overlap with the outcome (loneliness), and following the lead of an earlier study [37], we excluded the item on loneliness ('I felt lonely') that is included in the CES-D scale. Thus, scores from the remaining 19 items were summed to create a scale with values ranging from 0 to 57 where higher scores signified more depressive symptoms (Cronbach's alpha = 0.87). Previous studies have highlighted the validity of the CES-D scale as a measure of depression in community-dwelling older adults [38, 39].

Anxiety

The Hospital Anxiety and Depression Scale (HADS-A) [40] was used to assess anxiety symptoms. This scale measures the presence of anxiety symptoms without reference to a specific time frame. The scale consists of seven items rated on a four-point scale from 0 (not at all) to 3 (very often indeed), five of which are reverse coded. The scores from the individual items were summed to create a total score that ranged from 0 to 21, with higher scores indicating more anxiety (Cronbach's alpha = 0.65). Previous research has indicated that the HADS is a reliable measure in both younger and older persons [41].

Control variables

Social network index

The Berkman-Syme Social Network Index (SNI) was used to assess social networks. The SNI is a validated self-report questionnaire [42] that assesses the degree to which a person is socially integrated. Information is elicited on marital/partnership status (married/with partner versus not), sociability (number of children, close relatives, and close friends and the frequency of contact with them), and church group or community organization membership. A composite score is calculated that ranges from 0 to 4. In this study, we used what is regarded as the standard categorization [i.e., 0–1 (most isolated), 2 (moderately isolated), 3 (moderately integrated), and 4 (most integrated)] [42]. Further information on the psychometric properties of the SNI and evidence relating to its predictive validity has been provided elsewhere [43].

Chronic medical conditions

To assess chronic health conditions, participants were presented with a list of 17 medical conditions and asked, "has a doctor ever told you that you have any of the conditions on this card?" These conditions were: high blood pressure or hypertension; angina; heart attack (including myocardial or coronary thrombosis); congestive heart failure; diabetes or high blood sugar; stroke (cerebral vascular disease); ministroke or transient ischemic attack; high cholesterol; heart murmur; abnormal heart rhythm; any other heart trouble; chronic lung disease such as chronic bronchitis or emphysema; asthma; arthritis (including osteoarthritis, or rheumatism); osteoporosis; cancer or a malignant tumor (including leukemia or lymphoma but excluding minor skin cancers); cirrhosis or serious liver damage. The total number of chronic medical conditions was calculated and divided into three categories: 0 (none), 1, or ≥2.

Activities of daily living (ADL) disability

To assess ADL disability participants were asked to indicate whether they had difficulty performing six activities (dressing, walking, bathing, eating, getting in or out of bed, and using the toilet) [44]. Participants having difficulty with one or more ADLs were categorized as having an ADL disability.

Sociodemographic variables

Sociodemographic characteristics included age (50–59, 60–69, 70–79, and ≥80 years), sex, education, and wealth. Education was divided into three categories: primary (some primary/not complete; primary or equivalent); secondary (intermediate/junior/group certificate or equivalent; leaving certificate or equivalent); and tertiary (diploma/certificate; primary degree; postgraduate/higher degree). As more than 50% of the income values were missing, a proxy measure (financial strain) was used to assess wealth. Participants were thus asked to respond to the statement that a 'shortage of money stops me from doing the things I want to do' using one of the answer options, 'never', 'rarely', 'sometimes', and 'often'.

Statistical analysis

Stata version 14.1 (Stata Corp LP, College Station, Texas) was used to perform the analysis. In the first stage, descriptive statistics are presented of the study sample. The difference in sample characteristics by the presence of UI was tested by using Chi-square and Student's t-tests for categorical and continuous variables, respectively. Logistic regression analysis was then used to firstly assess the association between any UI (independent variable) and loneliness (dependent variable) based on the question 'During the last 12 months, have you lost any amount of urine beyond your control?'. A hierarchical analysis was conducted by including different variables sequentially in different models to assess how these variables influenced the

association between UI and loneliness. Six different models were thus constructed: Model 1: unadjusted; Model 2: adjusted for age, sex, education, financial strain, number of chronic conditions, and ADL disability; Model 3: adjusted for the variables in Model 2 and the SNI; Model 4: adjusted for the variables in Model 3 and depression; Model 5: adjusted for the variables in Model 3 and anxiety; Model 6: adjusted for the variables in Model 3, depression, and anxiety. The selection of the variables used for adjustment was based on past literature.

To assess the association between UI severity and loneliness, we repeated the analytic method described above but replaced the any UI variable with a three-category UI variable which incorporates the frequency of urinary inconsistence [UI (-); UI (+) once a month or less; UI (+) more than once a month], or activity limitations due to UI [UI (-); UI (+) but no activity limitations; UI (+) with

Table 1 Sample characteristics (overall and by urinary incontinence)

| Characteristic | Categories | Overall | Urinary incontinence | | P-value[a] |
			No	Yes	
Age (years)	50–59	40.5	41.9	30.3	<0.001
	60–69	30.7	30.9	29.8	
	70–79	20.0	19.2	25.1	
	≥80	8.8	7.9	14.9	
Sex	Male	47.9	51.4	23.8	<0.001
	Female	52.1	48.6	76.2	
Education	Primary	38.1	37.2	44.0	<0.001
	Secondary	43.3	44.1	38.3	
	Tertiary	18.6	18.8	17.6	
Financial strain	Never	23.1	23.4	20.7	<0.001
	Rarely	21.6	21.7	21.5	
	Sometimes	36.4	36.8	33.3	
	Often	18.9	18.1	24.6	
Number of	None	23.4	25.2	11.5	<0.001
chronic conditions	One	28.1	28.8	22.9	
	Two or more	48.5	46.0	65.6	
ADL disability	No	90.9	92.7	78.7	<0.001
	Yes	9.1	7.3	21.3	
Social Network Index	Most isolated	7.5	7.0	10.5	0.011
	Moderately isolated	28.8	28.9	27.4	
	Moderately integrated	41.0	41.1	40.3	
	Most integrated	22.7	22.9	21.9	
Depression	Mean (SD)	5.7 (6.8)	5.2 (6.4)	9.1 (8.6)	<0.001
Anxiety	Mean (SD)	5.5 (3.7)	5.3 (3.6)	6.7 (4.1)	<0.001

The data are column percentages unless otherwise stated
Estimates are based on weighted sample
Abbreviation: ADL Activities of daily living, SD Standard deviation
[a]The difference in sample characteristics by urinary incontinence was tested by Chi-square tests and Student's t-tests for categorical and continuous variables, respectively

activity limitations]. This analysis used 'no UI' as the reference category. Finally, we also performed this analysis while restricting it to those with UI to assess whether the frequency of UI or activity limitations due to UI confers an increased risk for loneliness among those with UI. All variables included in the models were categorical variables apart from depression and anxiety which were continuous variables. The dataset also included sampling weights that were created based on the age, sex and educational attainment values in the Quarterly National Household Survey 2010. In order to obtain nationally representative estimates, the sample weighting and the complex study design, including within household clustering, was taken into account in all analyses. Results are expressed as odds ratios (OR) and 95% confidence intervals (95% CIs). A p-value <0.05 was considered to be statistically significant.

Results

The mean age (standard deviation) of the sample was 63.6 (9.2) years and 52.1% were women. Overall, the prevalence of any UI was 12.4% (95% CI = 11.5–13.4%). Among those with UI, it occurred more than once a month in 76.6%, and 26.4% had activity limitations due to UI. The sample characteristics are shown in Table 1. Older age, female sex, lower education, financial strain, a higher number of chronic conditions, ADL disability, less social network integration, depression, and anxiety were all significantly associated with UI. The prevalence of any UI by the level of loneliness is illustrated in Fig. 1. Greater loneliness was associated with a higher prevalence of UI with the prevalence of UI ranging from 9.2%

(lowest level of loneliness) to 24.6% (highest level of loneliness). The results of the logistic regression analysis assessing the association between any UI and loneliness are shown in Table 2. In the unadjusted model, the OR (95% CI) was 1.74 (1.49-2.05) (Model 1). This was attenuated when the model was adjusted for sociodemographic factors, chronic conditions, and ADL disability but remained statistically significant (Model 2). Further adjustment for the SNI had little effect on the association (Model 3). The OR became non-significant when depression was included in the model (Model 4) but not when anxiety was included (Model 5). In the final model adjusting for all potential confounders the OR (95% CI) was 1.14 (0.94–1.37) (Model 6).

When the frequency of UI or activity limitations due to UI were taken into account, compared to no UI, having activity limitations due to UI was associated with particularly high odds for loneliness even in models adjusted for either depression or anxiety (Model 4 and 5) although the OR was no longer significant when depression and anxiety were included simultaneously in the model (Model 6). Frequency of UI was not as strongly associated with loneliness as activity limitations due to UI and became non-significant in the models where depression and anxiety were included (Table 3). Finally, in the analysis restricted to those with UI, a higher frequency of UI was not associated with elevated odds for loneliness, but activity limitations due to UI were associated with significantly higher odds for loneliness in all models except those which adjusted for depression (Table 4).

Discussion

Using data from a nationally representative sample of community-dwelling older Irish adults, this study showed that having any UI was associated with an increased risk for loneliness. When depression or anxiety was included in the analysis ORs were attenuated, particularly for depression, which suggests that this association is mainly explained by depression. Worse mental health was also important in the relation between UI severity and loneliness as depression fully attenuated the significant association between an increased frequency of UI and loneliness, while an association between activity limitations and loneliness became non-significant when both depression and anxiety were included in the fully adjusted model. When the analysis was restricted to those with UI, depression alone fully attenuated the significant association that was observed between activity limitations and loneliness.

The finding that UI was associated with loneliness when not adjusting for mental health conditions, accords with the results of earlier studies in Canada and the United States [22–24]. This result seems plausible given that UI has been linked to a range of 'safety-seeking

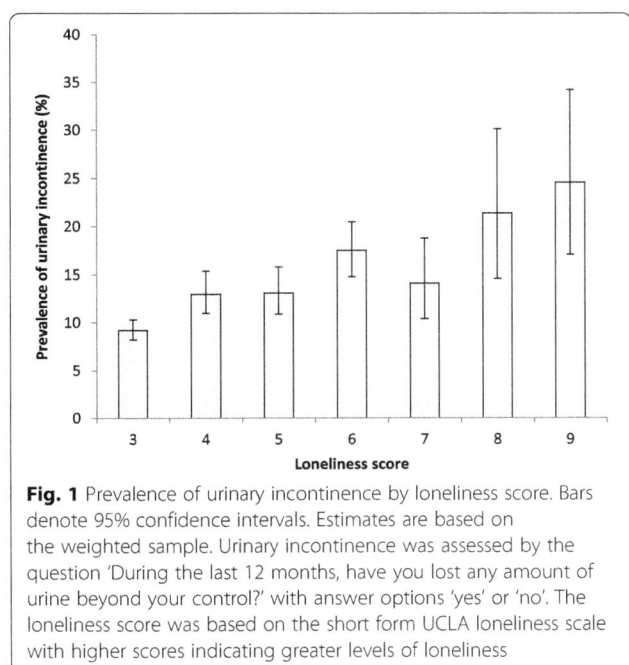

Fig. 1 Prevalence of urinary incontinence by loneliness score. Bars denote 95% confidence intervals. Estimates are based on the weighted sample. Urinary incontinence was assessed by the question 'During the last 12 months, have you lost any amount of urine beyond your control?' with answer options 'yes' or 'no'. The loneliness score was based on the short form UCLA loneliness scale with higher scores indicating greater levels of loneliness

Table 2 Association between urinary incontinence (independent variable) and loneliness (dependent variable) estimated by logistic regression

Characteristic	Categories	Model 1	Model 2	Model 3	Model 4	Model 5	Model 6
Urinary incontinence	No	Ref	Ref	Ref	Ref	Ref	Ref
	Yes	1.74***	1.50***	1.51***	1.20	1.27*	1.14
		[1.49,2.05]	[1.27,1.78]	[1.27,1.80]	[1.00,1.43]	[1.06,1.53]	[0.94,1.37]
Age (years)	50–59		Ref	Ref	Ref	Ref	Ref
	60–69		0.95	1.03	1.13	1.22**	1.27**
			[0.83,1.08]	[0.90,1.17]	[0.99,1.30]	[1.06,1.41]	[1.10,1.46]
	70–79		1.19*	1.30**	1.43***	1.74***	1.76***
			[1.01,1.40]	[1.10,1.53]	[1.20,1.70]	[1.46,2.07]	[1.47,2.10]
	≥80		1.46**	1.36*	1.53**	2.05***	2.06***
			[1.13,1.88]	[1.05,1.77]	[1.17,1.99]	[1.56,2.70]	[1.56,2.72]
Sex	Male		Ref	Ref	Ref	Ref	Ref
	Female		1.12*	1.10	0.98	0.92	0.87*
			[1.01,1.24]	[1.00,1.22]	[0.88,1.08]	[0.83,1.03]	[0.78,0.98]
Education	Primary		Ref	Ref	Ref	Ref	Ref
	Secondary		0.95	1.03	1.07	1.07	1.08
			[0.82,1.09]	[0.89,1.19]	[0.92,1.24]	[0.92,1.25]	[0.93,1.27]
	Tertiary		0.92	1.04	1.11	1.13	1.15
			[0.80,1.07]	[0.90,1.21]	[0.95,1.29]	[0.96,1.32]	[0.98,1.35]
Financial strain	Never		Ref	Ref	Ref	Ref	Ref
	Rarely		1.38***	1.41***	1.44***	1.21*	1.24*
			[1.18,1.62]	[1.20,1.66]	[1.21,1.70]	[1.02,1.43]	[1.04,1.48]
	Sometimes		1.87***	1.88***	1.80***	1.53***	1.54***
			[1.63,2.16]	[1.63,2.17]	[1.55,2.09]	[1.32,1.79]	[1.32,1.81]
	Often		3.66***	3.35***	2.66***	2.14***	1.99***
			[3.03,4.42]	[2.77,4.06]	[2.17,3.26]	[1.75,2.61]	[1.61,2.45]
Number of Chronic conditions	None		Ref	Ref	Ref	Ref	Ref
	One		1.01	1.04	1.02	1.03	1.02
			[0.86,1.18]	[0.89,1.22]	[0.87,1.20]	[0.87,1.22]	[0.87,1.21]
	Two or more		1.24**	1.25**	1.15	1.12	1.08
			[1.07,1.43]	[1.07,1.44]	[0.99,1.34]	[0.96,1.31]	[0.93,1.27]
ADL disability	No		Ref	Ref	Ref	Ref	Ref
	Yes		1.14	1.06	0.74**	0.94	0.76*
			[0.93,1.39]	[0.87,1.31]	[0.59,0.92]	[0.75,1.18]	[0.60,0.97]
Social Network Index	Mostly isolated			Ref	Ref	Ref	Ref
	Moderately isolated			0.59***	0.63**	0.60***	0.63**
				[0.45,0.77]	[0.47,0.83]	[0.45,0.80]	[0.46,0.84]
	Moderately integrated			0.40***	0.46***	0.40***	0.43***
				[0.31,0.52]	[0.35,0.60]	[0.30,0.52]	[0.32,0.57]
	Most integrated			0.26***	0.30***	0.25***	0.28***
				[0.20,0.34]	[0.23,0.40]	[0.19,0.33]	[0.21,0.37]
Depression	(per one-unit increase)				1.10***		1.06***
					[1.09,1.11]		[1.05,1.07]
Anxiety	(per one-unit increase)					1.24***	1.20***
						[1.21,1.26]	[1.17,1.22]

Data are odds ratio [95% confidence interval]
Models are adjusted for all the variables in the respective columns
Abbreviation: Ref Reference category, *ADL* Activities of daily living
*p < 0.05, **p < 0.01, ***p < 0.001

Table 3 Association between frequency of urinary incontinence or activity limitations due to urinary incontinence (independent variables) and loneliness (dependent variable) estimated by logistic regression with no urinary incontinence as the reference category

Characteristic	Categories	Model 1	Model 2	Model 3	Model 4	Model 5	Model 6
Frequency of	No urinary incontinence	Ref	Ref	Ref	Ref	Ref	Ref
Urinary incontinence	Once a month or less	1.62**	1.50*	1.53*	1.33	1.25	1.21
		[1.20,2.20]	[1.08,2.07]	[1.09,2.14]	[0.94,1.90]	[0.88,1.78]	[0.85,1.74]
	More than once a month	1.79***	1.51***	1.52***	1.16	1.29*	1.11
		[1.49,2.15]	[1.24,1.83]	[1.25,1.84]	[0.94,1.42]	[1.04,1.59]	[0.90,1.38]
Activity limitations	No urinary incontinence	Ref	Ref	Ref	Ref	Ref	Ref
Due to urinary	No activity limitations	1.53***	1.36**	1.37**	1.13	1.16	1.06
Incontinence		[1.28,1.84]	[1.12,1.64]	[1.12,1.67]	[0.92,1.39]	[0.94,1.43]	[0.86,1.32]
	Activity limitations	2.60***	2.07***	2.08***	1.46*	1.71**	1.41
		[1.91,3.55]	[1.51,2.84]	[1.50,2.88]	[1.03,2.05]	[1.20,2.45]	[0.98,2.04]

Data are odds ratio [95% confidence interval]
Model 1: Unadjusted
Model 2: Adjusted for age, sex, education, financial strain, number of chronic conditions, and ADL disability
Model 3: Adjusted for variables in Model 2 and the Social Network Index
Model 4: Adjusted for variables in Model 3 and depression
Model 5: Adjusted for variables in Model 3 and anxiety
Model 6: Adjusted for variables in Model 3, depression, and anxiety
Abbreviation: Ref Reference category
*p < 0.05, **p < 0.01, ***p < 0.001

behaviors' that are used to manage the condition and its effects, such as avoiding contact with others, intimacy and activities outside the home [45] that might all lead to social isolation among those with UI and give rise to feelings of loneliness. Moreover, the results from the analyses examining UI severity also seem to support this idea as activity limitations were strongly associated with loneliness in the whole sample and when the analysis was restricted to those with UI. Being treated differently by other people because of their condition [18] might also act to isolate those with UI and lead to feelings of loneliness, especially as a recent study from the United States has indicated that older women with daily UI often feel left out and that they lack companionship [23].

When the common mental disorder variables, in particular, depression, were entered into the analysis, however, the association between UI, UI severity and loneliness became non-significant. Together with our finding that those with UI are more likely to experience greater anxiety and depression, this suggests that poorer mental health might be an intervening variable between UI and loneliness. It can only be speculated what underlies the association between depression and loneliness among those with UI, as even though earlier research has indicated that they can both influence each other over time [28], as yet, there has been comparatively little research on the specific mechanisms linking depression to loneliness [27]. It is possible, for example, that certain psychological resources might be

Table 4 Association between frequency of urinary incontinence or activity limitations due to urinary incontinence (independent variables) and loneliness (dependent variable) restricted to individuals with urinary incontinence estimated by logistic regression

Characteristic	Categories	Model 1	Model 2	Model 3	Model 4	Model 5	Model 6
Frequency of	Once a month or less	Ref	Ref	Ref	Ref	Ref	Ref
Urinary incontinence	More than once a month	1.10	0.99	0.99	0.87	1.04	0.91
		[0.78,1.56]	[0.69,1.43]	[0.68,1.44]	[0.59,1.29]	[0.71,1.54]	[0.61,1.36]
Activity limitations	No activity limitations	Ref	Ref	Ref	Ref	Ref	Ref
Due to urinary	Activity limitations	1.70**	1.52*	1.54*	1.30	1.51*	1.34
Incontinence		[1.20,2.41]	[1.05,2.20]	[1.06,2.24]	[0.87,1.93]	[1.00,2.28]	[0.88,2.04]

Data are odds ratio [95% confidence interval]
Model 1: Unadjusted
Model 2: Adjusted for age, sex, education, financial strain, number of chronic conditions, and ADL disability
Model 3: Adjusted for variables in Model 2 and the Social Network Index
Model 4: Adjusted for variables in Model 3 and depression
Model 5: Adjusted for variables in Model 3 and anxiety
Model 6: Adjusted for variables in Model 3, depression, and anxiety
Abbreviation: Ref Reference category
*p < 0.05, **p < 0.01

important in this context. Specifically, a recent study has reported that a lower sense of mastery significantly contributes to the association between depression and (emotional) loneliness [27] while other research has indicated that UI is associated with a lower sense of mastery [46] and that there is an association between a poor sense of mastery and depression in those with UI [47]. One of the safety-seeking behaviors among those with UI – inquiring frequently if he or she smells [45] – might also be a factor that links depression and loneliness, as a more general connection has been shown to exist between seeking reassurance excessively and both depression and interpersonal rejection [48].

There are several limitations that should be borne in mind when considering this study's findings. UI data were self-reported in this study. Given the stigma and embarrassment that is associated with UI, it is possible that underreporting may have been an issue [4], although the prevalence estimate obtained fell within the range of those reported in other studies. We also lacked information on the type of UI that was experienced. This might be an important omission as there is some evidence that urge incontinence may affect well-being more than stress incontinence [11] and have a stronger association with worse mental health [49]. There may have also been a problem with one of the instruments used in this study. Specifically, a recent systematic review has questioned the ability of HADS to clearly differentiate between anxiety and depression and indicated that it might be better regarded as a measure of 'emotional distress' [50]. In addition, since individuals with cognitive impairment that was severe enough to preclude participation in the survey, and the institutionalized were not included in our study sample, the study results cannot be generalized to this population. Finally, as this study was cross-sectional, it was not possible to determine causality or the temporality of the observed associations.

Conclusion

This study, which used data from a nationally representative sample of almost 7000 community dwelling adults aged ≥ 50, has shown that UI and UI severity are linked to loneliness but that this association is largely dependent on the presence of comorbid depression. The results of this study and the detrimental (psychological/mental health) outcomes that have been reported in earlier studies, together with the fact that at least one-third of older adults with UI do not seek help [14], suggest that more effort is required to educate older respondents about this condition and its effects, as well as about the wide variety of treatment options that are available for it [51]. For patients, clinician screening for loneliness and then referral to agencies that run social programs (e.g. group

meals) that might help alleviate this phenomenon [52] may be one way to improve the quality of life in those individuals with UI. In addition, as poorer mental health is more prevalent among people with UI, and can affect the course and outcome of UI [49, 53], routine mental health screening and close collaboration with mental health professionals may also prove efficacious for patients with UI.

Abbreviations
95% CI: 95% confidence interval; ADL disability: Activities of daily living disability; CAPI: Computer-assisted personal interviewing; CES-D: Center for Epidemiologic Studies Depression scale; CMDs: Common mental disorders; HADS-A: The Hospital Anxiety and Depression Scale; OR: Odds ratio; SCQ: Self-completion questionnaire; SNI: The Berkman-Syme Social Network Index; TILDA: The Irish Longitudinal Study on Ageing; UCLA Loneliness Scale: University of California, Los Angeles Loneliness Scale; UI: Urinary incontinence

Acknowledgements
N/A.

Funding
ZIS's work has received funding from the People Programme (Marie Curie Actions) of the European Union's Seventh Framework Programme FP7/2007 – 2013 under REA grant agreement n° 316795. AK's work was supported by the Miguel Servet contract financed by the CP13/00150 and PI15/00862 projects, integrated into the National R + D + I and funded by the ISCIII - General Branch Evaluation and Promotion of Health Research - and the European Regional Development Fund (ERDF-FEDER).

Authors' contributions
AS had the study idea, designed the study and wrote the main text. AK and ZIS analyzed the data and commented on and wrote parts of the manuscript. All authors read and approved the final manuscript.

Competing interests
The authors declare that they have no competing interests.

Author details
[1]The Stockholm Center for Health and Social Change (SCOHOST), Södertörn University, Huddinge 141 89, Sweden. [2]The Danish National Institute of Public Health, University of Southern Denmark, Oester Farimagsgade 5A, 1353 Copenhagen, Denmark. [3]Parc Sanitari Sant Joan de Déu, Universitat de Barcelona, Fundació Sant Joan de Déu/CIBERSAM, Barcelona, Spain.

References
1. Abrams P, Cardozo L, Fall M, Griffiths D, Rosier P, Ulmsten U, van Kerrebroeck P, Victor A, Wein A. The standardization of terminology of lower urinary tract function: report from the standardization sub-committee of the International Continence Society. Neurourol Urodyn. 2002;21:167–78.
2. Bartoli S, Aguzzi G, Tarricone R. Impact on quality of life of urinary incontinence and overactive bladder: a systematic literature review. Urology. 2010;75:491–500.
3. Minassian VA, Drutz HP, Al-Badr A. Urinary incontinence as a worldwide problem. Int J Gynaecol Obstet. 2003;82:327–38.
4. Chang CH, Gonzalez CM, Lau DT, Sier HC. Urinary incontinence and self-reported health among the U.S. Medicare managed care beneficiaries. J Aging Health. 2008;20:405–19.
5. Van Oyen H, Van Oyen P. Urinary incontinence in Belgium; prevalence, correlates and psychosocial consequences. Acta Clin Belg. 2002;57:207–18.
6. Chapple CR, Manassero F. Urinary incontinence in adults. Surgery. 2005; 23:101–7.

7. Hannestad YS, Rortveit G, Sandvik H, Hunskaar S. A community-based epidemiological survey of female urinary incontinence: the Norwegian EPINCONT study. J Clin Epidemiol. 2000;53:1150–7.

8. Melville JL, Katon W, Delaney K, Newton K. Urinary incontinence in US women: a population-based study. Arch Intern Med. 2005;165:537–42.

9. Hunskaar S, Arnold EP, Burgio K, Diokno AC, Herzog AR, Mallett VT. Epidemiology and natural history of urinary incontinence. Int Urogynecol J Pelvic Floor Dysfunct. 2000;11:301–19.

10. Gavira Iglesias FJ, Caridad y Ocerín JM, Pérez del Molino Martín J, Valderrama Gama E, López Pérez M, Romero López M, Pavón Aranguren MV, Guerrero Muñoz JB. Prevalence and psychosocial impact of urinary incontinence in older people of a Spanish rural population. J Gerontol A Biol Sci Med Sci. 2000;55:M207–14.

11. Heidrich SM, Wells TJ. Effects of urinary incontinence: psychological well-being and distress in older community-dwelling women. J Gerontol Nurs. 2004;30:47–54.

12. Coyne KS, Wein A, Nicholson S, Kvasz M, Chen CI, Milsom I. Comorbidities and personal burden of urgency urinary incontinence: a systematic review. Int J Clin Pract. 2013;67:1015–33.

13. Gibson W, Wagg A. New horizons: urinary incontinence in older people. Age Ageing. 2014;43:157–63.

14. Farage MA, Miller KW, Berardesca E, Maibach HI. Psychosocial and societal burden of incontinence in the aged population: a review. Arch Gynecol Obstet. 2008;277:285–90.

15. Reigota RB, Pedro AO, de Souza Santos Machado V, Costa-Paiva L, Pinto-Neto AM. Prevalence of urinary incontinence and its association with multimorbidity in women aged 50 years or older: a population-based study. Neurourol Urodyn. 2016;35:62–8.

16. Felde G, Ebbesen MH, Hunskaar S. Anxiety and depression associated with urinary incontinence. A 10-year follow-up study from the Norwegian HUNT study (EPINCONT). Neurourol Urodyn. 2015. doi:10.1002/nau22921.

17. Kwak Y, Kwon H, Kim Y. Health-related quality of life and mental health in older women with urinary incontinence. Aging Ment Health. 2016;20:719–26.

18. Heintz PA, DeMucha CM, Deguzman MM, Softa R. Stigma and microaggressions experienced by older women with urinary incontinence: a literature review. Urol Nurs. 2013;33:299–305.

19. Teunissen D, Van Den Bosch W, Van Weel C, Lagro-Janssen T. "It can always happen": the impact of urinary incontinence on elderly men and women. Scand J Prim Health Care. 2006;24:166–73.

20. Luanaigh CO, Lawlor BA. Loneliness and the health of older people. Int J Geriatr Psychiatry. 2008;23:1213–21.

21. Luo Y, Hawkley LC, Waite LJ, Cacioppo JT. Loneliness, health, and mortality in old age: a national longitudinal study. Soc Sci Med. 2012;74:907–14.

22. Ramage-Morin PL, Gilmour H. Urinary incontinence and loneliness in Canadian seniors. Health Rep. 2013;24:3–10.

23. Yip SO, Dick MA, McPencow AM, Martin DK, Ciarleglio MM, Erekson EA. The association between urinary and fecal incontinence and social isolation in older women. Am J Obstet Gynecol. 2013;208:146e. 1-7.

24. Fultz NH, Herzog AR. Self-reported social and emotional impact of urinary incontinence. J Am Geriatr Soc. 2001;49:892–9.

25. Drageset J, Espehaug B, Kirkevold M. The impact of depression and sense of coherence on emotional and social loneliness among nursing home residents without cognitive impairment - a questionnaire survey. J Clin Nurs. 2012;21:965–74.

26. Losada A, Márquez-González M, Pachana NA, Wetherell JL, Fernández-Fernández V, Nogales-González C, Ruiz-Díaz M. Behavioral correlates of anxiety in well-functioning older adults. Int Psychogeriatr. 2015;27:1135–46.

27. Peerenboom L, Collard RM, Naarding P, Comijs HC. The association between depression and emotional and social loneliness in older persons and the influence of social support, cognitive functioning and personality: a cross-sectional study. J Affect Disord. 2015;182:26–31.

28. Cacioppo JT, Hughes ME, Waite LJ, Hawkley LC, Thisted RA. Loneliness as a specific risk factor for depressive symptoms: cross-sectional and longitudinal analyses. Psychol Aging. 2006;21:140–51.

29. Kearney PM, Cronin H, O'Regan C, Kamiya Y, Savva GM, Whelan B, Kenny R. Cohort profile: the Irish Longitudinal Study on Ageing. Int J Epidemiol. 2011; 40:877–84.

30. Whelan BJ, Savva GM. Design and methodology of the Irish Longitudinal Study on Ageing. J Am Geriatr Soc. 2013;61 Suppl 2:S265–8.

31. Richardson K, Kenny RA, Peklar J, Bennett K. Agreement between patient interview data on prescription medication use and pharmacy records in those aged older than 50 years varied by therapeutic group and reporting of indicated health conditions. J Clin Epidemiol. 2013;66:1308–16.

32. Russell D, Peplau LA, Cutrona CE. The revised UCLA Loneliness Scale: concurrent and discriminant validity evidence. J Pers Soc Psychol. 1980;39:472–80.

33. Hughes ME, Waite LJ, Hawkley LC, Cacioppo JT. A short scale for measuring loneliness in large surveys: results from two population-based studies. Res Aging. 2004;26:655–72.

34. Austin BA. Factorial structure of the UCLA Loneliness Scale. Psychol Rep. 1983;53:883–9.

35. Russell DW. UCLA Loneliness Scale (Version 3): reliability, validity, and factor structure. J Pers Assess. 1996;66:20–40.

36. Radloff LS. The CES-D scale: a self-report depression scale for research in the general population. Appl Psychol Meas. 1977;1:385–401.

37. Hawkley LC, Thisted RA, Cacioppo JT. Loneliness predicts reduced physical activity: cross-sectional & longitudinal analyses. Health Psychol. 2009;28:354–63.

38. Hertzog C, Van Alstine J, Usala PD, Hultsch DF, Dixon R. Measurement properties of the Center for Epidemiological Studies Depression Scale (CES-D) in older populations. Psychol Assess J Consult Clin Psychol. 1990;2:64–72.

39. Lewinsohn PM, Seeley JR, Roberts RE, Allen NB. Center for Epidemiologic Studies Depression Scale (CES-D) as a screening instrument for depression among community-residing older adults. Psychol Aging. 1997;12:277–87.

40. Zigmond AS, Snaith RP. The hospital anxiety and depression scale. Acta Psychiatr Scand. 1983;67:361–70.

41. Spinhoven P, Ormel J, Sloekers PPA, Kempen GI, Speckens AE, Van Hemert AM. A validation study of the Hospital Anxiety and Depression Scale (HADS) in different groups of Dutch subjects. Psychol Med. 1997;27:363–70.

42. Berkman LF, Syme SL. Social networks, host resistance, and mortality: a nine-year follow-up study of Alameda County residents. Am J Epidemiol. 1979; 109:186–204.

43. Berkman LF, Breslow L. Health and ways of living: the Alameda County study. New York: Oxford University Press; 1983.

44. Katz S, Ford AB, Moskowitz RW, Jackson BA, Jaffe MW. Studies of illness in the aged. The index of ADL: a standardized measure of biological and psychosocial function. JAMA. 1963;185:914–9.

45. Molinuevo B, Batista-Miranda JE. Under the tip of the iceberg: psychological factors in incontinence. Neurourol Urodyn. 2012;31:669–71.

46. Woods NF, Mitchell ES. Consequences of incontinence for women during the menopausal transition and early postmenopause: observations from the Seattle Midlife Women's Health Study. Menopause. 2013;20:915–21.

47. Chiverton PA, Wells TJ, Brink CA, Mayer R. Psychological factors associated with urinary incontinence. Clin Nurse Spec. 1996;10:229–33.

48. Starr LR, Davila J. Excessive reassurance seeking, depression, and interpersonal rejection: a meta-analytic review. J Abnorm Psychol. 2008;117:762–75.

49. Melville JL, Walker E, Katon W, Lentz G, Miller J, Fenner D. Prevalence of comorbid psychiatric illness and its impact on symptom perception, quality of life, and functional status in women with urinary incontinence. Am J Obstet Gynecol. 2002;187:80–7.

50. Cosco TD, Doyle F, Ward M, McGee H. Latent structure of the Hospital Anxiety And Depression Scale: a 10-year systematic review. J Psychosom Res. 2012;72:180–4.

51. Norton P, Brubaker L. Urinary incontinence in women. Lancet. 2006;367:57–67.

52. Perissinotto CM, Stijacic Cenzer I, Covinsky KE. Loneliness in older persons: a predictor of functional decline and death. Arch Intern Med. 2012;172:1078–83.

53. Stach-Lempinen B, Hakala AL, Laippala P, Lehtinen K, Metsänoja R, Kujansuu E. Severe depression determines quality of life in urinary incontinent women. Neurourol Urodyn. 2003;22:563–8.

2

Management of large renal stones: laparoscopic pyelolithotomy versus percutaneous nephrolithotomy

Yunjin Bai[†], Yin Tang[†], Lan Deng, Xiaoming Wang, Yubo Yang, Jia Wang and Ping Han[*]

Abstract

Background: Percutaneous nephrolithotomy (PCNL) remains the standard procedure for large (≥2 cm) renal calculi; however, laparoscopic pyelolithotomy (LPL) can be used as an alternative management procedure. The aim of present study was to compare LPL and PCNL in terms of efficacy and safety for the management of large renal pelvic stones.

Methods: A literature search was performed in Jan 2016 using electronic databases (Cochrane Central Register of Controlled Trials, Medline, and EMBASE) to identify relevant studies for the meta-analysis. Only comparative studies investigating LPL versus PCNL were included. Effect sizes were estimated by pooled odds ratio (ORs) and mean differences (MDs) with 95% confidence intervals (CIs).

Results: Five randomized and nine non-randomized studies were identified for analysis, involving a total of 901 patients. Compared with PCNL, LPL provided a significantly higher stone-free rate (OR 3.94, 95% CI 2.06–7.55, $P < 0.001$), lower blood transfusion rate (OR 0.28, 95% CI 0.13–0.61, $P = 0.001$), lower bleeding rate (OR 0.20, 95% CI 0.06–0.61, $P = 0.005$), fewer hemoglobin decrease(MD -0.80, 95% CI -0.97 to −0.63, $P < 0.001$), less postoperative fever (OR 0.38, 95% CI 0.21–0.68; $P = 0.001$), and lower auxiliary procedure rate (OR 0.24, 95% CI 0.12–0.46, $P < 0.001$) and re-treatment rate (OR 0.20, 95% CI 0.07–0.55, $P = 0.002$). However, LPL had a longer operative time and hospital stay. There were no significant differences in conversion to open surgery and prolonged urine leakage rates between LPL and PCNL.

Conclusions: Our present findings suggest that LPL is a safe and effective approach for management of patients with large renal stones. However, PCNL still suitable for most cases and LPL can be used as an alternative management procedure with good selection of cases.

Keywords: Laparoscopic pyelolithotomy, Percutaneous nephrolithotomy, Renal stone, Meta-analysis

Background

Percutaneous nephrolithotomy (PCNL) currently remains the first-line treatment for large or complex renal stones. Although it is a minimally invasive procedure with higher stone-free rate (SFR), there are still serious complications [1], such as bleeding and postoperative sepsis. Size of the stone was directly correlating with the overall incidence of complications after PCNL [2].

Therefore, treatment of large renal stones is still a challenging problem in urology.

The ideal procedure for large or complex renal stones would be the one that achieve complete stone free status with minimal morbidity and with the least number of procedures. The traditional standard procedure was open nephrolithotomy, which evolved into PCNL or retrograde intrarenal surgery [3]. With the recent development of technique in laparoscopic surgery, laparoscopic pyelolithotomy (LPL) has been frequently considered as an alternative procedure in the management of large or complex renal stones to PCNL or open surgery [4]. There are some advantages to LPL, the first

---
* Correspondence: hanpingwch@163.com
[†]Equal contributors
Department of Urology, Institute of Urology, West China Hospital, Sichuan University, Guoxue Xiang#37, Chengdu, Sichuan 610041, China

and most obvious advantage is that most of the stones can be removed integrally, in the next place, including the ability to minimize bleeding, lessen pain, and lower morbidity. Despite the potential advantages, its rare usage.

One prior meta-analysis [4] evaluated the efficacy and safety of LPL and PCNL in treating large renal stones and found that PCNL and LPL were effective and safe for managing this condition, but also found that LPL seems to be more advantageous. Recently, several additional clinical trials have been reported that compared PCNL and LPL for removal of large renal stones. Therefore, we perform an update meta-analysis to compare LPL and PCNL in terms of efficacy and safety for the management of large renal pelvic stones.

Methods

Literature search and article selection
An electronic search was performed in Jan 2016 using Medline, EMBASE, and the Cochrane Collaboration Central Register of Controlled Clinical Trials databases to identify relevant studies, using words related to percutaneous nephrolithotomy, laparoscopic pyelolithotomy, and renal calculi in all fields. Searches were restricted by English and in adult population. We also reviewed all the references of relevant articles, and recent reviews.

For studies to be included, they had to meet the following criteria: (1) patients with a large renal calculi (≥2 cm); (2) the comparison of LPL with PCNL;(3) report on at least one outcome or the data would allow the calculation; and (4) randomized controlled trial (RCT), quasi randomized controlled study, or case-control study(CCS). The most recent or complete report was used for multiple reports describing the same population. For example, when full article and conference abstract describing the same population, the former would be included. The final selection of the included studies was achieved through a consensus meeting of the reviewers.

Data extraction and quality assessment
Two authors independently confirmed study eligibility and extracted data. Any discrepancies were resolved by discussion. The following variables were extracted from each eligible study: characteristics, interventions, and outcome measures. Our outcomes were the SFR at 12 weeks after the procedure, auxiliary procedures rate, operative time, drop in hemoglobin level, length of stay, complication rate, blood transfusion rate, and postoperative fever. The methodological quality of the studies was assessed using the Newcastle-Ottawa Scale (NOS) for non-RCTs [5] and the Jadad scale for RCTs [6].

Data synthesis and analysis
Data analysis was performed with Review Manager version 5.1(Cochrane Collaboration, Oxford, UK). Odds

ratio (OR) was applied in dichotomous outcomes, and mean difference (MD) was used for the continuous variables. Respective 95% confidence intervals (CI) were calculated for each estimate. For studies presenting continuous data as means and range, standard deviations were calculated using the methodology described by Hozo and colleagues [7]. Pooled estimates were calculated with the fixed-effect model if no significant heterogeneity was detected; otherwise, the random-effect model was used. We assessed statistical heterogeneity among studies using the chi-square test and the degree of inconsistency (I^2). The pooled effects of OR/MD were determined by the z test, and $P < 0.05$ was considered to be statistically significant. Publication bias was evaluated by using a funnel plot.

Results

Study characteristics
The present study met the PRISMA statement (Additional file 1). The search identified 657 records, which were doubly screened. After study assessment, we identified 14 studies [8–21] fulfilled inclusion criteria (Fig. 1), 11 publications were full articles and three were conference abstracts [12, 13, 16]. Baseline characteristics and intervention protocols are summarized in Table 1. There were 901 patients involved in the 14 studies: 432 underwent LPL and 469 PCNL. Baseline information of study populations was comparable between LPL and PCNL groups. The types of imaging used in the studies included kidney-

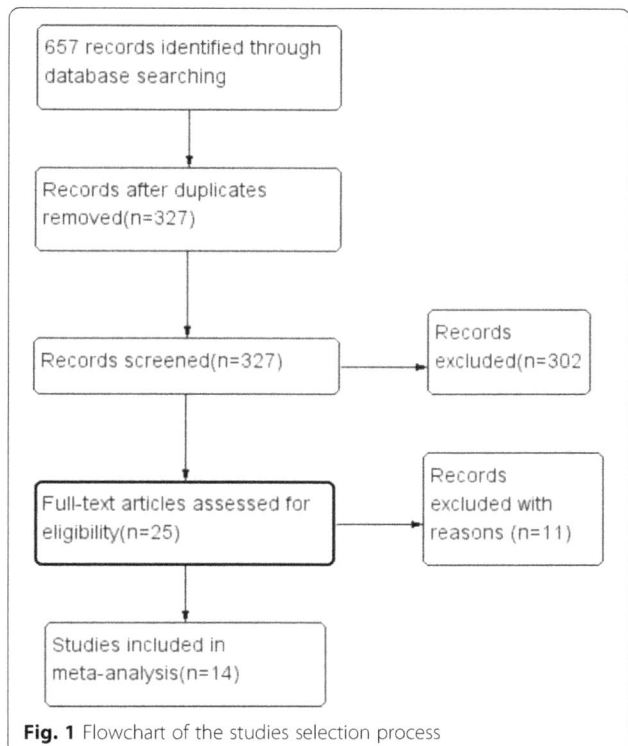

Fig. 1 Flowchart of the studies selection process

Table 1 The basic characteristic of included studies

Study/year	Study design	Study period	Surgical approach	Sample size	Age (year) (mean±SD)	Staghorn(%)	Stone feature	Stone burden (mean ±SD)	Study quality
Goel 2003 [11]	CCS	1995–2003	RLP	16	38.9(21–60)	NA	Solitary, Pelvis	3.6 cm(3.2–4.5)	5[a]
			PCNL	12	41.4(20–62)	NA		4.1 cm(3.5–5.2)	
Al-Hunayan 2011 [8]	RCT	2002–2010	RLP	55	41.2 ± 11.7	NA	Solitary, Pelvis	2.4 ± 0.4 cm	3[b]
			PCNL	50	38.9 ± 11.9	NA		2.5 ± 0.4 cm	
Perlin 2011 [12]	CCS	2009–2011	RLP	5	-	NA	Solitary, Pelvis	>2.3 cm	5[a]
			PCNL	20	-	NA		>2.3 cm	
Tefekli 2012 [9]	CCS	2006–2009	RLP	26	36.5 ± 11.1	NA	Solitary, Pelvis	>4 cm^2	6[a]
			PCNL	26	37.1 ± 10.0	NA		>4 cm^2	
Aminsharifi 2013 [10]	CCS	2009–2012	RLP	30	43.8 ± 15.0	NA	Solitary, Pelvis	3.53 ± 0.73 cm	5[a]
			PCNL	30	45.3 ± 14.8	NA		3.66 ± 0.7 cm	
Singh 2014 [14]	RCT	2010–2012	RLP	22	45.55 ± 14.22	NA	Solitary, Pelvis	>3 cm	3[b]
			PCNL	22	44.95 ± 13.81	NA		>3 cm	
Fawzi 2015 [13]	RCT	2012–2014	RLP	30	42.4 ± 12.1	NA	Solitary, Pelvis	3.2 ± 0.6 cm	2[b]
			PCNL	30	44.6 ± 11.4	NA		3.4 ± 0.5 cm	
Basiri 2014 [15]	RCT	2009–2012	TLP	30	38.5 ± 15.9	40	Pelvis	3.6 (2.8–4.4)cm	3[b]
			PCNL	30	42.1 ± 14.3	30		3.3 (2.7–4.2)cm	
Gaur 2001 [21]	CCS	–	RLP	42	39.12(8–65)	0	Multiple, Pelvis and calyx	2.0(1.0–4.8)cm	4[a]
			PCNL	47	34.4	0		2.9(2.0–3.8)cm	
Lee 2014 [19]	CCS	2004–2011	TLP	45	56.0 ± 13.7	4.4	Multiple, Pelvis and calyx	4.93 ± 3.03 cm	6[a]
			PCNL	39	54.3 ± 13.0	28		4.63 ± 1.65 cm	
Meria 2005 [17]	CCS	1999–2004	TLP	16	42 (21–63)	NA	Solitary, Pelvis	2.5 (2.0–3.3)cm	5[a]
			PCNL	16	45 (24–69)	NA		2.6 (2.0–4.0)cm	
Li 2014 [18]	RCT	2009–2013	RLP	89	55.63 ± 10.98	17	Pelvis	2.93 ± 1.02 cm	3[b]
			PCNL	89	53.15 ± 11.54	19		3.0 ± 0.96 cm	
Tepeler 2009 [16]	CCS	2006–2008	RLP	16	41.2 ± 16.8	NA	Pelvis	8.82 ± 3.2 cm2	3[a]
			PCNL	16	43.86 ± 14.11	NA		8.49 ± 2.6 cm2	
Haggag 2013 [20]	CCS	2009–2012	RLP	10	38.8 ± 12.17	NA	Pelvis	6.5 ± 1.20 cm2	4[a]
			PCNL	42	42.03 ± 13.17	NA		4.19 ± 2.03 cm2	

RCT randomized controlled trial, CCS case controlled study, PCNL percutaneous nephrolithotomy, NA not available, RLP retroperitoneal laparoscopic pyelolithotomy, TLP transperitoneal laparoscopic pyelolithotomy

[a] Using Newcastle-Ottawa Scale (score from 0 to 9)

[b] Using Jadad scale (score from 0 to 5)

ureter-bladder X-ray, ultrasonography, computer tomography, fluoroscopy, and nephrostogram. There are five RCTs [8, 13–15, 18], which information on method of randomization and allocation concealment was absent or unclear. The methodological quality of included studies was relatively high for four of the CCSs and medium for four RCTs and six CCSs, whereas relatively low were found to be of two studies (Table 1).

Meta-analysis outcomes

SFR

Two studies [16, 19] were not included in this meta-analysis as they did not assess patients' SFR at 3 months after treatment. The pooled analysis of 12 studies showed

that the SFR in the LPL and PCNL group was 97.57% (362/371) and 87.92% (364/414), respectively, and this difference was obvious (OR 3.94, 95% CI 2.06–7.55, $P < 0.001$) (Fig. 2). There was no evidence of statistical heterogeneity between studies as assessed by the Q statistic (Chi^2 = 6.95; I^2 = 0%).

Auxiliary procedures and retreatment rate

LPL provided a significantly lower auxiliary procedures rate (OR 0.24, 95% CI 0.12–0.46, $P < 0.001$) (Fig. 3a) and lower re-treatment rate compared with PCNL (OR 0.20, 95% CI 0.07–0.55, $P = 0.002$) (Fig. 3b). The pooled analysis showed that the extracorporeal shockwave lithotripsy rate in the LPL and PCNL group was 6.54% and

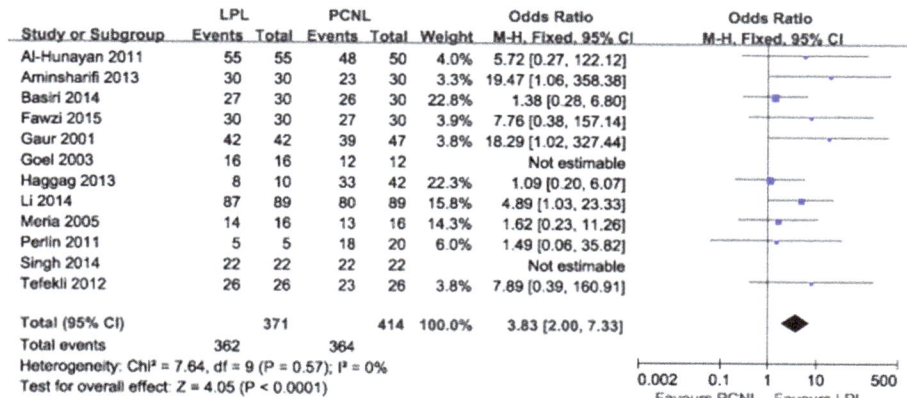

Fig. 2 Forest plot comparing stone-free rates between two groups at 3 months after treatment. LPL, laparoscopic pyelolithotomy; PCNL, percutaneous nephrolithotomy

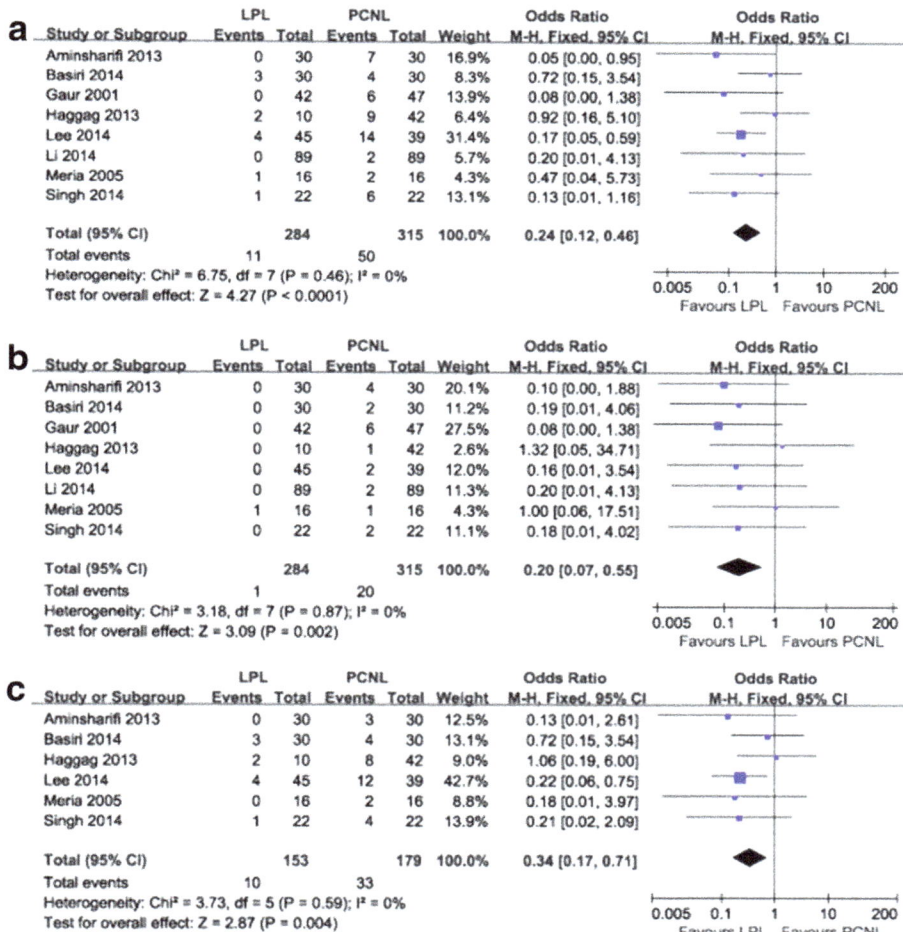

Fig. 3 Forest plot of LPL versus PCNL: **a** auxiliary procedures rate, **b** re-treatment rate, **c** extracorporeal shockwave lithotripsy rate. LPL, laparoscopic pyelolithotomy; PCNL, percutaneous nephrolithotomy

18.44%, respectively, and this difference was obvious (OR 0.34, 95% CI 0.17–0.71, P = 0.004) (Fig. 3c).

Hemorrhagic complications

The parameters assessed were postoperative hemoglobin drop, bleeding, and blood transfusion. LPL provided a significantly lower blood transfusion rate (OR 0.28, 95% CI 0.13–0.61, P = 0.001) (Fig. 4a), lower bleeding rate (OR 0.20, 95% CI 0.06–0.61, P = 0.005) (Fig. 4b), and fewer hemoglobin decrease (MD -0.80, 95% CI -0.97 to –0.63, P < 0.001) (Fig. 4c).

Postoperative fever and sepsis

There were seven studies comprising 596 patients included in the meta-analysis for postoperative fever. We found that the incidence of postoperative fever was lower in the LPL group than in the PCNL group (OR 0.38, 95% CI 0.21–0.68, P = 0.001) (Fig. 5a) with no heterogeneity between studies (I^2 = 0%). None of patients

from the included studies encountered sepsis or septic shock after the both procedures.

Conversion rate and prolonged urine leakage

There was no significant difference between the LPL and PCNL groups in terms of conversion rate (OR 1.35, 95% CI 0.65–2.81, P = 0.42) (Fig. 5b) and the incidence of prolonged urine leakage (OR 1.06, 95% CI 0.49–2.30, P = 0.88) (Fig. 5c). The reasons of conversion to open surgery included injury of renal vein [15] and peritoneum [21], uncontrolled bleeding [8, 18], stone migration into the calyx [11], and perirenal adhesions [11, 16, 17].

Operative time and hospital stay

Operative time was reported in all included studies. Heterogeneity was observed in the pooled analysis (Chi^2 = 250.73; I^2 = 95%). Meta-analysis of data showed that PCNL had significantly shorter operative time than LPL (random-effect model; MD 32.86, 95% CI 12.85–52.86,

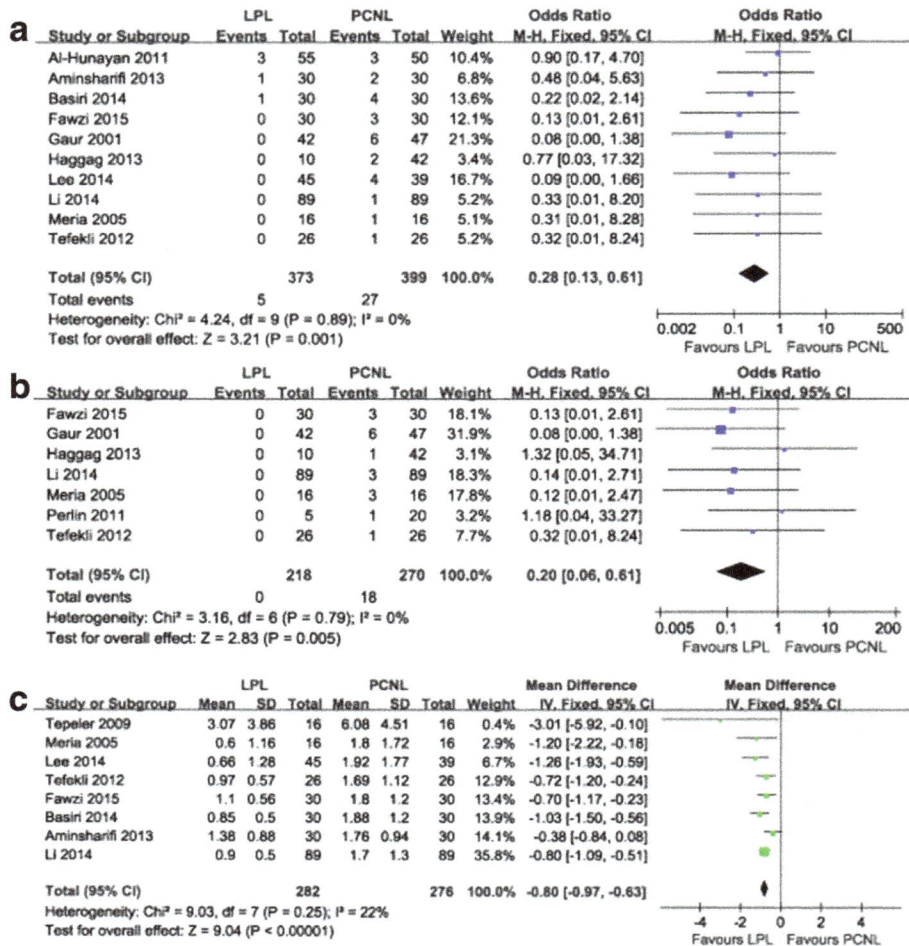

Fig. 4 Forest plot of LPL versus PCNL: **a** blood transfusion rate, **b** bleeding rate, **c** hemoglobin decrease. LPL, laparoscopic pyelolithotomy; PCNL, percutaneous nephrolithotomy

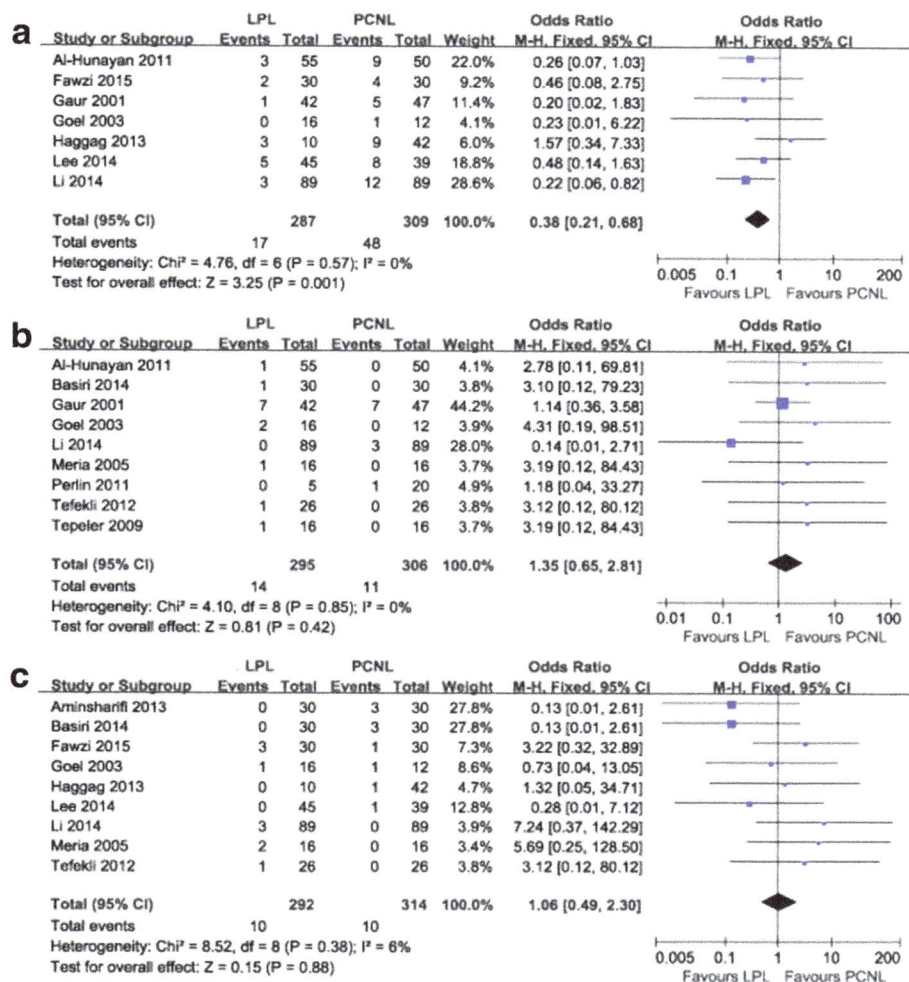

Fig. 5 Forest plot of LPL versus PCNL: **a** postoperative fever, **b** conversion rate, **c** prolonged urine leakage. LPL, laparoscopic pyelolithotomy; PCNL, percutaneous nephrolithotomy

$P = 0.001$). Sensitivity analysis was performed by sequentially removing each study, whereas this substantively did not affect the result. This result indicated that the meta-analysis was not influenced by any one study.

Thirteen studies reported the length of hospital. The results of meta-analysis of these studies indicated a benefit of shorter length of hospital stay in the PCNL group (random-effect model; MD 0.33, CI 95% -0.24 to 0.89, $P = 0.002$) with significant heterogeneity between studies (Chi^2 = 87.37; I^2 = 86%). We could not identify any plausible cause by sensitivity analysis.

Subgroup analyses
The subgroup analyses suggested that the results of this meta-analysis were relatively stable. When the studies

included patients with intra-renal pelvis and multiple stones (≥2) were removed [15, 16, 18–21], most of the outcomes including SFR (OR 5.10, 95% CI 1.79–14.51, $P = 0.002$, I^2 = 0%), auxiliary procedures rate (OR 0.13, 95% CI 0.03–0.52, $P = 0.004$, I^2 = 0%), conversion rate (OR 2.82, 95% CI 0.70–11.46, $P = 0.15$, I^2 = 0%), the incidence of prolonged urine leakage (OR 1.27, 95% CI 0.45–3.61, $P = 0.65$, I^2 = 4%), level of hemoglobin decrease(MD -0.71, 95% CI -0.90 to −0.51, $P < 0.0001$, I^2 = 0%), bleeding rate (OR 0.23, 95% CI 0.05–1.05, $P = 0.06$, I^2 = 0%), blood transfusion rate(OR 0.44, 95% CI 0.16–1.26, $P = 0.13$, I^2 = 0%), postoperative fever rate (OR 0.31, 95% CI 0.11–0.87, $P = 0.03$, I^2 = 0%), operative time (random-effect model; MD 39.39, 95% CI 21.33–57.45, $P < 0.0001$, I^2 = 87%), and hospital stay (random-effect model; MD 0.74, CI 95% 0.29–1.18, $P = 0.001$, $I^2 = 44\%$) were not greatly affected.

Publication bias analyses

We analyzed possible publication bias by generating funnel plots of the studies used for all of the evaluated comparisons of outcomes. No significant publication bias was observed in the above-mentioned analyses.

Discussion

One previous meta-analysis [4] included seven studies with 176 patients underwent LPL and 187 PCNL, showed equivalency for conversion rate, blood transfusion, prolonged urine leakage, and found higher SFR and lower incidence of bleeding and postoperative fever in the LPL group than PCNL group. In addition, the results of the previous study showed that operative time and length of hospital stay were shorter in the PCNL group, drop in hemoglobin level was fewer in the LPL group. In present study, we included 14 studies involving 432 patients underwent LPL and 469 PCNL, and found similar results from the previous meta-analysis regarding SFR, conversion rate, operative time, length of hospital stay, hemoglobin decrease, and postoperative fever. However, in term of blood transfusion rate, we found that there was a significantly lower blood transfusion rate in the LPL group than in the PCNL group, which was different to the previous meta-analysis result. We also found that LPL provided a significantly lower auxiliary procedures and re-treatment rate. The main reason for this difference might be due to the different sample sizes between previous and present studies, which also was the reason of our performed the present study.

Although the SFR was assessed in a different way in each study, the result revealed LPL provided a statistically higher SFR at 3 months after treatment than PCNL, regardless of the definition. The reason may be that most of the stones can be removed integrally in LPL. In the PCNL group, disintegration of the stone may have left some residual stones which can form nuclei for stone recurrence, and the scattering of stone fragments may reduce success rates, which associated with a significantly higher auxiliary procedures and re-treatment rate than LPL. Currently, PCNL is the recommended treatment option for patients with staghorn calculi. However, SFR after PCNL for staghorn calculi only ranges between 49 and 78% [22]. It is noteworthy that LPL can be considered an alternative and feasible technique to PCNL for patients with complex and large renal stones. Gandhi et al. [23] reported the 49 patients with staghorn stones (>3–4 cm) underwent LPL, the mean SFR in one session was 90% with lower complications, no blood transfusion and only two patients had urine

leak (Clavien-Dindo grade IIIa). However, the leak stopped after 10 days in both patients.

Our results showed that operative time was significantly shorter for PCNL than LPL. As known to all, the operative time is directly related with many variables such as the types of approach, surgeon's experience, individual differences of patients, and the different equipment used. In LPL procedure, closure of the pyelotomy incision requires advanced laparoscopic skills. Sometimes, delicate renal pelvis tissues, always caused by long-term chronic inflammation, brings many challenges for the closure of the pyelotomy incision [17] and prolongs the operative time. The longer time of LPL was usually related to the long learning curve as well as the time needed for intracorporeal suturing and delivery of the stone into the endobag [8]. However, Li et al. [18] randomized 178 patients with large renal pelvis stones into two groups found the mean operative time was significantly shorter in the LPL than PCNL, which is likely due to stones in LPL can be removed integrally. Indeed, retrieve stones is one of the major limitations of LPL. Lee et al. [19] used a flexible nephroscope to overcome this difficulty which enable easier approach. With the development of robot technology in urology, this interface maybe will improve the limits of tissue dissection, stone extraction during laparoscopy, intracorporeal reconstruction, and suturing, thereby having the potential to improve the outcomes and flattening the learning curve. However, much less is known about the relative outcomes and costs in robot-assisted pyelolithotomy, which is a major consideration in robotic surgery.

Although LPL have a longer operation time, this may be compensated by the lower complication and higher SFR. Postoperative fever secondary to an urinary tract infection (UTI) in patients with PCNL ranges between 2.8 and 32.1% [1]. Kidney stones are foreign bodies of the urinary tract and can allow bacteria to grow onto them and then become a reservoir for bacteria. They are disintegrated, bacteria are released from the stone into the collecting system, which tends to result in bacteriuria, bacteremia, and clinical UTI. Recently study demonstrated residual stone is a major contributing factor for the development of fever after tubeless PCNL [24]. This finding may translate into a clinical benefit for the patients in that stones removed integrally or the higher SFR of the LPL was associated to lower incidence of postoperative fever. Septic shock, the incidence after PCNL was 2.4% [25], is one of the most dangerous complications after lithotomy due to it can lead to significant mortality. The risk factors for septic shock includes positive urine culture, female gender, renal insufficiency, diabetes mellitus, high pressure of irrigation fluid during PCNL, staghorn calculus, infected stones, indwelling catheters, obstruction, and duration of the operation (>

90 min) [25, 26]. Positively, strict control of blood glucose and pre-operation antibiotics used could reduce the possibility of post-PCNL septic shock. Early recognition and timely comprehensive treatment of septic shock may decrease the mortality. In addition, infective or septic complications may be associated with laparoscopic approach. Transperitoneal approach could be more at risk about it due to this approach might lead to increase the interference of the abdominal organs, postoperative intra-abdominal infection, and the possibility of adhesions. Further prospective randomized controlled trials are needed to determine which approach should be favored.

Although LPL appears to be more invasive because three or four trocar punctures are needed compared with PCNL in which only a single percutaneous access was made, PCNL make renal parenchymal more susceptible to injury with it tends to result in various complications, such as nephron damage and bleeding. Bleeding after PCNL is common, which leads to a more frequent use of blood transfusion, according to previous reports, 1–12% of patients require [1]. With increasing stone burden, patients with PCNL, not only SFR decreased, but also the risk of blood transfusion increased [2]. Risk factors for severe bleeding were upper pole access, solitary kidney, staghorn stone, multiple punctures and inexperienced surgeon [27]. Therefore, PCNL should be performed by an experienced surgeon in patients at risk for severe bleeding. On the other hand, these patients might as well choose other alternative procedures. Our study found that LPL provided a significantly lower blood transfusion rate, lower bleeding rate, and fewer hemoglobin decrease. The reason was probably due to the fact that LPL harmlessness for renal parenchyma. Whatever the approaches, patients with bleeding tendencies needs careful preoperative, intra- and postoperative management because both the procedures may lead to a kidney loss.

For conversion rate and prolonged urine leakage, regardless of our or previous meta-analyses, the results were similar between the two groups. However, more incidence of prolonged urine leakage and longer hospital stay were found in the LPL group. Urine leakage can be attributed to incomplete closure of the pyelotomy incision after LPL, which can prolong hospital stay [8]. Closure of pyelotomy incision is technically difficult during laparoscopic surgery, advanced experience and high skills or robot-assisted surgery are needed. But urinary leakage has been minimized with advances in intracorporeal suturing techniques, such as barbed suture [28]. In addition, suture time was significantly decreased with barbed suture use during laparoscopic pyeloplasty [29], hence, this will shorten operative time.

However, the complications can be minimized with proper patient selection and sufficient preoperative preparation. LPL is certainly safe and feasible in experienced hands, but should not replace PCNL, which remains the gold standard for kidney stones greater than 2 cm. These procedures are technically challenging and should only be performed by experienced laparoscopic surgeons. According previous studies, LPL is more suitable for patients with urinary deformity require concomitant pyeloplasty.. Patients with previous history of open renal surgery always have significant perinephric adhesion which may affect the success or complication rate in LPL, does not in PCNL [30]. Therefore, PCNL is the first-selected treatment in such situation. LPL cannot be a feasible modality for renal stones with intrarenal pelvis, which increased the incidence of prolonged urine leakage. All in all, LPL is considered a successful alternative therapy for PCNL in selected cases with large renal stones like those in the extrarenal pelvis in patients without a history of previous surgery. In addition, LPL can be considered as a reasonable therapeutic option for large staghorn calculus which cannot be removed with a reasonable number of access and sessions of PCNL.

This study has some limitations. First, the present analysis was conducted using the currently available comparative studies. However, most of the studies were CCS, had a small sample number and quality ranged from low to moderate. Second, heterogeneity among studies was found to be high for several parameters. This heterogeneity can be explained by the difference in surgical practices, patient inclusion criteria, surgeons' experience, outcome definitions and standards. Third, the analysis did not incorporate stone shape and composition into the assessment, and either of these could have introduced bias into the analysis. Because of the above limitations might influence the interpretation of our findings, it highlights that large scale, multicenter RCTs are needed for a further robust conclusion.

Conclusion

Our present findings suggest that LPL is a safe and effective approach for management of patients with large renal pelvic stones with the merits of higher SFR, less blood loss, and lower auxiliary procedures rate. However, PCNL still suitable for most cases and LPL can be used as an alternative management procedure with good selection of cases.

Abbreviations
CCS: Case-control study; CI: Confidence interval; LPL: Laparoscopic pyelolithotomy; MD: Mean difference; NOS: Newcastle-Ottawa Scale; OR: Odds ratio; PCNL: Percutaneous nephrolithotomy; RCT: Randomized controlled trial; SFR: Stone-free rate; UTI: Urinary tract infection

Acknowledgments
None.

Funding

This work was collectively supported by grant (National Natural Science Foundation of China (No. 81270841)). The funder had no role in study design, data collection and analysis, decision to publish, or preparation of the manuscript.

Authors' contributions

Conceived and designed the experiments: PH and JW. Analyzed the data: JYB, LD and YBY. Contributed reagents/materials/analysis JYB and XMW. Wrote or revised the manuscript: JYB and YT. All authors have read and approved of the final manuscript.

Competing interests

The authors declare that they have no competing interests.

References

1. Seitz C, Desai M, Häcker A, Hakenberg OW, Liatsikos E, Nagele U, Tolley D. Incidence, prevention, and management of complications following percutaneous nephrolitholapaxy. Eur Urol. 2012;61(1):146–58.
2. Turna B, Umul M, Demiryoguran S, Altay B, Nazli O. How do increasing stone surface area and stone configuration affect overall outcome of Percutaneous Nephrolithotomy? J Endourol. 2007;21(1):34–43.
3. Zeng G, Zhu W, Li J, Zhao Z, Zeng T, Liu C, Liu Y, Yuan J, Wan SP. The comparison of minimally invasive percutaneous nephrolithotomy and retrograde intrarenal surgery for stones larger than 2 cm in patients with a solitary kidney: a matched-pair analysis. World J Urol. 2015;33(8):1159–64.
4. Wang X, Li S, Liu T, Guo Y, Yang Z. Laparoscopic pyelolithotomy compared to percutaneous nephrolithotomy as surgical management for large renal pelvic calculi: a meta-analysis. J Urol. 2013;190(3):888–93.
5. Wells GA, Shea B, O'Connell D, Peterson J, Welch V, Losos M, Tugwell P. The Newcastle-Ottawa Scale (NOS) for assessing the quality of nonrandomized studies in metaanalyses. Applied Engineering in Agriculture. 2014;18(6):727-34.
6. Clark HD, Wells GA, Huet C, McAlister FA, Salmi LR, Fergusson D, Laupacis A. Assessing the quality of randomized trials: reliability of the Jadad scale. Control Clin Trials. 1999;20(5):448–52.
7. Hozo SP, Djulbegovic B, Hozo I. Estimating the mean and variance from the median, range, and the size of a sample. BMC Med Res Methodol. 2005;5:13.
8. Al-Hunayan A, Khalil M, Hassabo M, Hanafi A, Abdul-Halim H. Management of Solitary Renal Pelvic Stone: laparoscopic retroperitoneal Pyelolithotomy versus Percutaneous Nephrolithotomy. J Endourol. 2011;25(6):975–8.
9. Tefekli A, Tepeler A, Akman T, Akcay M, Baykal M, Karadag MA, Muslumanoglu AY, de la Rosette J. The comparison of laparoscopic pyelolithotomy and percutaneous nephrolithotomy in the treatment of solitary large renal pelvic stones. Urol Res. 2012;40(5):549–55.
10. Aminsharifi A, Hosseini MM, Khakbaz A. Laparoscopic pyelolithotomy versus percutaneous nephrolithotomy for a solitary renal pelvis stone larger than 3 cm: a prospective cohort study. Urolithiasis. 2013;41(6):493–7.
11. Goel A, Hemal AK. Evaluation of role of retroperitoneoscopic pyelolithotomy and its comparison with percutaneous nephrolithotripsy. Int Urol Nephrol. 2003;35(1):73–6.
12. Perlin D, Alexandrov I, Zipunnikov V, Kargin K. Laparoscopic retroperitoneal pyelolithotomy for management of solitary renal stones: our experience. J Endourol. 2011;25:A336.
13. Fawzi AMAA, Shello HE, Khalil SA, El Kady SAM, Kamel HM, Desoky EAE. Retroperitoneal laparoscopic pyelolithotomy versus percutaneous nephrolithotomy for treatment of renal pelvis stones: a prospective randomized study. Eur Urol Suppl. 2015;14(2):e588.
14. Singh V, Sinha RJ, Gupta DK, Pandey M. Prospective randomized comparison of retroperitoneoscopic pyelolithotomy versus percutaneous nephrolithotomy for solitary large pelvic kidney stones. Urol Int. 2014;92(4):392–5.
15. Basiri A, Tabibi A, Nouralizadeh A, Arab D, Rezaeetalab GH, Hosseini Sharifi SH, Soltani MH. Comparison of safety and efficacy of laparoscopic pyelolithotomy versus percutaneous nephrolithotomy in patients with renal pelvic stones: a randomized clinical trial. Urol J. 2014;11(6):1932–7.
16. Tepeler ABM, Sari E, Akcay M, Berberoglu Y, Ahmet Yaser AY, Ahmet Hamdi AH. The comparison of laparoscopic pyelolithotomy versus percutaneous nephrolithotomy in the management of large renal pelvic stones. Eur Urol Suppl. 2009;8(4):261.
17. Meria PMS, Desgrandchamps F, Mongiat-Artus P, Duclos JM, Teillac P. Management of Pelvic Stones Larger than 20 mm: laparoscopic Transperitoneal Pyelolithotomy or Percutaneous Nephrolithotomy? Urol Int. 2005;75(4):322–6.
18. Li S, Liu TZ, Wang XH, Zeng XT, Zeng G, Yang ZH, Weng H, Meng Z, Huang JY. Randomized controlled trial comparing retroperitoneal laparoscopic Pyelolithotomy versus Percutaneous Nephrolithotomy for the treatment of large renal pelvic calculi: a pilot study. J Endourol. 2014;28(8):946–50.
19. Lee JW, Cho SY, Jeong CW, Yu J, Son H, Jeong H, Oh SJ, Kim HH, Lee SB. Comparison of surgical outcomes between laparoscopic Pyelolithotomy and Percutaneous Nephrolithotomy in patients with multiple renal stones in various parts of the Pelvocalyceal system. J Laparoendosc Adv S. 2014; 24(9):634–9.
20. Haggag YM, Morsy G, Badr MM, Al Emam AB, Farid M, Etafy M. Comparative study of laparoscopic pyelolithotomy versus percutaneous nephrolithotomy in the management of large renal pelvic stones. Can Urol Assoc J. 2013;7(3–4):E171–5.
21. Gaur DDPH, Madhusudhana HR, Rathi SS. Retroperitoneal laparoscopic pyelolithotomy: how does it compare with percutaneous nephrolithotomy for larger stones? Minim Invasive Ther Allied Technol. 2001;10(2):105–9.
22. Soucy F, Ko R, Duvdevani M, Nott L, Denstedt JD, Razvi H. Percutaneous nephrolithotomy for staghorn calculi: a single center's experience over 15 years. J Endourol. 2009;23(10):1669–73.
23. Gandhi HR, Thomas A, Nair B, Pooleri G. Laparoscopic pyelolithotomy: an emerging tool for complex staghorn nephrolithiasis in high-risk patients. Arab J Urol. 2015;13(2):139–45.
24. Jou YC, Lu CL, Chen FH, Shen CH, Cheng MC, Lin SH, Chuang SC, Li YH. Contributing factors for fever after tubeless percutaneous nephrolithotomy. Urology. 2015;85(3):527–30.
25. Wang Y, Jiang F, Wang Y, Hou Y, Zhang H, Chen Q, Xu N, Lu Z, Hu J, Lu J, et al. Post-percutaneous nephrolithotomy septic shock and severe hemorrhage: a study of risk factors. Urol Int. 2012;88(3):307–10.
26. Liu C, Zhang X, Liu Y, Wang P. Prevention and treatment of septic shock following mini-percutaneous nephrolithotomy: a single-center retrospective study of 834 cases. World J Urol. 2013;31(6):1593–7.
27. El-Nahas AR, Shokeir AA, El-Assmy AM, Mohsen T, Shoma AM, Eraky I, El-Kenawy MR, El-Kappany HA. Post-percutaneous nephrolithotomy extensive hemorrhage: a study of risk factors. J Urol. 2007;177(2):576–9.
28. Shah HN, Nayyar R, Rajamahanty S, Hemal AK. Prospective evaluation of unidirectional barbed suture for various indications in surgeon-controlled robotic reconstructive urologic surgery: Wake Forest University experience. Int Urol Nephrol. 2012;44(2):775–85.
29. Amend B, Muller O, Bedke J, Leichtle U, Nagele U, Kruck S, Stenzl A, Sievert KD. Biomechanical proof of barbed sutures for the efficacy of laparoscopic pyeloplasty. J Endourol. 2012;26(5):540–4.
30. Ozgor F, Kucuktopcu O, Sarılar O, Toptas M, Simsek A, Gurbuz ZG, Akbulut MF, Muslumanoglu AY, Binbay M. Does previous open renal surgery or percutaneous nephrolithotomy affect the outcomes and complications of percutaneous nephrolithotomy. Urolithiasis. 2015;43(6):541–7.

3

Assessing health-related quality of life in urology – a survey of 4500 German urologists

A. Schmick[1,2]* (iD), M. Juergensen[1,3], V. Rohde[4], A. Katalinic[1,5] and A. Waldmann[1]

Abstract

Background: Urological diseases and their treatment may negatively influence continence, potency, and health-related quality of life (HRQOL). Although current guidelines recommend HRQOL assessment in clinical urology, specific guidance on how to assess HRQOL is frequently absent. We evaluated whether and how urologists assess HRQOL and how they determine its practicality.

Methods: A random sample of 4500 (from 5200 identified German urologists) was drawn and invited to participate in a postal survey (an initial letter followed by one reminder after six weeks). The questionnaire included questions on whether and how HRQOL is assessed, general attitudes towards the concept of HRQOL, and socio-demographics. Due to the exploratory character of the study we produced mainly descriptive statistics. Chi^2-tests and logistic regression were used for subgroup-analysis.

Results: 1557 urologists (85% male, with a mean age of 49 yrs.) participated. Most of them (87%) considered HRQOL assessment as 'important' in daily work, while only 7% reported not assessing HRQOL. Patients with prostate carcinoma, incontinence, pain, and benign prostate hyperplasia were the main target groups for HRQOL assessment. The primary aim of HRQOL assessment was to support treatment decisions, monitor patients, and produce a 'baseline measurement'. Two-thirds of urologists used questionnaires and interviews to evaluate HRQOL and one-quarter assessed HRQOL by asking: 'How are you?'. The main barriers to HRQOL assessment were anticipated questionnaire costs (77%), extensive questionnaire length (52%), and complex analysis (51%).

Conclusions: The majority of German urologists assess HRQOL as part of their clinical routine. However, knowledge of HRQOL assessment, analysis, and interpretation seems to be limited in this group. Therefore, urologists may benefit from a targeted education program.

Keywords: Health-related quality of life, Assessment, Urology, Survey

Background

The most widely-accepted definition of health-related-quality-of-life (HRQOL) is that from the World Health Organization (WHO), which organisation defines this as an 'individual's perception of their position in life in the context of the culture and value systems in which they live and in relation to their goals, expectations, standards and concerns'. Consequently, physical and mental health, the measure of one's independence, social relationships and spiritual/religious beliefs influence the broad concept of HRQOL [1].

Over the last few decades, standardized generic and disease-specific instruments for the assessment of HRQOL have been developed and widely used in research – i.e. HRQOL has been commonly used as a clinical endpoint of therapy-comparing studies. Furthermore, HRQOL has recently gained increased relevance in clinical practice as the

* Correspondence: antonschmick@gmail.com
[1]Institute for Social Medicine and Epidemiology, University Luebeck, Ratzeburger Allee 160 (Hs 50), 23562 Luebeck, Germany
[2]Department of Emergency Medicine, Klinik Hirslanden, Witellikerstrasse 40, 8032 Zurich, Switzerland
Full list of author information is available at the end of the article

guidelines of most medical associations consider the enhancement of HRQOL as one of the primary therapeutic endpoints.

To the best of our knowledge, only a few studies have explored the view of clinicians regarding the concept of HRQOL and its potential for the clinical routine. In an earlier survey, 154 oncologists were interviewed about their attitudes toward HRQOL assessment. While 93.5% of participants reported being familiar with HRQOL research, 64% had assessed HRQOL for research purposes. Moreover, while 28% had used standardized questionnaires, 20% preferred self-made instruments. The research group identified the latter as patient-reported-outcome (PRO) scales [2]. Thus, the difference between HRQOL and patient-reported-outcome measures (PROMs) may not have been clear.

Another group surveyed 89 data managers from the EORTC-Trials regarding their attitude towards HRQOL assessment and found that not only financial and time resources, but also insufficient knowledge about the concept were substantial barriers to the integration of HRQOL assessment in clinical routine [3].

A review of older studies suggests that HRQOL is rarely measured in clinical settings due to a lack of financial and time resources, bureaucratic effort, and insufficient methodical knowledge (know-how) of HRQOL assessment [4].

A more recent survey of 309 Italian clinicians reported that 73.5% would like to assess HRQOL and 94.3% would be willing to prescribe expensive drugs to increase HRQOL. Again, the barriers to doing this were cited as insufficient methodical knowledge accompanied by restrained financial and time resources. Nonetheless, the number of clinicians who routinely measured HRQOL remains unclear [5].

Most studies on HRQOL assessments have investigated relatively small populations of oncologists [2–4]. The study participants were often familiar with HRQOL research and so they may not have been representative. Some of them did not differentiate between PROs and HRQOL [2].

The guidelines of the German Society of Urology (DGU) declare HRQOL as the principal therapeutic aim [6]. Nevertheless, many researchers continue to question the importance of HRQOL in clinical urology [7]. To our knowledge, thus far no studies have been conducted to explore physicians' proficiency in and attitudes towards HRQOL. Furthermore, the methods of HRQOL assessment in clinical urology remain uncertain.

The objectives of this study are to determine the importance of HRQOL in the clinical setting and to survey how useful, comprehensive, and accessible clinicians estimate HRQOL assessment to be. Moreover, we aim to ascertain the patient cohorts where HRQOL is frequently measured

and to assess which methods and HRQOL instruments are regularly applied.

Methods
Questionnaire development
In numerous successive expert meetings (A.W., V.R, A.K.) we developed the survey and, to test its usability, conducted two subsequent pre-tests, improving the design after the first pre-test ($n = 16$) and, due to satisfactory results, finalizing it following the second pre-test ($n = 10$).

The final survey consisted of three parts:

(1) 15 closed questions about the attitude towards HRQOL (Likert-scales),

(2) eight questions concerning the assessment of HRQOL in clinical routine (30 items in total for multiple choice questions and extra space for comments),

(3) demographic data (year of birth, year of specialty certification, working environment) and the last two items from the EORTC-QLQ-C30 to assess the HRQOL of the study participants [8–10] as well as extra space for comments.

Postal survey
We conducted a cross-sectional, nationwide postal survey of German urologists. The addresses were previously obtained from the register of the Association of the Statutory Health Insurance for Physicians and the German Association of Urologists. Our financial resources were capable of covering a survey of 4500; as such, after the revision of the database, a random sample of 4500 out of 5200 urologists was drawn.

The questionnaire was sent out with a post-paid return envelope. We identified non-respondents and sent them a reminder, containing the survey, six weeks after the initial dispatch.

Statistics
We hypothesized that the HRQOL played an essential role in clinical practice if more than 30% of participants were employing validated questionnaires for recorded HRQOL assessment.

Besides the hypothesis, our study had a mainly exploratory character and we produced primarily descriptive statistics. Additionally, to provide finer distinctiveness, Likert-scale items were added as follows: 'absolutely disagree' and 'slightly disagree' were condensed into 'disagree'; consequently, 'fairly agree' and 'absolutely agree' were subsumed into the category 'agree'. One question had a different scale so that 'absolutely not important' and 'slightly important' became 'not important', 'fairly important', 'very important' and 'important', while 'more or less important' was not included in either category.

Participants were divided into subgroups by gender, age, working environment and status of specialty training to investigate possible group differences. The subgroup analysis was calculated using Chi-square tests and logistic regression. The complete data analysis was accomplished using SPSS 20.0 software.

Results

Sample description

We contacted 4500 German urologists. The response rate was 37.9%. Accordingly, there were no statistically significant differences between the socio-demographics of respondents and non-respondents.

The mean age of respondents was 49 years (SD: 9.8) and a significant majority was male (85%). Slightly more than half of them were working in private practices (55.3%) and, consequently, most respondents had completed their specialty training in urology (94.6%; Table 1).

Attitude towards HRQOL

Relevance of HRQOL assessment in the clinical routine

HRQOL assessment was recognized as an important part of the clinical routine by most urologists (86.5%; Table 2). The perceived importance was reported more frequently with ascending age in respondents ($p = 0.124$, Chi^2-test). Consequently, consultants venerated HRQOL assessments more than urologists in training ($p = 0.009$, Chi^2-test). Nevertheless, gender and workplace did not significantly influence the perceived value of HRQOL assessment in the clinical routine.

Perception of HRQOL

The statement 'HRQOL is a vague term' was acknowledged by the majority of doctors (93.3%, Table 2). Moreover, private practice urologists approved the statement

more frequently than those from hospitals (OR = 1.77; 95% CI: 1.10–2.83).

Furthermore, the difference between symptom rating and HRQOL assessment was apparent for most of the respondents (87.9%). With increasing age, however, this difference became slightly less definite (OR = 0.97, 95% CI: 0.96–0.99).

Consequently, HRQOL assessments were considered suitable for daily use by more than 62 % (62.1%, Table 2). Notwithstanding, doctors from private practices found HRQOL assessments less suitable for everyday use than those doctors working in hospitals (OR = 1.46; 95% CI: 1.14–1.86).

Integrity of HRQOL in clinical routine

Numerous physicians deemed HRQOL assessments as valuable in consultations (94.8%) and therapy follow-ups (95.4%; Table 2). Additionally, verbal HRQOL assessment was considered sufficient by slightly more than half of the physicians (55.2%). Moreover, urologists from private practices (OR = 3.05; 95% CI: 2.40–3.87) preferred verbal HRQOL assessment compared to those from hospitals.

Concurrently, almost three-quarters of physicians approved standardized measures for HRQOL assessment as useful (72.4%, Table 2), whereas urologists occupied in private practices, and those advancing in age, reported the use of validated instruments less frequently (age: OR = 0.98; 95% CI 0.96–0.99 / private practice: OR = 0.37; 95% CI: 0.28–0.49).

Predominantly, urologists stated that their patients would ordinarily accept questionnaires for HRQOL assessment (87.3%). Notwithstanding, patients approved

Table 1 Description of study participants

	Female $n = 239$	Male $n = 1318$	Total $n = 1557$
Age[a]			
Mean age in years (SD) Range	43.8 (8.1) 31–72	50.4 (9.8) 27–90	49.4 (9.8) 27–90
Consultant			
Consultants (%)	88.3	95.8	94.6
Number of years as Consultant (mean (SD))[b]	11 (8.2)	17 (10.0)	16.2 (10.0)
Working Environment[c]			
Private Practice (%) [eigene Niederlassung][d]	19.8	32.0	30.1
Group (private) Practice (%)[Gemeinschaftspraxis][d]	20.3	26.1	25.2
Certified Prostate Centers (%)[zertifiziertes Prostatazentrum][d]	6.9	8.7	8.4
District hospital (%) [Maximalversorger][5]	34.9	20.0	22.3
Community hospital (%) [Schwerpunktversorger][d]	15.1	16.3	16.1
General hospital (%) [Regelversorger][d]	12.9	12.4	12.5

[a]6 (4 females and 32 males) have not provided their age
[b]118 (34 females und 84 males) have not provided the year of their consultant exam
[c]Percentages based on 1.515 due to missing information
[d]German translation

Table 2 Attitudes towards HRQOL assessment

Clinical Importance		Not important		Important		More or less important
		Absolutely not important	Slightly important	Fairly important	Very important	
Is HRQOL assessment important for clinical work?	% (N)	0.3 (5)	2.0 (29)	44.8 (659)	41.7 (614)	11.2 (165) [9.6–12.8]
	%Σ	2.3 [1.5–3.1]		86.5 [84.7–88.3]		
Perception of HRQOL		Disagree	Slightly disagree	Agree	Absolutely agree	Cannot estimate
		Absolutely disagree		Fairly agree		
To me HRQOL is a vague term.	% (N)	0.6 (9)	5.4 (84)	29.2 (453)	64.0 (992)	0.7 (11) [0.3–1.1]
	%Σ	6.0 [4.8–7.2]		93.3 [92.1–94.5]		
The difference between HRQOL assessment and symptom rating is not apparent.	% (N)	55.1 (849)	32.4 (499)	8.0 (123)	2.7 (42)	1.9 (29) [1.2–2.6]
	%Σ	87.4 [85.7–89.1]		10.7 [9.2–12.2]		
I regard HRQOL assessment as not suitable for daily use.	% (N)	15.7 (243)	46.4 (717)	28.1 (435)	5.5 (85)	4.3 (66) [3.3–5.3]
	%Σ	62.1 [59.7–64.5]		33.6 [31.2–36.0]		
Integrity of HRQOL						
HRQOL assessments are valuable in patient consultations.	% (N)	0.5 (8)	3.3 (51)	23.6 (366)	71.2 (1.103)	1.4 (22) [0.8–2.0]
	%Σ	3.8 [2.8–4.8]		94.8 [93.7–95.9]		
HRQOL assessments are valuable in therapy follow-ups.	% (N)	0.9 (14)	2.8 (43)	24.2 (375)	71.2 (1.106)	0.9 (14) [0.4–1.4]
	%Σ	3.7 [2.8–4.6]		95.4 [94.4–96.4]		
Verbal HRQOL assessment is generally sufficient.	% (N)	5.9 (92)	37.7 (585)	36.1 (559)	19.1 (296)	1.2 (18) [0.7–1.7]
	%Σ	43.6 [41.1–46.1]		55.2 [52.7–57.7]		
Validated HRQOL instruments are useful for HRQOL assessment.	% (N)	2.7 (42)	21.7 (337)	32.9 (511)	39.5 (613)	3.2 (50) [2.3–4.1]
	%Σ	24.4 [22.3–26.5]		72.4 [70.2–74.6]		
Barriers for HRQOL assessment						
My patients do not accept HRQOL questionnaires.	% (N)	36.0 (558)	43.6 (675)	10.0 (155)	2.7 (41)	7.7 (120) [6.4–9.0]
	%Σ	79.6 [77.6–81.6]		12.7 [11.0–14.4]		
I prefer not to pay for HRQOL questionnaires.	% (N)	5.0 (77)	5.8 (90)	13.1 (203)	64.1 (989)	12.0 (185) [10.4–13.6]
	%Σ	10.8 [9.3–12.3]		77.2 [75.1–79.3]		
The effort is too extensive to assess HRQOL in clinical routine.	% (N)	10.4 (161)	37.7 (585)	34.7 (538)	16.2 (251)	1.0 (16) [0.5–1.5]
	%Σ	48.1 [45.6–50.6]		50.9 [48.4–53.4]		
HRQOL questionnaires are disadvantageous due to their length.	% (N)	4.2 (66)	23.5 (363)	36.8 (569)	15.5 (240)	20.0 (309) [18.0–22.0]

Table 2 Attitudes towards HRQOL assessment (Continued)

	%∑	27.7 [25.5–29.9]		52.3 [49.8–54.8]		
HRQOL questionnaires are disadvantageous due to the complexity of their interpretation.	% (N)	5.2 (81)	25.0 (386)	34.2 (528)	13.9 (214)	21.7 (335) [19.6–23.8]
	%∑	30.2 [27.9–32.5]		48.1 [45.6–50.6]		
I am not sufficiently trained to assess HRQOL.	% (N)	39.7 (617)	46.5 (722)	9.6 (149)	1.9 (29)	2.3 (36) [1.6–3.0]
	%∑	86.2 [84.5–87.9]		11.5 [9.9–13.1]		
I cannot invoice HRQOL assessment due to a missing number in the medical-fee schedule.	% (N)	6.9 (105)	5.5 (84)	8.0 (122)	40.7 (619)	38.9 (593) [36.5–41.3]
	%∑	12.4 [10.7–14.1]		48.7 [46.2–51.2]		

%∑ = composite score in percent
[…] = 95% CI

HRQOL surveys in private practices less often (OR = 0.53; 95% CI: 0.37–0.76) than patients in hospitals.

Barriers to HRQOL assessment

The payment for HRQOL questionnaires was regularly considered inadmissible (77.2%, Table 2). Half of the physicians considered the effort of HRQOL assessment as too voluminous (50.2%). Furthermore, urologists from private practices reported this more frequently (OR = 1.43; 95% CI: 1.14–1.80) than those working in hospitals.

The HRQOL questionnaires were regarded by half of the physicians as disadvantageous due to their length (52.3%) and the complexity of their interpretation (48.1%). Both disadvantages were reported more frequently by physicians in private practice (length: OR = 1.50; 95% CI: 1.14–1.97 / complexity: OR = 1.64; 95% CI: 1.26–2.19) compared with their colleagues from hospitals.

A significant number of urologists regarded themselves to be adequately trained to assess HRQOL (86.2%). Conversely, those from private practices considered themselves less sufficiently trained (OR = 0.62; 95% CI: 0.44–0.88) than those doctors from hospitals.

Most urologists said it was impossible to invoice the HRQOL assessment due to a missing number in the medical-fee schedule (79.7%, Table 2). Nonetheless, this has been our survey's most frequently unanswered question. Consequently, private practice physicians tended to answer it twice as often (OR = 2.32; 95% CI: 1.60–3.37) when compared with hospital doctors.

Clinical implementation of HRQOL

The second part of our survey examined the clinical implementation of HRQOL. Almost every urologist assessed HRQOL (93.5%). There were no differences between subgroups.

Patient cohorts

Urologists most frequently assessed HRQOL in prostate cancer patients (63.5%) followed by those with incontinence (53.2%). Conversely, only a few doctors assessed HRQOL in patients with testosterone deficiency (31.8%; Fig. 1).

Aims for HRQOL assessment

The motivation for HRQOL assessment was primarily to support a therapy choice (82.8%), evaluate a follow-up (82.1%) and survey a baseline (75.2%). Urologists rarely assessed HRQOL for research purposes (17.2%).

Methods of HRQOL-assessment

Most urologists used combined recorded and verbal HRQOL assessment (61.8%), followed by verbal-only (22.0%) and written-only (10.8%). Consequently, female urologists used the combined approach more regularly (75,9% vs. 64,7%, p = 0,003; Chi^2-Test). Nevertheless, males, private practice urologists, and consultants favored the verbal-only assessment (Table 3).

The oral HRQOL assessment was frequently reduced to the single question: 'How are you?' (53.7%), and it was rarely carried out with validated questionnaires in the sense of a structured interview (20.6%). Private practice and female physicians tended to assess HRQOL by asking: 'How are you?', more commonly. Conversely, urologists from hospitals and those of a younger age preferred validated questionnaires for verbal HRQOL assessment (Table 3).

More than 65 % of urologists (65.9%) applied validated questionnaires for recorded HRQOL-assessment. Notwithstanding, female urologists tended to use validated questionnaires less often (OR = 0.54; 95% CI: 0.31–0.95). Moreover, with advancing age the probability of validated questionnaire use slightly decreased (OR = 0.96, 95% CI: 0.93–0.98).

Urologists most frequently applied the International Prostate Symptom Score (IPSS) (96.1%) followed by the International Index of Erectile Function (IIEF) (78.7%), the Karnofsky-Index (44.7%), and Aging Male Symptoms (AMS) (36.8%). Conversely, the Eastern Cooperative Oncology Group Score (ECOG) was infrequently used (1.7%). Surprisingly, the EORTC-QLQ-C30, which is recommended by the German Society of Urology for HRQOL assessment in prostate-cancer-patients, was administered rather scarcely (4.5%). Other rarely-used scores included the International Consultation on Incontinence Questionnaire (ICIQ) (4.1%) and the International Continence Society on Quality of Life (ICSQoL) (1.8%). In a bivariate analysis, younger physicians preferred the IPSS (p < 0.001, Chi^2-Test). Multivariate analysis showed female urologists to administer IPSS and IIEF significantly less than their male counterparts (OR: 0.65; 95%CI: 0.38–1.08; OR: 0.61; 95%CI: 0.61; 0.42–0.89). Older and hospital physicians preferred IIEF (each: p < 0.001, Chi^2-Test) both in bi- and multivariate analysis. The Karnofsky-Index was used significantly less often by females (p = 0.044, Chi^2-Test). However, in multivariate analysis the gender difference was less prominent (OR: 0.76; 95%CI: 0.54–1.07). Males, older physicians, consultants and those in private practice applied AMS more frequently (males: p = 0.017; others: p < 0.001; Chi^2-Test). In multivariate analysis, AMS administration was significantly higher in private practice (OR: 6.30; 95%CI: 4.58–8.66). Table 4 shows the results of the multivariate analysis.

Discussion

The principal aims of the study were to determine the importance of HRQOL in a clinical setting, to evaluate

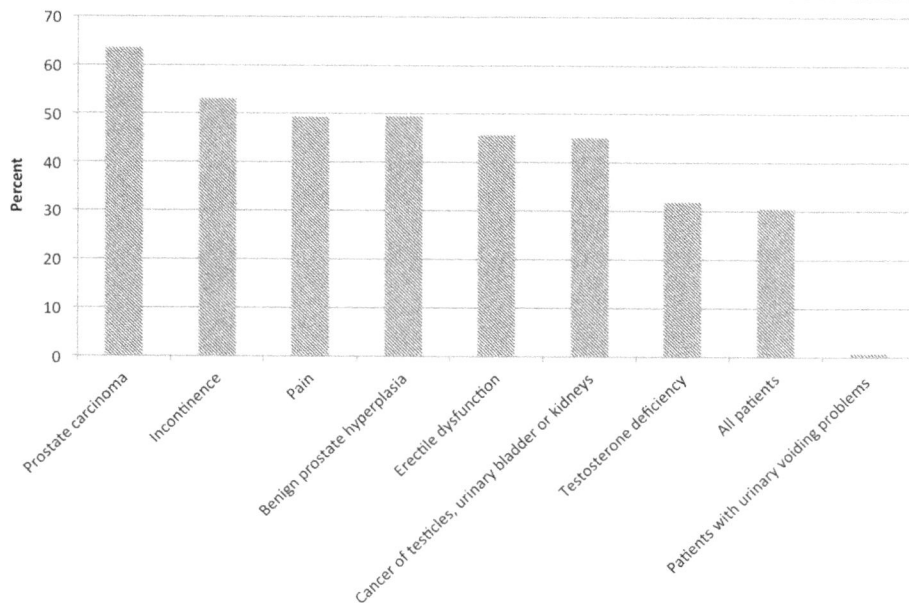

Fig. 1 Frequency of HRQOL assessment in different patient groups, according to diagnosis

how useful, comprehensive and feasible clinicians find HRQOL assessment, to ascertain the most significant patient cohorts and aims for HRQOL assessment, and to describe the methods and instruments used.

Among our 1557 study participants, the attitude towards HRQOL was mainly positive, and most urologists considered HRQOL necessary as part of their clinical routine. The barriers towards the implementation of routine HRQOL assessment were constraints on time and financial resources. The length and complexity of questionnaires also had an adverse impact on HRQOL assessment. Our respondents regularly measured HRQOL in prostate cancer patients and patients with incontinence. Furthermore, they predominantly assessed HRQOL to determine a therapy, evaluate a follow-up or measure a baseline.

The central hypothesis of the survey was that HRQOL achieved an essential role in clinical practice if more than 30% of participants were employing validated questionnaires for recorded HRQOL assessment. These results suggest that the hypothesis was proven to be correct. While almost every respondent assessed HRQOL, more than 60 % employed validated questionnaires for recorded HRQOL assessment.

General attitudes towards HRQOL and its clinical use

In general, urologists expressed interest in HRQOL assessment and were positive towards its clinical implementation, as had been found in other studies [5, 15, 16]. The positive image of HRQOL in urological guidelines [6] may have generated additional interest in the subject.

Most urologists agreed that the understanding of HRQOL among people might alternate. The WHO defines HRQOL as: 'individuals' perception of their position in life in the context of the culture and value systems in which they live and in relation to their goals, expectations, standards and concerns' [1]. HRQOL can change at different stages of both disease and therapy as various concerns may arise [17].

HRQOL assessment enhances doctor-patient communication, facilitates the discussion of the psychosocial impact of the disease and ultimately improves the patient's HRQOL [17–19]. In our study urologists perceived HRQOL assessment as valuable and suitable for daily use, while earlier surveys indicated that only a minority of physicians recognized the assessment of HRQOL as useful in clinical practice. Overall, there may have been a change of perception regarding HRQOL [2, 20].

In our study urologists felt confident to assess HRQOL, while in a different study pediatricians did not consider themselves to be sufficiently trained to assess HRQOL [15]. The different opinions may have been caused by the higher complexity of HRQOL assessment for children (including the intricacy of proxy methods) [21, 22].

The majority of urologists disapproved of the length and complexity of HRQOL questionnaires, while in another study physicians requested simplified scales for better applicability [16]. Notwithstanding, simplified scales may entail the risk of reductionism and the multidimensional construct of HRQOL could lose its significance. For an improved usability and easier HRQOL

Table 3 Methods of HRQOL assessment in subgroup analysis (Chi[2]-Test and logistic regression analysis)

HRQOL assessment	Recorded and verbal Cells-% (N)	Verbal only Cells-% (N)	Recorded only Cells-% (N)	"How are you?" Cells-% (N)	Verbal Standardized HRQOL Instruments Cells-% (N)	Recorded Non-Standardized Cells-% (N)	Recorded Standardized HRQOL Instruments		
							Cells-% (N)	Multivariate OR[a] [95% CI]	Multivariate Significance[a] (Logistic Regression)
Total	61.8 (960)	22.0 (342)	10.8 (143)	53.7 (833)	20.6 (320)	13.5 (209)	65.9 (1023)		
Gender									
Male	64.7[b] (790)	24.6[b] (300)	10.7[b] (131)	52.5[e] (690)	20.7 (272)	13.0 (171)	65.2 (857)	1	P = 0.033
Female	75.9 (170)	18.8 (42)	5.4 (12)	59.8 (143)	20.1 (48)	15.9 (38)	69.5 (166)	0.54 [0.31–0.95]	
Working Environment									
Hospital	63.3[c] (433)	12.5[c] (81)	18.1[c] (117)	48.2[c] (432)	17.3[c] (126)	12.8 (89)	77.6[c] (541)	1	P = 0.178
Private practice	69.3 (448)	33.8 (231)	2.9 (20)	5.2 (336)	24.5 (170)	14.2 (104)	55.9 (408)	0.64 [0.29–1.44]	
Age									
25-44y	74.1[c] (386)	13.4[c] (70)	12.5[c] (65)	56.6 (318)	24.4[f] (137)	12.3 (69)	77.6[c] (436)	0,96[h] [0.93–0.98]	P < 0.001[h]
45-59y	64.2 (433)	26.9 (181)	8.9 (60)	52.9 (379)	18.7 (134)	13.8 (99)	62.8 (450)		
60-90y	55.0 (120)	38.5 (84)	6.4 (14)	50.0 (121)	16.9 (41)	14.5 (35)	47.5 (115)		
Qualification									
Consultant	66.4 (909)	24.1[d] (330)	9.4[d] (129)	53.3 (785)	20.5 (302)	13.5 (199)	65.3[g] (962)	1	P = 0.981
In Training	66.2 (51)	15.6 (12)	18.2 (14)	59.3 (48)	22.2 (18)	12.3 (10)	76.5 (62)	0.99 [0.34–2.88]	

[a]controlled for gender, working environment, age and qualification
[b]p = 0.003 Chi[2]-Test
[c]p < 0.001 Chi[2]-Test
[d]p = 0.019 Chi[2]-Test
[e]p = 0.036 Chi[2]-Test
[f]p = 0.014 Chi[2]-Test
[g]p = 0.038 Chi[2]-Test
[h]linear age model

Table 4 Factors influencing the choice of questionnaires used for HRQOL assessment (logistic regression analysis)

	IPSS OR (95% CI)	IIEF OR (95% CI)	Karnofsky-Index OR (95% CI)	AMS OR (95% CI)
Age[a]	0.95 (0.93–0.97)	0.96 (0.95–0.98)	1.01 (0.99–1.03)	0.99 (0.97–1.01)
Gender				
Male	1	1	1	1
Female	0.65 (0.38–1.08)	0.61 (0.42–0.89)	0.76 (0.54–1.07)	0.72 (0.48–1.08)
Working Environment				
Hospital	1	1	1	1
Private practice	1.10 (0.72–1.69)	0.67 (0.49–0.92)	0.78 (0.59–1.03)	6.30 (4.58–8.66)
Qualification				
Consultant	1	1	1	1
In Training	0.95 (0.39–2.33)	0.77 (0.41–1.43)	1.01 (0.59–1.72)	0.34 (0.14–0.81)

[a]In years as continuous variable

assessment in clinical routine, the employment of ten visual analogous scales was suggested [23].

Constraints of both time and financial resources were mentioned in our study. Nonetheless, these results did not differ much from previous findings [2, 24, 25]. However, the deficit of economic resources may be expedited by the impossibility of invoice for HRQOL assessment due to the German medical-fee schedule [26]. Consequently, to facilitate patient-centered care, the medical-fee schedule may have to be changed.

Practical use of HRQOL in clinical routine

Urologists mostly assessed HRQOL in patients with prostate cancer, incontinence, and benign prostate hyperplasia. It may be that, out of all German urological guidelines, only those concerning these three conditions recommend strategies for HRQOL assessment [6]. Moreover, German urologists are likely to follow national guidelines, as has been proven in a recent survey [27]. Consequently, the enhancement of strategies for HRQOL assessment in guidelines for other diseases may aid HRQOL implementation.

HRQOL was assessed to support a therapy choice, create a baseline measure, and evaluate a follow-up status. It was least frequently evaluated for research purposes. This finding is especially interesting as most other studies have shown that HRQOL was primarily obtained for research purposes [5]. Supporting a therapy choice, creating a baseline measure, and evaluating a follow-up status are altogether important in patient-centered care. However, we believe that patients may benefit more from a continuous HRQOL assessment as proposed by Velikova et al. [17].

Evaluation of recorded and verbal HRQOL assessment

The standardized, recorded HRQOL assessment is shown to influence doctor-patient communication positively and ultimately enhance the patient's HRQOL [17–19]. It is evident that physicians must verbalize HRQOL and hence the differentiation of recorded and verbal approaches may seem academic. Consequently, less than 10 % used a recorded-only approach. However, it was important to investigate the use of standardized measures, which in turn are predominantly designed for recorded use. Most urologists used combined (verbal and written) HRQOL assessment.

Standardization of such a personal, individual and subjective measure as HRQOL raised skepticism among Wilm et al. [28], who argued that standardized measures would fail to incorporate individualized concepts of disease and bring a 'scientific bias' in approaching patients. Furthermore, proxy measures would raise unsolved methodological and ethical questions. Hence Wilm et al. advocated an open question: 'How are you?', to address HRQOL [28]. Our

survey showed, however, that less than a quarter of urologists have exclusively asked this question.

Among numerous factors, doctor-patient communication is relationship based. Therefore, 'How are you?' is a question that may fail to address the multiple dimensions of HRQOL [29], whereas standardized HRQOL measurement proved to facilitate the doctor-patient relationship and, furthermore, enhance patients' HRQOL [17–19].

An open question has reportedly failed to address important HRQOL issues, ascribed to a discrepancy in the topics of most importance to patients, who preferred to address social, psychological and spiritual issues, and doctors, who preferred to discuss the physical functioning and wellbeing [30]. Consequently, a standardized measure provides a chance to integrate all dimensions of HRQOL.

Wilson et al. investigated possible inadequacies of the standardized HRQOL measures [31]. However, contrary to Wilm et al., the Wilson group did not advise against their use but encouraged it in combination with an open discussion of HRQOL [31]. The same recommendations were given based on the results of other studies [16, 32].

Used questionnaires

In our study, the IPSS had been the most frequently reported instrument used for HRQOL assessment. The German Society of Urology (DGU) recommends the use of IPSS for HRQOL assessment in patients with benign prostate hyperplasia [33]. It consists of a few symptom questions and a 'bother score' [34]. Although it is recommended for HRQOL assessment, it does not cover the psychosocial and spiritual dimensions of HRQOL, and hence important aspects of HRQOL may get lost. However, similarly to the 'distress thermometer' [35], clinicians could use the IPSS (and similar 'bother scores') as a screening for HRQOL impairment to decide whether to refer patients to a psychologist or a psycho-oncologist.

Compared to IPSS the EORTC-QLQ-C30 is a rather extensive HRQOL score. It is recommended by DGU for HRQOL assessment in patients with prostate cancer [36]. However, less than 5 % of our study participants have applied it in their clinical routine. More frequently, they reported using the Karnofsky Index and IIEF to assess HRQOL. However, these instruments are not capable of determining HRQOL. Similar to ECOG, the Karnofsky Index has been developed to evaluate general performance status [7, 37]. While these scores consist of single scales, the structure of IIEF is more complex. IIEF assesses Patient Reported Outcomes (PROs) related to erectile dysfunction using 15 Likert-scales. However, it does not measure the multidimensional concept of HRQOL [38]. These findings suggest that study participants may not have distinguished between Patient Reported Outcome Measures (PROMs) and HRQOL. Another study found that urologists were, in general, more accurate in recording sexual and incontinence symptoms (PROMs) than HRQOL [37].

PROMs and HRQOL are also frequently confused in the literature. For example, Doehn and Jocham discussed ECOG and the Karnofsky Index extensively in their review article on HRQOL assessment in urology, yet left unmentioned that both scores are incapable of measuring HRQOL [7]. Using the Karnofsky Index, urologists failed to detect significant role limitations [37].

Another example of the misrepresentation of HRQOL assessment is the recently published 'Expanded Prostate Cancer Index Composite for Clinical Practice' (EPIC-CP). It consists of 16 scales, each assessing the intensity of prostate-cancer-related symptoms [39]. Not a single scale evaluates psychosocial (or spiritual) aspects of the disease, hence failing to address the multidimensional concept of HRQOL as defined by the WHO [39].

Clinical implications

Our findings are important for clinicians as they illustrate a typical pattern of clinical HRQOL assessment. The fact that over 60 % claim to assess HRQOL, while most of them use symptom-screening scales such as IPSS and some only ask an open question ('How are you?'), is of particular importance for the clinical routine. Following either of the above strategies may lead to failure to assess the full spectrum of HRQOL [30, 34]. To avoid this, distinguishing separate PROMs from HRQOL is crucial. Furthermore, physicians tend to underestimate the impact of disease on patients' HRQOL and hence should administer appropriate questionnaires [37].

We propose the use of validated instruments to investigate the impact of HRQOL on the disease, successional to an open discussion of HRQOL [16, 31, 32]. Consequently, along with Velikova et al., we recommend putting the emphasis of HRQOL assessment on the complaints that affect particular HRQOL dimensions according to the stages of chronic disease [17].

Importance and limitations

Primarily, HRQOL has achieved an essential role in clinical practice. This conclusion is supported by the fact that over 60 % of urologists reported frequent use of validated HRQOL questionnaires.

Nevertheless, a response bias may be a limitation, as respondents may have been more interested in the study topic than non-respondents [11]. Response bias can be calculated by estimating the difference between the demographics of respondents and non-respondents [12–14], as demographics can be associated with the attitude towards the survey topic. In our subgroup analysis, females were

associated with lesser use of validated HRQOL instruments. However, this has not affected the response bias as no significant differences between the demographics of respondents and non-respondents were found.

A qualitative interrogation of non-respondents could have provided a better understanding of the non-respondents and helped to weigh the non-response bias. However, due to lack of fiscal and personnel resources such qualitative analysis could not be determined.

The use of a non-validated instrument could be considered a limitation. Therefore, ahead of the survey, the instrument's feasibility was examined with two subsequent pre-tests. It was the first explorative study of its kind and the use of the questionnaire seems to be justified.

The survey was concluded nationwide, had a comparatively high response rate compared to other surveys among physicians and the socio-demographics of respondents did not differ significantly from non-respondents. Consequently, the chance of a response bias seems to be low.

Our survey addressed a general population of urologists and, therefore, the results could be considered generalizable, while other studies [3, 5] were based on rather specific populations and may have suffered from a selection bias.

To our knowledge, this is the first survey of German urologists on HRQOL in clinical routine. It provides detailed insights on the integration of HRQOL.

Conclusions

Most urologists assess HRQOL in their daily clinical routine. Interestingly, the most ordinarily reported instruments were capable of rating symptoms, hence evaluating PROMs instead of measuring the complex concept of HRQOL. Conclusively, urologists' knowledge concerning HRQOL assessment, analysis, and interpretation appears to be limited. To further integrate HRQOL into their clinical routine, urologists could benefit from a targeted education program.

Abbreviations
AMS: Aging Male Symptoms; CI: Confidence interval; DGU: German Society of Urology; ECOG : East cooperative oncology group (Score); EORTC-QLQ-C30: European Organization for Research and Treatment of Cancer Quality of Life Questionnaire for Cancer patients; EPIC-CP: Expanded Prostate Cancer Index Composite for Clinical Practice; HRQOL : Health related quality of life; ICIQ: International Consultation on Incontinence Questionnaire; ICSQoL: International Continence Society on Quality of Life; IIEF: International Index of Erectile Function; IPSS : International prostate syndrome score; OR: Odds ratio; PRO: Patient related outcome; PROM: Patient related outcome measure; WHO: World Health Organization

Acknowledgments
We would like to express our gratitude to Jessica Lückert, who co-created the electronic database and helped with data entry. We thank Takeda GmbH for the unrestricted grant.

Sponsor
Takeda Pharma GmBH funded the research project with an unrestricted grant. The sponsor had no influence on the design and conduct of the study, nor on the analysis or interpretation of data.

Funding
Takeda Pharma GmBH funded the study with an unrestricted grant. The sponsor had no influence on either the design or conduct of the study or on the analysis and interpretation of the data.

Authors' contributions
AS carried out the postal survey, co-created the electronic database, was responsible for data entry, statistical analysis and interpretation of data and drafted the manuscript. MJ participated in finalizing the questionnaire as well as in statistical analysis and interpretation of data and has been revising the manuscript critically for important intellectual content. VR participated in the design and development of the questionnaire and has been revising the manuscript critically for important intellectual content. AK participated in the design and development of the survey and has been revising the manuscript critically for important intellectual content. AW participated in the design and development of the questionnaire, supervised the creation of the database, data entry, analysis, and interpretation of data and has been revising the manuscript critically for important intellectual content. All authors read and approved the final manuscript and agreed to be accountable for all aspects of the work in ensuring that questions related to the accuracy or integrity of any part of the work are appropriately investigated and resolved.

Competing interests
All authors declare that they have no conflict of interest.

Author details
[1]Institute for Social Medicine and Epidemiology, University Luebeck, Ratzeburger Allee 160 (Hs 50), 23562 Luebeck, Germany. [2]Department of Emergency Medicine, Klinik Hirslanden, Witellikerstrasse 40, 8032 Zurich, Switzerland. [3]Institute for History of Medicine and Science Studies, University Luebeck, Koenigstr. 42, 23552 Luebeck, Germany. [4]Medical Practice of Urology, Auguststr. 4, 23611 Bad Schwartau, Germany. [5]Institute for Cancer Epidemiology, University Luebeck, Ratzeburger Allee 160 (Hs 50), 23562 Luebeck, Germany.

References
1. WHOQOL-Group (1997). WHOQOL: Measuring the Quality of Life.1;1–2.
2. Morris J, Perez D, McNoe B. The use of quality of life data in clinical practice. Qual Life Res. 1998;7(1):85–91.
3. Young T, Maher J. Collecting quality of life data in EORTC clinical trials—what happens in practice? Psycho-Oncology. 1999;8(1):260–3.
4. Davis K, Cella D. Assessing quality of life in oncology clinical practice: a review of barriers and critical success factors. JCOM. 2002;9(6):327–32.
5. Bossola M, Murri R, Onder G, Turriziani A, Fantoni M, Padua L. Physicians' knowledge of health-related quality of life and perception of its importance in daily clinical practice. Health Qual Life Outcomes. 2010;43(8):1–7.
6. Schmick A. (2016). Attitudes of Urologists towards HRQOL and its Clinical Use. Doctoratethesis. University of Luebeck. 11–15.
7. Doehn C, Jocham D. Neues zur Lebensqualität in der urologischen Onkologie. Onkologie. 2002;26(4):30–4.
8. Aaronson NK, Ahmedzai S, Bergman B. The European Organization for Research and Treatment of cancer QLQ-C30: a quality-of-life instrument for use in international clinical trials in oncology. J Natl Cancer Inst. 1993;85(5):365–76.
9. Osoba D, Rodrigues G, Myles J, Zee B, Pater J. Interpreting the significance of changes in health-related quality-of-life scores. J Clin Oncol. 1998;16(1):139 44.
10. Waldmann A, Schubert D, Katalinic A. Normative data of the EORTC QLQ-C30 for the German population: a population-based survey. PLoS One. 2013;8(9):e74149. https://doi.org/10.1371/journal.pone.0074149.
11. Dillman DA. The design and administration of mail surveys. Annu Rev Sociol. 1991;17(1):225–49.
12. Kellerman S, Herold J. Physician response to surveys a review of the literature. Am J Prev Med. 2001;20(1):61–7.
13. McFarlane E, Olmsted M, Murphy J, Hill C. Nonresponse bias in a mail survey of physicians. Eval Health Prof. 2007;30(2):170–85.
14. van Goor H, Stuiver B. Can weighting compensate for Nonresponse bias in a dependent variable? An Evaluation of weighting methods to correct for substantive bias in a mail survey among Dutch municipalities. Soc Sci Res. 1998;27(4):481–99.
15. Baars RM, van der Pal SM, Koopman HM, Wit JM. Clinicians' perspective on quality of life assessment in paediatric clinical practice. Acta Paediatr. 2004; 93(10):1356–60.
16. Skevington SM, Day R, Chisholm A, Trueman P. How much do doctors use quality of life information in primary care? Testing the trans-theoretical model of behaviour change. Qual Life Res. 2005;14(4):911–22.
17. Velikova G, Awad N, Coles-Gale R, Penny Wright E, Brown J, Selby P. The clinical value of quality of life assessment in oncology practice - a qualitative study of patient and physician views. Psycho-Oncology. 2008; 17(7):690–8.
18. Velikova G, Booth L, Smith AB, Brown PM, Lynch P, Brown JM, et al. Measuring quality of life in routine oncology practice improves communication and patient well-being: a randomized controlled trial. J Clin Oncol. 2004;22(4):714–24.
19. Detmar SB, Muller MJ, Schornagel NH, Wever LD, Aaronson NK. Health-related quality of life assessments and patient-physician communication. JAMA. 2002;288(23):3027–34.
20. Bezjak A, Ng P, Skeel R, DePetrillo AD, Comis R, Taylor KM. Oncologists' use of quality of life information: results of a survey of eastern cooperative oncology group physicians. Qual Life Res. 2001;10(1):1–13.
21. Bianchini J, da Silva D, Nardo C, Carolino I, Hernandes F, Nardo N. Parent-proxy perception of overweight adolescents' health-related quality of life is different according to adolescent gender and age and parent gender. Eur J Pediatr. 2013;172(10):1371–7.
22. Rotsika V, Coccossis M, Vlassopoulos M, Papaeleftheriou E, Sakellariou K, Anagnostopoulos D, et al. Does the subjective quality of life of children with specific learning disabilities (SpLD) agree with their parents' proxy reports? Qual Life Res. 2011;20(8):1271–8.
23. Rosenzveig A, Kuspinar A, Daskalopoulou SS, Mayo NE. Toward patient-centered care: a systematic review of how to ask questions that matter to patients. Baltimore Med. 2014;93(22):e120.
24. Straus SE, Sackett DL. Getting research findings into practice: using research findings in clinical practice. Br Med J. 1998;317(7154):339–42.
25. Osoba D. Health-related quality of life and cancer clinical trials. Ther Adv Med Oncol. 2011;3(2):57–71.
26. Kassenärztliche Bundesvereinigung. (2016) EBM - Einheitlicher Bewertungsmaßstab; http://www.kbv.de/html/online-ebm.php; accessed: 5 Aug 2016.
27. Fröhner M, Khan C, Koch R, Schorr S, Wirth M. Implementierung der S3-Leitlinie Prostatakarzinom im klinischen Alltag. Urologe. 2014;53(10):1500–3.
28. Wilm S, Leve V, Santos S. Is it quality of life that patients really want? Assessment from a general practitioner's perspective. Z Evid Fortbild Qual Gesundhwes. 2014;108(2–3):126–9.
29. Arora NK, Jensen RE, Sulayman N, Hamilton AS, Potosky AL. Patient-physician communication about health related quality of life problems: are non-Hodgkin lymphoma survivors willing to talk? J Clin Oncol. 2013;31(31):3964–70.
30. Rodriguez KL, Bayliss N, Alexander SC. How oncologists and their patients with advanced cancer communicate about health-related quality of life. Psychooncology. 2010;19(5):490–9.
31. Wilson T, Birks Y, Alexander D. Pitfalls in the interpretation of standardised quality of life instruments for individual patients? A qualitative study in colorectal cancer. Qual Life Res. 2013;22(7):1879–88.
32. Detmar SB. Use of HRQOL questionnaires to facilitate patient–physician communication. Expert Rev Pharmacoecon Outcomes Res. 2003;3(3):215–7.
33. Oelke M, Berges R, Tunn U. Diagnostik und Differenzialdiagnostik des benignen Prostatasyndroms (BPS). AWMF. 2009;1(1):1–16.
34. O'Leary M. Validity of the "bother score" in the Evaluation and treatment of symptomatic benign prostatic hyperplasia. Rev Urol. 2005;7(1):1–10.
35. Zwahlen D, Hagenbuch N, Jenewein J, Carley M, Buchi S. Adopting a family approach to theory and practice: measuring distress in cancer patient–partner dyads with the distress thermometer. Psycho-Oncology. 2011;20(4):394–403.

Symptom clusters and related factors in bladder cancer patients three months after radical cystectomy

Hongyan Ren[1], Ping Tang[2], Qinghua Zhao[3] and Guosheng Ren[4*]

Abstract

Background: To identify symptom distress and clusters in patients 3 months after radical cystectomy and to explore their potential predictors.

Methods: A cross-sectional design was used to investigate 99 bladder cancer patients 3 months after radical cystectomy. Data were collected by demographic and disease characteristic questionnaires, the symptom experience scale of the M.D. Anderson symptom inventory, two additional symptoms specific to radical cystectomy, and the functional assessment of cancer therapy questionnaire. A factor analysis, stepwise regression, and correlation analysis were applied.

Results: Three symptom clusters were identified: fatigue-malaise, gastrointestinal, and psycho-urinary. Age, complication severity, albumin post-surgery (negative), orthotropic neobladder reconstruction, adjuvant chemotherapy and American Society of Anesthesiologists (ASA) scores were significant predictors of fatigue-malaise. Adjuvant chemotherapy, orthotropic neobladder reconstruction, female gender, ASA scores and albumin (negative) were significant predictors of gastrointestinal symptoms. Being unmarried, having a higher educational level and complication severity were significant predictors of psycho-urinary symptoms. The correlations between clusters and for each cluster with quality of life were significant, with the highest correlation observed between the psycho-urinary cluster and quality of life.

Conclusions: Bladder cancer patients experience concurrent symptoms that appear to cluster and are significantly correlated with quality of life. Moreover, symptom clusters may be predicted by certain demographic and clinical characteristics.

Keywords: Bladder cancer, Quality of life, Radical cystectomy, Symptom cluster, Symptom distress

Background

Radical cystectomy (RC) with urinary diversion is currently the standard treatment for muscle-invasive bladder cancer and is recommended for high-risk non-muscle-invasive bladder cancers. In China, bladder cancer is the eighth most common cancer in men and has recently increased in frequency [1]. Among diagnosed patients, 20% are candidates for RC [2]. However, bladder cancer itself and its treatment, such as surgery and chemotherapy, may cause symptom distress in patients, including fatigue, pain, appetite loss, nausea, vomiting, insomnia, diarrhea, colostomy problems, urine leakage, sexual dysfunction, and

emotional distress [3–5]. Notably, clinical experiences have shown that multiple symptoms are clustered in cancer patients in disease trajectories [6]. Kim et al. [7] refined the definition of a symptom cluster (SC) as consisting of two or more symptoms that are related to each other and that occur together. The existence of SCs appears to exert a complex and synergistic detrimental effect on quality of life (QoL). Exploring the mechanics of concurrent symptoms such as SCs may facilitate the development of effective strategies to reduce the impact of treatment- and disease-related symptoms to improve patient QoL.

However, few studies have reported systematic, patient-reported symptom distress data, particularly at 3 months after operation, which is important for patient transition from post-surgery to long-term recovery.

* Correspondence: rengs726@126.com
[4]Molecular Oncology and Epigenetics Laboratory, The First Affiliated Hospital of Chongqing Medical University, No. 1 Youyi Road, Yuzhong District, Chongqing 400016, China
Full list of author information is available at the end of the article

Based on previous studies, we hypothesized that patient symptoms might appear concurrently in a clustered manner and might be influenced by several demographic and disease variables. Therefore, the aims of this study were to (1) describe symptom experiences, (2) explore whether symptoms were clustered, (3) explore the potential predictors of each SC, and (4) analyze the correlations between SCs and QoL in bladder cancer patients 3 months after RC with an ileal conduit (IC) or orthotopic neobladder (ONB) reconstruction.

Methods
Patients and design
A cross-sectional design was used. The participants were consecutively enrolled from March 2013 to December 2015 at the first affiliated hospital of Chongqing medical university, China. The participant inclusion criteria included the following: (1) histologically confirmed bladder cancer and (2) treatment with RC combined with IC or ONB. The exclusion criteria included the following: (1) psychosis or cognitive impairment and (2) loss of contact or death during the study.

Data collection
The clinical trial was approved by the university institutional review board. The demographic data were collected using an interview tool; the clinical information was collected by reviewing the patients' medical records. Complications were defined as those occurring within 3 months after surgery. All events leading to a prolonged hospital stay or requiring medication or surgical intervention were scored as a complication. According to the Accordion Severity Grading System of surgical complications, complications were classified as minor, moderate or major.

The symptom questionnaires and the QoL assessments were completed through telephone or face-to-face interviews with the patients by trained oncology nurses 3 months after the operation. Data integration was reviewed immediately after the interviews, and any missing data were captured.

Instruments
Patient symptoms were assessed using the revised symptom severity scale of the M.D. Anderson symptom inventory (MDASI) [8]. This original section of this scale has 13 items used to measure the severity of each symptom (item) in the previous 24 h, and the score ranges from 0 ("symptom not present") to 10 ("as bad as you can imagine"). The Chinese version translated and tested by Wang et al. [9] was used. For our objectives, two disease-specific symptoms were added: one to measure urinary function (urinary control for ONB and urostomy management for IC) and the other to gauge patient dissatisfaction with one's appearance. In the current study,

the internal consistency coefficient (Cronbach's alpha) for this 15-item scale was 0.803, and the content validity index determined by five urology experts was 0.855.

The QoL was measured using the self-administered Functional Assessment of Cancer Therapy-General (FACT-G) [10]; a higher score indicated a better QoL.

Statistical analyses
Descriptive statistics were used to summarize the demographic and clinical characteristics and the prevalence and severity of symptoms. The SCs were identified by exploratory factor analysis using principal axis factoring. Similar to the method of Chen and Tseng [11], three items with inter-item correlations <0.40 (numbness, shortness of breath and dry mouth) were excluded from the factor analysis. Following the Kaiser-Meyer-Olkin measure (0.819) and Bartlett's test of sphericity ($P < 0.001$), varimax rotation was used to simplify the factor structure, and the communality of remain items was 0.600 (standard deviation 0.120) which was adequately high to allow 99 samples to suffice for factor analysis. The internal reliability of each cluster was assessed by Cronbach's alpha.

The association of SCs and QoL was determined using Pearson's coefficient. Subsequently, each SC was regarded as a dependent variable, while the variables listed in Table 1 were regarded as independent variables. With an entrance criterion of 0.05 and a removal criterion of 0.1, stepwise multivariate linear regressions were applied to analyze which characteristics might be predictors of the independent variables. All tests were two-tailed, and $P < 0.05$ was considered significant. All analyses were performed using SPSS 20.0 software.

Results
Patient characteristics
In total, 101 patients met the eligibility criteria, except two of them lost contacts, 99 patients participated in the study. As shown in Table 1, most patients were male, married, and had stage II bladder cancer.

Symptom distress and SCs
The descriptive statistics regarding the symptom severity of the items and the prevalence of the symptoms 3 months after RC are presented in Table 2. The most severe symptom was distress, followed by fatigue and urinary dysfunction. Notably, pain ranked only eighth in symptom severity. Overall, all the participants experienced ten or more symptoms, and almost half of the participants (56.6%) reported more than four concurrent symptoms at moderate and severe levels.

Using an eigenvalue >1.0 as the criterion for retaining factors, a three-factor solution emerged, with 60.0% of the variance explained. Inspection of the items in each factor led us to name the clusters as the fatigue-malaise,

Table 1 Demographic and clinical characteristics of the participants

Characteristics	N (%) or Mean (SD)
Sex	
Male	93 (93.9%)
Female	6 (6.1%)
Cancer stage [b]	
I/Tis	22 (22.2%)
II	64 (64.6%)
III	13 (13.1%)
Urinary diversion	
IC	67 (67.7%)
ONB	32 (32.3%)
Adjuvant chemotherapy	
No	54 (54.5%)
Yes	45 (45.5%)
ASA score [a]	
1	51 (51.5%)
2	37 (37.4%)
3-4	11 (11.1%)
Postoperative complications, severity	
None	50 (50.5%)
Mild	21 (21.2%)
Moderate	19 (19.2%)
Severe	9 (9.1%)
Education level	
≤ 5 years	34 (34.3%)
6-11 years	50 (50.5%)
≥ 12 years	15 (15.2%)
Marital status	
Unmarried	24 (24.2%)
Married	75 (75.8%)
Albumin (mg/dl)	24.86 (5.00)
Age	61.85 (9.48)

[a]ASA score: American Society of Anesthesiologists score
[b]The total percentage is 99.9% with 0.1% error

Table 2 Descriptive statistics for symptom prevalence and severity

Symptoms	Severity Mean (SD)	Moderate [a] N (%)	Severe [b] N (%)
Distress	6.58 (1.43)	38 (38.4)	54 (54.5)
Fatigue	5.75 (1.77)	47 (47.5)	29 (29.3)
Urinary dysfunction	5.53 (1.38)	53 (53.5)	23 (23.2)
Loss of appetite	5.05 (1.66)	41 (41.4)	17 (17.2)
Sleep disturbance	4.74 (1.67)	43 (43.4)	12 (12.1)
Sadness	4.71 (1.21)	54 (54.5)	5 (5.1)
Body image dissatisfaction	4.62 (1.51)	40 (40.4)	9 (9.1)
Pain	4.14 (1.75)	30 (30.3)	7 (7.1)
Memory problems	4.10 (1.82)	27 (27.3)	10 (10.1)
Drowsiness	3.91 (1.90)	25 (25.3)	10 (10.1)
Nausea	3.62 (1.84)	17 (17.2)	8 (8.1)
Shortness of breath	2.17 (1.95)	9 (9.1)	4 (4.0)
Dry mouth	1.64 (2.21)	11 (11.1)	3 (3.0)
Vomiting	1.53 (1.17)	1 (1.0)	0
Numbness	1.46 (2.31)	8 (8.1)	5 (5.1)

[a]Score 5-6
[b]Score 7-10

Table 3 Factor analysis of symptoms

Cluster	Factor Loading		
	Factor 1	Factor 2	Factor 3
Fatigue-malaise			
Fatigue	0.828		
Drowsiness	0.828		
Pain	0.811		
Memory problems	0.783		
Loss of appetite	0.536		0.484
Psycho-urinary			
Sleep disturbance		0.725	
Body image impairment		0.725	
Urinary dysfunction		0.654	
Sadness		0.646	
Distress		0.487	
Gastrointestinal			
Nausea			0.842
Vomiting			0.803
Explained variance	26.347	18.959	14.688
Cumulative variance	26.347	45.306	59.994

Extraction method: Principal component analysis. Rotation method: Varimax with Kaiser normalization

gastrointestinal, and psycho-urinary SCs. Cronbach's alpha for each of the clusters was 0.863, 0.625, and 0.701, respectively. The factor analysis results are shown in Table 3.

Predictors of SCs

The results of the stepwise multiple regression analysis to predict SCs are presented in Table 4. Age, complication severity, plasma albumin after operation (negative), ONB, adjuvant chemotherapy and American Society of Anesthesiologists (ASA) score were significant predictors of fatigue-malaise distress and explained 38.5% of

Table 4 Stepwise regression model of predictors for symptom clusters

Model	B	SE	Sta. B	t	P	Adj R^2
Fatigue-malaise						
(Constant)	10.209	5.298		1.927	0.057	
Age	0.257	0.065	0.341	3.944	0.000	0.133
Complication severity	1.084	0.604	0.156	1.794	0.076	0.221
Albumin	- 0.408	0.120	−0.278	−3.394	0.001	0.273
Urinary diversion(0 = IC, 1 = ONB)	3.716	1.308	0.244	2.842	0.006	0.311
Adjuvant chemotherapy (0 = no, 1 = yes)	3.138	1.143	0.220	2.744	0.007	0.346
ASA score	2.355	0.894	0.225	2.636	0.010	0.385
Gastrointestinal						
(Constant)	4.421	1.299		3.404	0.001	
Adjuvant chemotherapy (0 = no, 1 = yes)	2.511	0.438	0.478	5.740	0.000	0.178
Urinary diversion (0 = IC, 1 = ONB)	1.614	0.472	0.288	3.420	0.001	0.233
Sex (0 = male, 1 = female)	2.312	0.924	0.211	2.503	0.014	0.274
ASA score	0.829	0.319	0.216	2.599	0.011	0.310
Albumin	−0.094	0.045	−0.173	−2.086	0.040	0.334
Psycho-urinary						
(Constant)	24.918	1.627		15.312	0.000	
Marital status (0 = unmarried, 1 = married)	−3.884	1.019	−0.343	−3.813	0.000	0.154
Education level	1.893	0.644	0.264	2.938	0.004	0.213
Complication severity	0.879	0.419	0.185	2.097	0.039	0.240

the total variance. Adjuvant chemotherapy, ONB, female gender, ASA score and albumin (negative) were significant predictors of gastrointestinal distress and explained 33.4% of the total variance. Being unmarried and having a higher educational level and complication severity level were significant predictors of psycho-urinary distress and explained 24.0% of the total variance.

Correlation of SCs with QoL
As shown in Table 5, the mean score of psycho-urinary problems was higher than that of fatigue-malaise and gastrointestinal symptoms. According to the percentage of the total score, the QoL score (50.39 ± 12.39) was low. The correlations between clusters and each cluster with quality of life were significant, and the maximum correlation observed was between psycho-urinary

symptoms and QoL ($r = 0.685$), while the minimum correlation observed was between psycho-urinary symptoms and gastrointestinal symptoms ($r = 0.268$).

Discussion
This study revealed that patients with RC experienced multiple symptoms simultaneously 3 months after RC from which three significant SCs were derived: fatigue-malaise, gastrointestinal, and psycho-urinary symptoms. Compared with the most commonly reported SCs from a systematic review, notwithstanding slight differences in the composition of items, the core symptoms tended to remain the same, such as fatigue, drowsiness and pain for fatigue-malaise, nausea and vomiting for gastrointestinal, and anxiety and depression for psycho-urinary symptoms [12]. The difference may be due to

Table 5 Bivariate correlations between symptom clusters and QoL

Variable	Mean (SD)	Fatigue-malaise	Gastrointestinal	Psycho-urinary
Fatigue-malaise (0-50)	22.95 (7.15)	1.00		
Gastrointestinal (0-20)	5.14 (2.63)	0.398**	1.00	
Psycho-urinary (0-50)	26.16 (4.88)	0.429**	0.268**	1.00
QoL (0-108)	50.39 (12.39)	−0.595**	−0.311**	−0.685**

**: $P < 0.01$

incongruous used scales, analytical techniques or the disease stage of the objects, and suggested that the SC composition or prevalence may change with the cancer type and stage.

When interpreting the results of factor analysis, consideration of the underlying commonality of the symptoms is important because one symptom may be a cause of another symptom or the symptoms may share a cause [13]. Therefore, we further explored the possible related factors. These findings will aid our understanding of the symptoms experienced by patients and facilitate further patient-centered symptom management in advanced bladder cancer for the period of transitional care from the prolonged peri-operative phase to long-term rehabilitation.

Fatigue-malaise

The fatigue-malaise SC consisted of non-specific symptoms, including fatigue, drowsiness, pain, memory problems and lack of appetite. It is similar to the "sickness cluster" reported by Chen and Tseng [11], with which four items were found in common (i.e., fatigue, pain, lack of appetite, and drowsiness). We also found that this cluster is well matched to the concept of systemic exertion intolerance disease (SEID), which was defined as a substantial reduction or impairment in the ability to engage in pre-illness levels of occupational, educational, social, or personal activities; post-exertional malaise and unrefreshing sleep; and at least one of the following two symptoms: cognitive impairment and orthostatic intolerance [14].

Researchers have attempted to explain the mechanism of this cluster. Chen and Tseng [11] observed that this SC is mediated by proinflammatory cytokines (e.g., interleukin-1, interleukin-6, TNF-α, and interferon-α). In this study, proinflammatory cytokines and hypothalamic-pituitary-adrenal (HPA) function were not directly measured; however, the regression analysis revealed that physiological factors, such as postoperative complications, albumin and ASA scores, were significant predictors of such symptom distress. These factors also provided evidence supporting the conceptual meaning of the "fatigue-malaise cluster".

Nausea-vomiting

Similar to previous studies, nausea and vomiting combined to form an independent and robust cluster [8, 13, 15]. Although Cronbach's coefficient was only 0.625, this value was acceptable considering the underlying commonality; however, whether loss of appetite was involved remains debatable. In some studies, such as the study by Sarna and Brecht [13] on lung cancer, loss of appetite was combined with nausea-vomiting. In the present study, loss of appetite overlapped with both the fatigue-malaise and nausea-vomiting clusters, while the loading coefficient was lower for the nausea-vomiting cluster than the former. As indicated by Molassiotis et al. [16],

the presence of a symptom in more than one cluster is clinically meaningful, contributes to an increase in the internal consistency of the cluster, and may potentially indicate the biological outcome or other link between the two clusters. Indeed, the overlapping of loss of appetite in the gastrointestinal and fatigue-malaise clusters reflects the link between these two clusters.

The regression analysis showed that adjuvant chemotherapy, ONB surgery, female gender, and ASA scores significantly increased the burden of nausea and vomiting. Nausea and vomiting are generally considered side effects of chemotherapy. Additionally, female gender is well established as the most important predictor of post-operative- and chemotherapy-related nausea and vomiting [17, 18]. Nevertheless, in this study, ONB surgery was also shown to be a predictor of nausea and vomiting. Published studies have compared ONB and IC surgeries using a variety of indices; however, to date, no data account for this gastrointestinal symptom difference in such a transitional phase. Conditions associated with this difference may include a longer operative time and more complications of prolonged ileus obstruction after ONB surgery. Additionally, in accordance with Sarna and Brecht [13] we found that the comorbidities of systemic disease (ASA scores) significantly increase the distress of nausea-vomiting. Although gastrointestinal motility disorders associated with diabetes mellitus primarily due to autonomic nervous dysfunction have been well established [19], the evidence of an association of nausea and vomiting with other systemic diseases, such as cardiovascular disease, has not been determined. Rather, patients with a longer duration of illness are more likely to be poly-symptomatic, which may partly explain this finding [20].

Psycho-urinary

Distress, sadness, urinary dysfunction, body image, and sleep disturbance comprised the psycho-urinary cluster. The grouping of distress and sadness as a cluster in cancer patients has already been shown in several studies [11, 21]. However, in this study, impaired urinary function, body image dissatisfaction, and sleep disturbance were highly linked to emotional symptoms and comprised a cluster considered unique to patients with RC. In accordance with the results of Punnen et al. [22], when urinary function worsened, individuals experienced more body image impairment and depressive symptoms. Furthermore, due to a decrease in the tone of the external sphincter, the urethral pressure is reduced during sleep, causing more severe nighttime urinary dysfunction, which could exacerbate sleep disturbance, emotional distress, and sadness. Zahran et al. [23] also compared people with and without nocturnal incontinence, and the results showed that the latter group had worse emotional and social function than the former group. The results suggest that urinary function is an important factor to consider in symptom management for depression.

Two demographic factors, educational level and marital status, correlated with the severity of psycho-urinary cluster symptoms. As reported by Xiao et al. [24], a positive relationship between a higher education level and symptom distress was found; moreover, as they discussed, patients who are more highly educated may seek more health care assistance and have a higher potential and willingness to report more symptoms. Sarna and Brecht [13] also reported that distress was associated with the educational level, with the greatest distress found among those with the most education. In this study, the patients with a higher education may have had higher expectations regarding the therapeutic effects and their QoL; therefore, they might have been more sensitive to psycho-urinary symptoms at this early rehabilitation stage. The relationship between marital status and psycho-urinary symptoms may be due to the intermediate function of social support, including medical help and emotional support, which was previously confirmed to be positively related to disease outcome in other chronic diseases [25].

Correlation of SCs and QoL

The results of this study further confirmed that symptom distress was a reliable predictor of QoL. Greater symptom distress resulted in a poor QoL. Sun et al. [26] demonstrated that the symptom experience, such as nausea, appetite, and insomnia, significantly impacted QoL, particularly aspects of health and psychosocial behavior in bladder cancer patients. The possible SCs and their impact on QoL have also been explored in other diseases. Hwang et al. [21] reported that in ovarian cancer patients, the SCs of abdominal discomfort, psychological distress, fatigue-pain, and flu-like symptoms explained 46.0%, 40.0%, 38.0%, and 37.0% of the total variance in QoL, respectively, which partially supports our results. However, Somani et al. [27] systematically reviewed the association between body image distress and QoL and obtained different results, which suggests that this factor may not always be important for the QoL of RC patients. These contradictory results may be due to the different post-RC study period investigated. Our research targeted the early rehabilitative period, which was characterized by adaptation and adjustment, and during this period, QoL was worse and influenced by many factors.

Among the three clusters, the psycho-urinary cluster had the strongest association with QoL. This result is in agreement with a previous study by Kim et al. [28], which indicated that psychological distress was the most

significant predictor of QoL and explained 20.1% of the total variation. Dong et al. [29] found that the emotional cluster (tense-worried-irritable-depressed) was a stronger predictor of overall QoL compared with other clusters, and this result reinforces the significant effect of psycho-urinary symptoms on QoL.

It should be noted the sexual symptom didn't assessment in this research because the response rate was too low during the preliminary experiment. Further inquiry revealed the attitude of Chinese to it were much conservative, since most of them neither had sexual activity before surgery nor believed such activity was applicable during such stage of disease.

This study has some limitations. First, this was a single-centered research study that occurred in China and notwithstanding a consecutive enrolling method, the female enrollment rate was very low. Second, except for IC and ONB, other methods of urinary diversion such as cutaneous ureterostomy, for which comparable peri-operative outcomes in high-risk older adults were recently reported [30], were not included in this study. Therefore, the results must be carefully interpreted for females and patients who undergo other types of urinary diversion.

Conclusion

Based on the aforementioned results, medical staff should be aware of the symptom management of patients with bladder cancer 3 months after RC and focus on three areas: fatigue-malaise improvement, nausea-vomiting control, and psycho-urinary adjustment. The fatigue-malaise management should begin with the diligent recognition and treatment of postoperative complications and comorbidities, along with the prevention of malnutrition. Nausea-vomiting management should be focused more on females and those with ONB surgery and comorbidities. Besides, the most important goal should be emotional adjustment and urinary function restoration. Since urinary incontinence or urostomy management and emotional disorders coexist within the same cluster, the diagnosis and management of any symptom in this cluster should not be formulated in isolation. A combination of strategies that target both aspects in a cluster should be administered simultaneously or in an orderly manner, while the demographic and clinical characteristics should be considered to relieve symptom distress and improve QoL in this transitional phase.

Abbreviations
ASA: American Society of Anesthesiologists; IC: Ileal conduit; MDASI: M.D. Anderson symptom inventory; ONB: Orthotropic neobladder; QoL: Quality of life; RC: Radical cystectomy

Acknowledgments
We acknowledge the assistance of statisticians Zhongxiaoni and Pengbin.

Funding
Funding was provided by the nursing research project of the First Affiliated Hospital of Chongqing Medical University, HLJJ2012-28.

Authors' contributions
HR, GR designed the study. HR, PT, QZ acquired the data. HR, PT performed the statistical analysis of the data. HR drafted the manuscript. GR provided a critical revision of the manuscript. All authors read and approved the final manuscript.

Competing interests
The authors declare that they have no competing interests.

Author details
[1]Department of Urology, The First Affiliated Hospital of Chongqing Medical University, No. 1 Youyi Road, Yuzhong District, Chongqing 400016, China. [2]Department of Cardiology, The First Affiliated Hospital of Chongqing Medical University, No. 1 Youyi Road, Yuzhong District, Chongqing 400016, China. [3]Department of Nursing, The First Affiliated Hospital of Chongqing Medical University, No. 1 Youyi Road, Yuzhong District, Chongqing 400016, China. [4]Molecular Oncology and Epigenetics Laboratory, The First Affiliated Hospital of Chongqing Medical University, No. 1 Youyi Road, Yuzhong District, Chongqing 400016, China.

References
1. Chen W, Zheng R, Baade PD, Zhang S, Zeng H, Bray F, et al. Cancer statistics in China, 2015. CA Cancer J Clin. 2016;66:115–32.
2. Patel MI, Bang A, Gillatt D, Smith DP. Contemporary radical cystectomy outcomes in patients with invasive bladder cancer: a population-based study. BJU Int. 2015;116(Suppl 3):18–25.
3. Benner C, Greenberg M, Shepard N, Meng MV, Rabow MW. The natural history of symptoms and distress in patients and families following cystectomy for treatment of muscle invasive bladder cancer. J Urol. 2014; 191:937–42.
4. Huang Y, Pan X, Zhou Q, Huang H, Li L, Cui X, et al. Quality-of-life outcomes and unmet needs between ileal conduit and orthotopic ileal neobladder after radical cystectomy in a Chinese population: a 2-to-1 matched-pair analysis. BMC Urol. 2015;15:1–7.
5. Singh V, Yadav R, Sinha RJ, Gupta DK. Prospective comparison of quality-of-life outcomes between ileal conduit urinary diversion and orthotopic neobladder reconstruction after radical cystectomy: a statistical model. BJU Int. 2014;113:726–32.
6. Patrick DL, Ferketich SL, Frame PS, Harris JJ, Hendricks CB, Levin B, et al. National Institutes of Health state-of-the-science conference statement: symptom management in cancer: pain, depression, and fatigue, July 15-17, 2002. J Natl Cancer Inst Monogr. 2003;95:1110–7.
7. Kim HJ, McGuire DB, Tulman L, Barsevick AM. Symptom clusters: concept analysis and clinical implications for cancer nursing. Cancer Nurs. 2005;28: 270–82. quiz 83-4
8. Cleeland CS, Mendoza TR, Wang XS, Chou C, Harle MT, Morrissey M, et al. Assessing symptom distress in cancer patients: the M.D. Anderson symptom inventory. Cancer. 2000;89:1634–46.
9. Wang XS, Wang Y, Guo H, Mendoza TR, Hao XS, Cleeland CS. Chinese version of the M. D. Anderson symptom inventory: validation and application of symptom measurement in cancer patients. Cancer. 2004;101: 1890–901.
10. Cella DF, Tulsky DS, Gray G, Sarafian B, Linn E, Bonomi A, et al. The functional assessment of cancer therapy scale: development and validation of the general measure. J Clin Oncol 1993;11:570-9.
11. Chen ML, Tseng HC. Symptom clusters in cancer patients. Support Care Cancer. 2006;14:825–30.
12. Kirkova J, Walsh D, Aktas A, Davis MP. Cancer symptom clusters: old concept but new data. Am J Hosp Palliat Care. 2010;27:282.
13. Sarna L, Brecht ML. Dimensions of symptom distress in women with advanced lung cancer: a factor analysis. Heart Lung. 1997;26:23 30.
14. Institute of Medicine (U.S.), Committee on the Diagnostic Criteria for Myalgic Encephalomyelitis/Chronic Fatigue Syndrome, Board on the Health of Select Populations Institute of Medicine. Beyond myalgic encephalomyelitis/chronic fatigue syndrome: redefining an illness. Washington, DC: National Academies Press; 2015.
15. Stapleton SJ, Holden J, Epstein J, Wilkie DJ. Symptom clusters in patients with cancer in the hospice/palliative care setting. Support Care Cancer. 2016;24:3863–71.
16. Molassiotis A, Wengstrom Y, Kearney N. Symptom cluster patterns during the first year after diagnosis with cancer. J Pain Symptom Manag. 2010;39: 847–58.
17. Aapro MS, Grunberg SM, Manikhas GM, Olivares G, Suarez T, Tjulandin SA, et al. A phase III, double-blind, randomized trial of palonosetron compared with ondansetron in preventing chemotherapy-induced nausea and vomiting following highly emetogenic chemotherapy. Ann Oncol. 2006;17:1441–9.
18. Gan TJ. Risk factors for postoperative nausea and vomiting. Anesth Analg. 2006;102:1884–98.
19. Feldman M, Schiller LR. Disorders of gastrointestinal motility associated with diabetes mellitus. Ann Intern Med. 1983;98:378–84.
20. Collin SM, Nikolaus S, Heron J, Knoop H, White PD, Crawley E. Chronic fatigue syndrome (CFS) symptom-based phenotypes in two clinical cohorts of adult patients in the UK and The Netherlands. J Psychosom Res. 2016;81:14–23.
21. Hwang KH, Cho OH, Yoo YS. Symptom clusters of ovarian cancer patients undergoing chemotherapy, and their emotional status and quality of life. Eur J Oncol Nurs. 2016;21:215–22.
22. Punnen S, Cowan JE, Dunn LB, Shumay DM, Carroll PR, Cooperberg MR. A longitudinal study of anxiety, depression and distress as predictors of sexual and urinary quality of life in men with prostate cancer. BJU Int. 2013;112:E67–5.
23. Zahran MH, El-Hefnawy AS, Zidan EM, El-Bilsha MA, Taha DE, Ali-El-Dein B. Health-related quality of life after radical cystectomy and neobladder reconstruction in women: impact of voiding and continence status. Int J Urol. 2014;21:887–92.
24. Xiao C, Hanlon A, Zhang Q, Movsas B, Ang K, Rosenthal DI, et al. Risk factors for clinician-reported symptom clusters in patients with advanced head and neck cancer in a phase 3 randomized clinical trial: RTOG 0129. Cancer. 2014; 120:848–54.
25. Heo S, Lennie TA, Moser DK, Kennedy RL. Types of social support and their relationships to physical and depressive symptoms and health-related quality of life in patients with heart failure. Heart Lung. 2014;43:299–305.
26. Sun J, Tsai J, Lin C. The quality of life, social support, and symptom distress among patients with bladder cancer. NewTaibei Nursing. 2006;8:11–9.
27. Somani BK, Gimlin D, Fayers P, N'Dow J. Quality of life and body image for bladder cancer patients undergoing radical cystectomy and urinary diversion–a prospective cohort study with a systematic review of literature. Urology. 2009;74:1138–43.
28. Kim SH, Oh EG, Lee WH. Symptom experience, psychological distress, and quality of life in Korean patients with liver cirrhosis: a cross-sectional survey. Int J Nurs Stud. 2006;43:1047–56.
29. Dong ST, Costa DS, Butow PN, Lovell MR, Agar M, Velikova G, et al. Symptom clusters in advanced cancer patients: an empirical comparison of statistical methods and the impact on quality of life. J Pain Symptom Manag. 2016;51:88–98.
30. Longo N, Imbimbo C, Fusco F, Ficarra V, Mangiapia F, Di LG, et al. Complications and quality of life in elderly patients with several comorbidities undergoing cutaneous ureterostomy with single stoma or ileal conduit after radical cystectomy. BJU Int. 2016;118:521–6.

5

A gonadotropin-releasing hormone antagonist reduces serum adrenal androgen levels in prostate cancer patients

Yoshiyuki Miyazawa[*], Yoshitaka Sekine, Takahiro Syuto, Masashi Nomura, Hidekazu Koike, Hiroshi Matsui, Yasuhiro Shibata, Kazuto Ito and Kazuhiro Suzuki

Abstract

Background: Adrenal androgens play an important role in the development of castration-resistant prostate cancer therapeutics. The effect of gonadotropin-releasing hormone (GnRH) antagonists on adrenal androgens has not been studied sufficiently. We measured testicular and adrenal androgen levels in patients treated with a GnRH antagonist.

Methods: This study included 47 patients with histologically proven prostate cancer. All of the patients were treated with the GnRH antagonist degarelix. The mean patient age was 73.6 years. Pre-treatment blood samples were collected from all of the patients, and post-treatment samples were taken at 1, 3, 6, and 12 months after starting treatment. Testosterone (T), dihydrotestosterone (DHT), dehydroepiandrosterone (DHEA), 17β-estradiol (E2), and androstenedione (A-dione) were measured by liquid chromatography-mass spectrometry. Dehydroepiandrosterone-sulfate (DHEA-S), luteinizing hormone, and follicle-stimulating hormone levels were measured by electro-chemiluminescence immunoassays.

Results: A significant reduction in T level (97.3% reduction) was observed in the patients 1 month after initiating treatment. In addition, levels of DHT, E2, DHEA-S, and A-dione decreased 1 month after initiating treatment (93.3, 84.9, 16.8, and 35.9% reduction, respectively). T, DHT, E2, DHEA-S, and A-dione levels remained significantly suppressed (97.1, 94.6, 85.3, 23.9, and 40.5% reduction, respectively) 12 months after initiating treatment. A significant decrease in DHEA level (15.4% reduction) was observed 12 months after initiating treatment.

Conclusions: Serum adrenal androgen levels decreased significantly in patients treated with a GnRH antagonist. Thus, long-term GnRH antagonist treatment may reduce serum adrenal androgen levels.

Keywords: Prostate cancer, GnRH antagonist, Adrenal androgen

Background

Prostate cancer has become one of the most prevalent diseases among men in Western countries, and its incidence has increased in Japan [1]. The disease is dependent on androgens; therefore, patients are often treated with androgen deprivation therapy [2]. Gonadotropin-releasing hormone (GnRH) antagonists block receptors directly, thereby rapidly suppressing testosterone (T) without the T surge and flare. No clinical studies on the GnRH antagonist degarelix have reported evidence of a T surge or flare [3–6]. Various drugs that interact with androgen receptors (ARs) have been developed and used clinically. In addition

to "conventional" AR inhibitors such as flutamide [7] and bicalutamide [8], enzalutamide prolongs survival time before and after chemotherapy [9, 10]. Abiraterone, an androgen biosynthetic enzyme inhibitor, also improves patient prognosis [11]. Adrenal androgens are important hormones for developing therapy for castration-resistant prostate cancer. Although circulating adrenal androgens are mainly secreted from the adrenal glands, the testes secrete about 10% of the total [12]. In addition, the role of aberrant luteinizing hormone (LH) receptor expression in the adrenal glands has been studied in patients with adrenocorticotropic hormone (ACTH)-independent Cushing's syndrome [13–15]. We previously reported that long-term luteinizing hormone-releasing hormone (LH-RH) agonist treatment reduced adrenal androgen levels via LH

* Correspondence: miya.yoshi@hotmail.co.jp
Department of Urology, Gunma University Graduate School of Medicine, 3-9-22 Showa-machi, Maebashi, Gunma 371-8511, Japan

receptors in the adrenal cortex [16]. However, the effects of GnRH antagonists on adrenal androgens have not been studied sufficiently. In this study, we evaluated the effects of a GnRH antagonist on changes in serum adrenal androgen levels.

Methods

Patients

We studied 47 patients diagnosed with prostate cancer pathologically at Gunma University Hospital (Maebashi, Japan). Table 1 shows the clinical characteristics of the enrolled patients, who ranged in age from 60 to 87 years (mean, 73.6 years). The clinical stages of the patients were T1cN0M0 ($n = 8$), T2N0M0 ($n = 14$), T3N0M0 ($n = 9$), T4N0M0 ($n = 2$), TanyN1M0 ($n = 4$), TanyN0M1 ($n = 5$), and TanyN1M1 ($n = 5$). Ten patients had distant metastases; seven had a bone metastasis and three had a visceral metastasis. All patients were administered degarelix as a monthly subcutaneous injection (240 mg for the first month followed by 12 maintenance doses of 80 mg). Four patients were treated with bicalutamide as a combined antiandrogen blockade. Of the 33 TanyN0M0 patients, 12 (mean age, 69.3; range, 60–77 years) underwent curative radiation therapy in combination with hormone therapy: 7 patients received intensity-modulated radiation therapy, 4 patients received carbon-ion radiotherapy, and 1 patient received high-dose brachytherapy. The other 21 patients of the 33 TanyN0M0 patients received hormone

Table 1 Clinical characteristics of the patients

Characteristic		
No. of patients	47	
Age (year, mean ± SD)	73.6 ± 7.02	
Initial PSA (median ± SD)	11.1 ± 489.1 ng/ml	
Stage	No. of patients	
T1cN0M0	8	17%
T2N0M0	14	29.8%
T3N0M0	9	19.1%
T4N0M0	2	4.3%
TanyN1M0	4	8.5%
TanyN0M1	5	10.6%
TanyN1M1	5	10.6%
Metastasis		
All distant metastasis	10	21.2%
Bone metastasis	7	14.9%
Visceral metastasis	3	6.4%
Gleason Score		
GS 6	4	9%
GS 7	15	32%
GS≧8	28	59%

Abbreviations: PSA Prostate Specific Antigen

therapy either because of their age or their wishes (mean age, 76.8; range, 62–84 years). All 14 patients who had lymph node metastasis or distant metastasis (TanyN1M0: $n = 4$, TanyN0M1: $n = 5$, and TanyN1M1: $n = 5$) were treated with hormonal therapy. The Ethical Committee for Clinical Study of Gunma University Graduate School of Medicine approved this study, and written consent was obtained from all of the enrolled patients. We registered this clinical trial with the University Hospital Medical Information Network (UMIN ID: UMIN000011990).

Blood samples and measurement of hormone levels

Pre-treatment blood samples were collected from all of the patients, and post-treatment samples were taken at 1, 3, 6, and 12 months after starting the treatment. All serum samples were stored at –80 °C prior to testing. T, dihydrotestosterone (DHT), 17β-estradiol (E2), dehydroepiandrosterone (DHEA), and androstenedione (A-dione) were measured by liquid chromatography-mass spectrometry. Dehydroepiandrosterone-sulfate (DHEA-S), LH, and follicle-stimulating hormone (FSH) were measured by electro-chemiluminescence immunoassays. To investigate the rapid T-lowering effect of degarelix, additional tests were conducted using serum 1 ($n = 39$) and 2 ($n = 36$) weeks after degarelix administration by electro-chemiluminescence immunoassays.

Statistical analysis

All values are expressed as the mean ± standard deviation and were compared using Student's t-test. A p-value <0.05 was considered significant. We used an analysis of variance (ANOVA) and the Tukey-Kramer method to analyze the changes in LH and FSH levels between the nadir and other time points.

Results

Table 2 shows the changes in hormone levels during treatment. T levels decreased significantly (97.3% reduction) in GnRH antagonist-treated patients 1 month after initiating treatment compared to those at baseline. In addition, the lower T level was maintained until 12 months after initiating treatment (97.1% reduction). DHT and E2 decreased 1 month after initiating treatment (DHT, 93.2%; E2, 84.9% reduction, respectively) and these levels were maintained until 12 months after initiating treatment. DHEA-S and A-dione levels decreased significantly 1, 3, 6, and 12 months after initiating treatment and remained low until 12 months after the start of treatment (DHEA-S, 23.9%; A-dione, 40.5% reduction, respectively). We did not observe a decrease in DHEA levels 1, 3, or 6 months after initiating treatment, but the DHEA level was significantly lower 12 months after treatment compared to baseline (15.4% reduction). LH and FSH levels decreased 1 month after initiating treatment compared to baseline (LH, 96.0%; FSH,

Table 2 Changes of hormone levels in prostate cancer patients treated GnRH antagonist

	Pre	1 w	2 w	1 mo	3 mo	6 mo	12 mo	Statistics
T								$p < 0.05$
Measurement, ng/dL percentile change	376.66 ± 161.71	19.4 ± 9.11[†] −94.8% (n = 39)	11.8 ± 7.13[†] −96.7% (n = 36)	10.23 ± 5.09 −97.3%	10.09 ± 3.98 −97.3%	10.49 ± 4.52 −97.2%	10.81 ± 5.36 −97.1%	Pre vs 1 w, 2 w, 1 mo, 3 mo, 6 mo, 12 mo
DHT								$p < 0.05$
Measurement, pg/mL percentile change	442.76 ± 256.68			29.95 ± 15.89 −93.2%	27.09 ± 15.28 −93.9%	25.30 ± 14.48 −94.3%	24.12 ± 14.01 −94.6%	Pre vs 1 mo, 3 mo, 6 mo, 12 mo
E_2								$p < 0.05$
Measurement, pg/mL percentile change	23.58 ± 12.81			3.56 ± 2.58 −84.9%	3.25 ± 2.21 −86.2%	3.32 ± 2.01 −85.9%	3.46 ± 2.37 −85.3%	Pre vs 1 mo, 3 mo, 6 mo, 12 mo
DHEA-S								$p < 0.05$
Measurement, µg/dL percentile change	125.47 ± 62.48			104.38 ± 56.03 −16.8%	103.7 ± 52.52 −17.3%	104.17 ± 57.03 −17.0%	95.47 ± 58.23 −23.9%	Pre vs 1 mo, 3 mo, 6 mo, 12 mo
DHEA								$p < 0.05$
Measurement, ng/mL percentile change	2.50 ± 1.46			2.19 ± 1.52 −12.0%	2.27 ± 1.45 −8.7%	2.23 ± 1.57 −10.8%	2.11 ± 1.69 −15.4%	Pre vs 12 mo
A-dione								$p < 0.05$
Measurement, ng/mL percentile change	0.715 ± 0.348			0.458 ± 0.278 −35.5%	0.472 ± 0.231 −33.9%	0.448 ± 0.230 −37.4%	0.426 ± 0.220 −40.5%	Pre vs 1 mo, 3 mo, 6 mo, 12 mo
LH								$p < 0.05$
Measurement, mIU/mL percentile change	7.20 ± 7.31			0.285 ± 0.385 −96.0%	0.255 ± 0.306 −96.5%	0.303 ± 0.355 −95.8%	0.453 ± 0.479 −93.7%	Pre vs 1 mo, 3 mo, 6 mo, 12 mo
FSH								$p < 0.05$
Measurement, mIU/mL percentile change	14.56 ± 14.47			0.889 ± 1.100 −93.9%	0.993 ± 0.100 −93.2%	1.224 ± 1.135 −91.6%	1.83 ± 1.424 −87.4%	Pre vs 1 mo, 3 mo, 6 mo, 12 mo

Abbreviations: *T*, Testosterone, *DHT* dihydrotestosterone, *E_2* Estradiol, *DHEA* dehydroepiandrosterone, *DHEA-S* Dehydroepiandrosterone-sulfate, *A-dione* androstene-dione, *LH* Luteinizing hormone, *FSH* Follicle Stimulating Hormone, *Pre* pretreatment, *1,2 w* 1,2 weeks after initiation of GnRH antagonist treatment, *1,3,6,12 mo*, 1,3,6,12 months after initiation of GnRH antagonist treatment

Percentile change indicates changes in comparison with pretreatment levels. Values are expressed as mean ± SD

†: Data of testosterone after 1 week (n = 39) and 2 weeks (n = 36) were measured by the ECLIA, and all other data were measured by LC-MS/MS

93.9% reduction, respectively), and they reached the nadir 1 month after initiating treatment. An ANOVA detected no change between the nadir LH level and levels measured 3, 6, and 12 months after initiating treatment (p = 0.065). FSH levels increased gradually from 1 to 12 months after initiating treatment. We found a significant change between the FSH nadir level and the level 12 months after initiating treatment (p = 0.0006). In addition, we found a significant change between the levels 3 and 12 months after initiating treatment. The changes and statistical results for the nadir LH and FSH levels and the levels at the other time points are shown in Table 3. Examining the early decline in T using an electro-chemiluminescence immunoassay, the mean T level was 19.4 ± 9.11 ng/mL at 1 week after treatment (n = 39) and 11.8 ± 7.13 ng/mL at 2 weeks after (n = 36) treatment (Data is shown in Table 2).

Discussion

The serum adrenal androgen levels decreased significantly after treatment with a GnRH antagonist. To our

Table 3 The changes and statistical processing in LH and FSH levels of nadir and other points

	1 mo (nadir)	3 mo	6 mo	12 mo	Statistics
LH					
Measurement, mIU/mL	0.285 ± 0.385	0.255 ± 0.306	0.303 ± 0.355	0.453 ± 0.479	There were no significant changes between nadir and other points. ANOVA; $p = 0.065$
FSH					
Measurement, mIU/mL	0.889 ± 1.100	0.993 ± 0.100	1.224 ± 1.135	1.83 ± 1.424	There were significant changes between nadir and 12 mo, 3 mo and 12 mo.Tukey-Kramer methods; $p = 0.0006$

Abbreviations: *LH* Luteinizing hormone, *FSH* Follicle Stimulating Hormone. Values are expressed as mean ± SD

knowledge, this is the first report to show a significant decrease in adrenal androgen levels in patients with prostate cancer treated long-term with a GnRH antagonist. Some studies have shown a relationship between LH-RH agonist therapy and changes in adrenal androgen levels. The DHEA-S levels decreased slightly albeit not significantly in patients with prostate cancer treated with a LH-RH agonist for 28 days [17]. Eri et al. [18] showed that the A-dione and DHEA-S levels of patients treated with a LH-RH agonist for 6 months for benign prostate hyperplasia decreased by 48 and 24%, respectively. Those authors showed that reduced testicular secretion of both hormones contributed to the decrease.

DHEA-S and A-dione are secreted from the adrenal glands and testes. No more than 10% of DHEA-S is of testicular origin [12]. Similarly, Kroboth et al. [19] showed that 5% of DHEA-S is secreted by the testes. Weinstein et al. [20] compared serum levels of sex steroids in peripheral veins and spermatic veins and found that the DHEA, A-dione, and T levels in the spermatic vein were 73.1, 30.7, and 751 ng/mL, respectively. These findings prove that DHEA and A-dione are secreted from the testes. Further, de Ronde et al. [21] measured adrenal androgen levels and estimated the percentage contributed by the testes. They stratified cases according to serum DHEA-S level and found that 0–14% of A-dione originated from the testes. In this study, DHEA-S decreased by about 24%, DHEA decreased by about 15%, and A-dione decreased by about 40%. These findings made us consider the role of the adrenal glands in the decrease in adrenal androgen levels after long-term GnRH antagonist treatment.

Several researchers have reported cases of ACTH-independent adrenal hyperplasia [12, 13], and the presence of functional LH receptors has been demonstrated in patients with ACTH-independent Cushing's syndrome [13, 14]. These findings demonstrate that LH-RH agonist treatment reduces serum cortisol levels and reveal a relationship between the presence of LH receptors in the adrenal glands and cortisol production. LH receptors were identified on the reticular layer of adrenal cortex cells and demonstrated the presence of the cytochrome P450 side-chain cleavage enzyme in the same cells [22]. These results suggest that LH-positive adrenal cortex cells are steroidogenic. DHEA-S is produced in H295R adrenal cortical cells via functional LH receptors [23]. These findings suggest that LH affects the function of the adrenal glands and regulates the secretion of adrenal hormones.

Our group previously found a significant decrease in serum adrenal androgen levels in patients with a prostate carcinoma treated with a LH-RH agonist [16]. Using immunohistochemistry, we also discovered the presence of LH receptors on adrenal cortex cells in the reticular layer in patients treated with a LH-RH agonist. Furthermore, we found that the correlation between ACTH and DHEA-S levels shifted to an inverse relationship during the treatment period. These results show that reduced adrenal synthesis of androgens stimulates ACTH secretion through a feedback mechanism. Therefore, long-term GnRH antagonist treatment might reduce serum adrenal androgen levels via LH receptors.

We speculated the existence of another mechanism by which GnRH antagonists inhibit adrenal androgen production directly via GnRH receptor protein in the adrenal glands. In addition to its expression in the pituitary gland, GnRH receptor is expressed in lymphocytes and many extra-pituitary tissues, including breast, ovarian, and prostate [24]. Ziegler et al. [25] demonstrated that GnRH receptor is present in the adrenal glands at the mRNA and protein levels in normal human adrenal tissues, adrenocortical and adrenomedullary tumors, and adrenal cell lines. Although the presence of GnRH receptor in the adrenal glands suggests that adrenal androgen production was suppressed via GnRH receptor, it is unclear how the receptor works in the adrenal glands.

Bashin et al. [26] demonstrated that FSH levels began to rise towards pretreatment levels despite continued administration of a LH-RH agonist after achieving an initial nadir in young healthy men. They called this effect "FSH escape" but the mechanism is unknown. Santen et al. [27] reported the same increase in FSH after the administration of a LH-RH agonist in patients with prostate cancer. Crawford et al. [28] investigated the efficacy and safety of the GnRH antagonist degarelix compared to the LH-RH agonist leuprolide in the main trial CS21 and extension trial CS21A. The authors showed that the median FSH levels were 1.20 and 4.40 IU/L in the degarelix 240/80 mg and leuprolide groups, respectively ($p < 0.0001$) 1 year after initiating treatment. In this study, the serum LH and FSH levels reached a nadir 1 month after initiating treatment (LH: 0.285 ± 0.385, FSH: 0.889 ± 1.100; mean $\pm$ standard deviation). After reaching the nadir, the FSH levels began to rise gradually until 12 months after treatment started. We found a significant change between the FSH nadir and the level 12 months after initiating treatment. We observed very little "FSH escape", but the FSH levels 12 months after initiating treatment were similar to data reported by Crawford et al. [28]. Continuous suppression of FSH caused by a GnRH antagonist has been discussed and its therapeutic advantage is under discussion [29]. Radu et al. [30] showed that FSH receptors are expressed by endothelial cells in a wide range of tumors, including prostate carcinomas. We are continuing to study the relationship between FSH and the prognosis of the patients examined in this study.

Conclusions

In summary, we found a significant decrease in adrenal androgen levels in patients treated with a GnRH antagonist for 12 months. Considering the existence of functional LH receptors in cases of ACTH-independent Cushing's syndrome or in human adrenal cortex cells, long-term GnRH antagonist administration may reduce serum adrenal androgen levels via LH receptors.

Abbreviations
ACTH: Adrenocorticotropic hormone; A-dione: Androstenedione; DHEA: Dehydroepiandrosterone; DHT: Dihydrotestosterone; E_2: 17β-estradiol; FSH: Follicle-stimulating hormone; GnRH: Gonadotropin-releasing hormone; LH: Luteinizing hormone; LH-RH: Luteinizing hormone-releasing hormone; T: Testosterone

Acknowledgements
None.

Funding
This research received grant from Astellas Pharma Inc.

Authors' contributions
YM and KS performed the design of the study and drafted the manuscript. YM, TS, YS, MN, HK, HM and YS contributed experiments and data analysis, KI and KS helped the experiments and data analysis. KS conceived of and supervised the work. All authors read and approved the final manuscript.

Competing interests
Yoshiyuki Miyazawa, Takahiro Syuto, Yoshitaka Sekine, Masashi Nomura, Hidekazu Koike, Hiroshi Matsui, Yasuhiro Shibata and Kazuto Ito declare that there are no conflicts of interest that could be perceived as prejudicing the impartiality of the research reported. Kazuhiro Suzuki is a recipient of research grants and honoraria from Takeda Pharmaceutical Co. Ltd. and Astellas Pharma Inc.

References
1. Ito K. Prostate cancer in Asian man. Nat Rev Urol. 2014;11:197–212.
2. Mohler JL, Kantoff PW, Armstrong AJ, et al. Prostate cancer, version 2.2014. J Natl Compr Cancer Netw. 2014;12:686–718.
3. Gittelman M, Pommerville P, Persson B, et al. A 1-year, open label, randomized phase II dose finding study of degarelix for the treatment of prostate cancer in North America. J Urol. 2008;180:1986–92.
4. Klotz L, Miller K, Crawford ED, et al. Disease control outcomes from analysis of pooled individual patient data from five comparative randomised clinical trials of degarelix versus luteinising hormone-releasing hormone agonists. Eur Urol. 2014;66:1101–8.
5. Van Poppel H, Tombal B, De La Rosette J, et al. Degarelix: a novel gonadotropin-releasing hormone (GnRH) receptor blocker-results from a 1-yr, multicentre, randomised, phase 2 dosage-finding study in the treatment of prostate cancer. Eur Urol. 2008;54:805–13.
6. Ozono S, Ueda T, Hoshi S, et al. The efficacy and safety of degarelix, a GnRH antagonist: a 12-month, multicentre, randomized, maintenance dose-finding phase II study in Japanese patients with prostate cancer. Jpn J Clin Oncol. 2012;42:477–84.
7. Crawford ED, Eisenberger MA, McLeod DG, et al. A controlled trial Leuprolide with and without Flutamide in prostatic carcinoma. N Engl J Med. 1989;321:419–24.
8. Schellhammer PF, Sharifi R, Block NL, et al. A controlled trial of bicalutamide versus flutamide, each in combination with luteinizing hormone-releasing hormone analogue therapy, in patients with advanced prostate carcinoma. Analysis of time to progression. CASODEX combination study group. Cancer. 1996;78(10):2164–9.
9. Scher HI, Fizzazi K, Saad F, et al. Increased survival with Enzalutamide in prostate cancer after chemotherapy. N Engl J Med. 2012;367:1187–97.
10. Beer TM, Armstrong AJ, Rathkopf DE, et al. Enzalutamide in metastatic prostate cancer before chemotherapy. N Engl J Med. 2014;371:424–33.
11. Ryan CJ, Smith MR, Fizazi K, et al. Abiraterone acetate plus prednisone versus placebo plus prednisone in chemotherapy-naive men with metastatic castration-resistant prostate cancer (COU-AA-302): final overall survival analysis of a randomised, double-blind, placebo-controlled phase 3 study. Lancet Oncol. 2015;16:152–60.
12. Braunstein DG. Testes. In: Greenspan FS, editor. Basic and clinical endocrinology. 3rd ed. Englewood Cliffs, NJ: Prentice Hall; 1991. p. 407–41.
13. Lacroix A, Mamet P, Boutin JM. Leuprolide acetate therapy in luteinizing hormone-dependent Cushing's syndrome. N Engl J Med. 1999;341:1577–81.
14. Feelders RA, Lamberts WJ, Hofland LJ, et al. Luteinizing hormone (LH)-responsive Cushing's syndrome: the demonstration of LH receptor messenger ribonucleic acid in hyperplastic adrenal cells, which respond to chorionic gonadotropin and serotonin agonists in vitro. J Clin Endocrinol Metab. 2003;88:230–7.
15. de Groot JWB, Links TP, Themmen APN, et al. Aberrant expression of multiple hormone receptors in ACTH-independent macronodular adrenal hyperplasia causing Cushing's syndrome. Eur J Endocrinol. 2010;163:293–9.
16. Nishii M, Nomura M, Sekine Y, et al. Luteinizing hormone (LH)-releasing hormone agonist reduces serum adrenal androgen levels in prostate cancer patients: implications for the effect of LH on the adrenal glands. J Androl. 2012;33:1233–8.
17. Ayub M, Jevell MJ. Suppression of plasma androgens by the antiandrogen flutamide in prostatic cancer patients treated with zoladex, a GnRH analogue. Clin Endocrinol. 1990;32:329–39.
18. Eri LM, Haug E, Tveter KJ. Effects on the endocrine system of long- term treatment with the luteinizing hormone-releasing hormone agonist leuprolide in patients with benign prostatic hyperplasia. Scand J Clin Lab Invest. 1996;56:319–25.
19. Kroboth PD, Salek FS, Pittenger AL, et al. DHEA and DHEA-S: a review. J Clin Pharmacol. 1999;39:237–348.
20. Weinstein RL, Kelch RP, Jenner MR, et al. Secretion of unconjugated androgens and estrogens by the normal and abnormal human testis before and after human chorionic gonadotropin. J Clin Invest. 1974;53:1–6.
21. de Ronde W, Hofman A, Pols HAP, et al. A direct approach to the estimation of the origin of oestrogens and androgens in elderly men by comparison with hormone levels in postmenopausal women. Eur J Endocrinol. 2005;152:261–8.
22. Pabon JE, Li X, Lei ZM, et al. Novel presence of luteinizing hormone/ chorionic gonadotropin receptors in human adrenal glands. J Clin Endocrinol Metab. 1996;81:2397–400.

23. Rao CV, Zhou XL, Lei ZM. Functional luteinizing hormone/chorionic gonadotropin receptors in human adrenal cortical H295R cells. Biol Reprod. 2004;71:579–87.

24. Cheng CK, Leung PC. Molecular biology of Gonadotropin-releasing hormone (GnRH)-I, GnRH-II, and their receptors in humans. Endocr Rev. 2005;26:283–306.

25. Ziegler CG, Brown JW, Schally AV, et al. Expression of neuropeptide hormone receptors in human adrenal tumors and cell lines: Antiproliferative effects of peptide analogues. PNAS. 2009;106:15879–84.

26. Bashin S, Berman N, Swerdloff RS. Follicle-stimulating hormone (FSH) escape during chronic Gonadotropin-releasing hormone (GnRH) agonist and testosterone treatment. J Andol. 1994;15:386–91.

27. Santen RJ, Demers LM, Max DT, et al. Long term effects of administration of a gonadotropin-releasing hormone superagonist analog in men with prostatic carcinoma. J Clin Endocrinol Metab. 1984;58:397–400.

28. Crawford ED, Thombal B, Miller K, et al. A phase III extension trial with a 1-arm crossover from Leuprolide to Degarelix: comparison of Gonadotropin-releasing hormone agonist and antagonist effect on prostate cancer. JUrol. 2011;186:889–97.

29. Porter AT, Ben-Josef E. Humoral mechanisms in prostate cancer: a role for FSH. Urol Oncol. 2001;6:131–8.

30. Radu A, Pichon C, Camparo P, et al. Expression of follicle-stimulating hormone receptor in tumor blood vessels. N Engl J Med. 2010;363:1621–30.

Anti-proliferative potential of Glucosamine in renal cancer cells via inducing cell cycle arrest at G0/G1 phase

Long-sheng Wang[†], Shao-jun Chen[†], Jun-feng Zhang, Meng-nan Liu, Jun-hua Zheng[*] and Xu-dong Yao[*]

Abstract

Background: Renal cell carcinoma (RCC) is one of the most common types of cancer in urological system worldwide. Recently, the anticancer role of Glucosamine has been studied in many types of cancer. The aim of this study was to investigate the effects of Glucosamine on RCC.

Methods: The effects of Glucosamine on RCC cell proliferation and apoptosis were investigated by MTT assay and Annexin V-FITC Apoptosis assay, respectively in vitro. Cell cycle was detected by flow cytometry after treatment with Glucosamine. Protein levels of several cell cycle associated markers were examined by Western Blot.

Results: Our data showed that Glucosamine significantly inhibited the proliferation of renal cancer 786-O and Caki-1 cells in a dose-dependent manner. Besides, Glucosamine treatment resulted in cell cycle arrest at G0/G1 phase in both cell lines. Meanwhile, the expression of several regulators that contribute to G1/S phased transition, such as Cyclin D1, CDK4 and CDK6, were significantly down-regulated with the up-regulation of cell cycle inhibitors, p21 and p53, after treatment with glucosamine. However, the apoptosis rate of RCC cells was down-regulated when treatment with Glucosamine at 1 mM and 5 mM, while up-regulated at 10 mM.

Conclusions: Our findings indicated that Glucosamine inhibited the proliferation of RCC cells by promoting cell cycle arrest at G0/G1 phase, but not promoting apoptosis. The present results suggested that Glucosamine might be a potential therapeutic agent in RCC treatment in the future.

Keywords: Renal cell carcinoma, Glucosamine, Proliferation, Cell cycle

Background

D-Glucosamine (2-amino-2-deoxy-d-glucose), a naturally occurring amino monosaccharide, is used to synthesize UDP-GlcNAc in the body via the hexosamine biosynthetic pathway (HBP) [1]. UDP-GlcNAc is the principal substrate for the glycosylation of proteins [2, 3]. Because it is highly water soluble and nontoxic, Glucosamine has been widely used as a nutritional supplement in both humans and dogs [4]. The most famous use of glucosamine is to treat human osteoarthritis [5, 6]. Except for its chondroprotective action, glucosamine has been demonstrated to have many other functions, such as anti-cancer.

Glucosamine was first demonstrated as an anticancer pharmaceutical more than 60 years ago [7]. Recently, more attentions have been attracted to its antitumor properties. Glucosamine is an effective lytic agent for several types of tumors with little toxicity to normal cells [8]. It has been reported that glucosamine suppresses the proliferation of human prostate cancer DU145 cells through STAT3 signaling pathway [9]. Glucosamine can also play anti-cancer activity through the inhibition of N-linked glycosylation [10]. In retinal pigment epithelial cells, glucosamine exhibits its antitumor role through the inhibition of epidermal growth factor-induced proliferation and cell-cycle progression [11]. However, the effects of Glucosamine on renal cancer cells remain unclear, let alone the mechanisms.

It is well-known that cell cycle deregulation is one of the most prevalent characteristics of all cancers [12].

* Correspondence: zhengjunhua2016@163.com; yaoxudong1967@163.com
[†]Equal contributors
Department of Urology, Shanghai Tenth People's Hospital, Tongji University, School of Medicine, Shanghai 200072, China

Cyclins, cyclin-dependent kinases (CDKs) and various kinds of cyclin-dependent kinase inhibitors (CDKIs) are closely involved in cell cycle distribution [13]. Cyclin D1, which is responsible for the transition from G1 phase to S phase via forming complexes with CDK4 and CDK6, is one of the most important cell cycle regulators in the process of tumor development [14, 15]. M. S. Lima et al. reported that Cyclin D1 was overexpressed in RCC and can be used as an prognostic factor in RCC patients [16]. P21 protein is a well-known CDK inhibitor, participating in cell-cycle regulation via the inhibition of cyclin-CDK complex activity in G1 phase [15]. Tumor suppressor p53 also takes part in regulating the cell cycle process and p21 acts as a major downstream effector of p53 in G1 phase [17, 18]. The deficiency of p21 along with p53 may lead to unrestricted cell cycle progression and carcinogenesis.

Renal cell carcinoma, which accounts for about 3% of all cancers in adults, is one of the most common diagnosed cancers in urological system in the world [19]. About 62,700 cases of kidney cancer and renal pelvis cancer are expected to occur and lead to more than 14,240 deaths in the United States in 2016 [20]. Among all the subtypes of RCC, about 70% is clear cell histopathology [21]. It is estimated that approximate 25% of patients with RCC have encountered metastases at the time of diagnosis and another 25% have locally advanced disease [22]. RCC was reported inherently resistant to cytotoxic therapy, hormone therapy or radiation [23, 24].

The aim of the present study was to investigate the effects of D-Glucosamine on RCC cells. Our results show that Glucosamine inhibited the proliferation of renal cancer cells in a dose-dependent manner. Meanwhile, we tried to explore how Glucosamine exert its anti-proliferation effect. The apoptosis assay revealed that RCC cells apoptosis was down-regulated when treatment with Glucosamine at low concentration, while up-regulated at very high concentration. Moreover, Glucosamine treatment resulted in cell-cycle arrest in G0/G1 phase. Mechanically, Cyclin D1 was dramatically repressed by Glucosamine, while the expression of p53 and p21 was significantly up-regulated. These results suggested that Glucosamine inhibited the proliferation of renal cancer cells by promoting cell-cycle arrest.

Methods
Cell culture and reagents
Human renal cancer cell lines 786-O and caki-1 were purchased from the Cell Bank of Type Culture Collection of Chinese Academy of Sciences (CCCAS, China) and were cultured in RPMI-1640 medium (HyClone) supplemented with 10% fetal bovine serum (Gibco). All cells were cultured in a humidified incubator with 5% CO_2 at 37 °C. D-glucosamine was purchased from Sigma Chemical Co (sigma A3286). All the antibodies were purchased from Abcam.

MTT assay
Five groups of RCC cells were plated in 96-well culture plates in triplicate at a concentration of about 2×10^3/ well. 200 μl culture medium containing various concentrations of glucosamine (0 mM, 1 mM, 5 mM and 10 mM) was added into 96-well culture plates, respectively. After incubated for different time perious (12, 24, 48 and 72 h), 200 μl MTT solution was added to each well. Then, cells were incubated at 37 °C for 4 h and the medium was discarded from each well. After that, 200 μl DMSO was used and thoroughly mixed for 15 min. The optical density (OD) of each well was measured at 490 nm using a micro-plate reader (Bio-Rad). All experiments were performed three times and three replicates in each repeat.

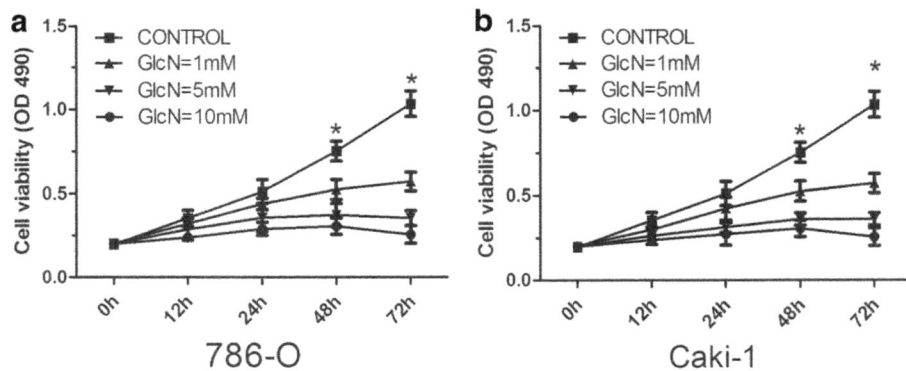

Fig. 1 Glucosamine induces growth inhibition in 786-O (a) and Caki-1 cells (b). Cells were treated with various concentrations of Glucosamine (0 mM, 1 mM, 5 mM and 10 mM), and cell viability was analyzed using MTT assay at different time points (0 h,12 h, 24 h, 48 h and 72 h). * $P < 0.05$ compared with the control group (0 mM)

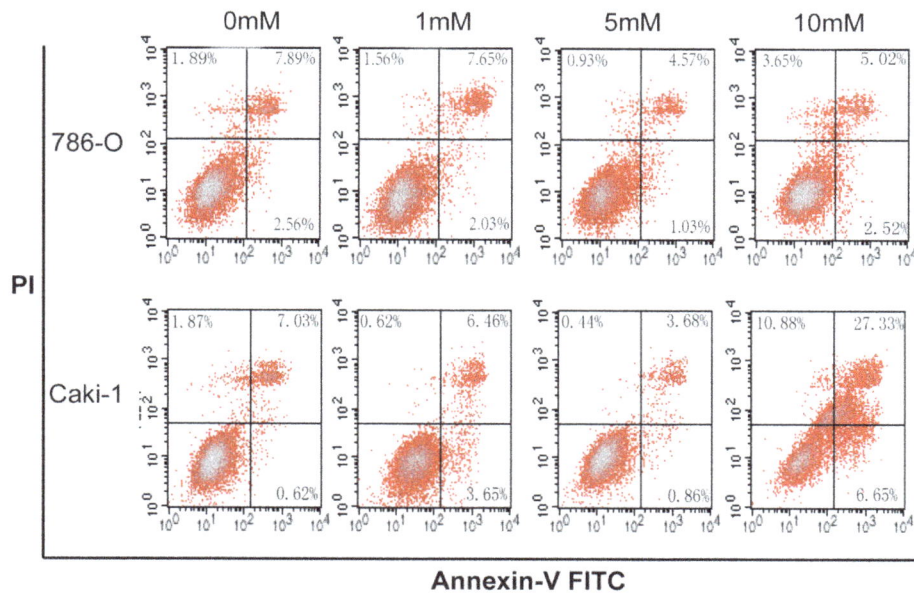

Fig. 2 Effects of Glucosamine on the apoptosis of 786-O and Caki-1 cells as shown by Annexin V-FITC/PI analysis. 786-O and Caki-1 cells were treated for 24 h with various doses of Glucosamine under serum-free conditions, and apoptotic cells were measured as the percentage of Annexin V-positive/PI-negative cells. The representative images were shown. Three independent experiments were performed and the trend is the same

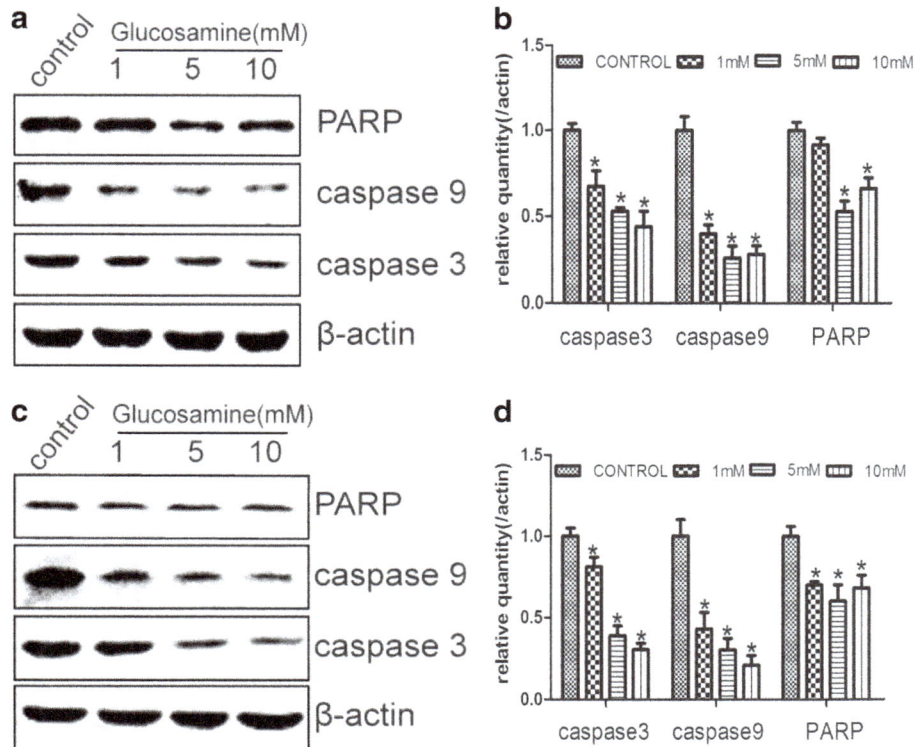

Fig. 3 Effects of Glucosamine on the expression of apoptosis regulators caspase 3/9 and PARP. 786-O and Caki-1 cells were deprived of serum for 24 h and cultured with various doses of Glucosamine for 24 h. Afterward, the total protein was collected and the expression of caspase 3/9 and PARP was detected with Western Blot. The expression of these three proteins was obviously down-regulated in both 786-O (**a**) and Caki-1(**c**) cells. Columns show the mean values of three experiments of 786-O (**b**) and Caki-1(**d**) (± SD). *$P < 0.05$ compared with the control group (0 mM)

Western blot assay

Total protein was extracted using precooled RIPA lysis buffer with protease inhibitors. The concentration of total protein was measured using a Bio-Rad protein assay system. Equal amount of protein was separated by 10% SDS-PAGE for electrophoresis and transferred to nitrocellulose membranes (Bio-Rad). Afterward, the membrane was incubated at 4 °C for 12 h with specific primary antibodies (Bioworld, Nanjing, China). After incubation with secondary antibodies for 1 h at room temperature, signals were visualized.

Cell cycle assays

To measure cell cycle distribution, the cells were harvested after addition with different concentrations of glucosamine for 24 h and fixed in 70% ice-cold ethanol overnight. Then, the cells were washed by PBS and stained with propidium iodide (PI; BD Biosciences) in PBS added with RNase (100 µg/ml) and Triton X-100 (0.2%) for 30 min. Afterward, cell cycle distribution was analyzed by flow cytometry according to the manufacturer's guidelines (FACS, BD Biosciences). Tests were performed three times for each sample.

Apoptosis assay

For the apoptosis assay, the Annexin V-FITC Apoptosis Detection kit (BD Biosciences) was used according to manufacturer's protocol. Cells were serum starved for 24 h, and treated with various doses of glucosamine (0 mM, 1 mM, 5 mM and 10 mM) for 24 h. RCC cells were collected and washed twice with PBS. Then, cells were re-suspended, stained with (FITC)-Annexin V/PI for 15 min and analyzed by flow cytometry (FACS, BD Biosciences).

Statistical analysis

SPSS version 18.0 software was used for all statistical analyses of this study. Data are expressed as mean ± SD from at least three independent experiments. The differences between each experimental group was analyzed by Student's t-test or chi-square test. P-value of <0.05 was treated as statistically significant.

Results

Glucosamine inhibits renal cancer cell proliferation

To examine the effects of Glucosamine on the proliferation of human renal cancer cells, 786-O and Caki-1 cells were treated with Glucosamine at different doses and

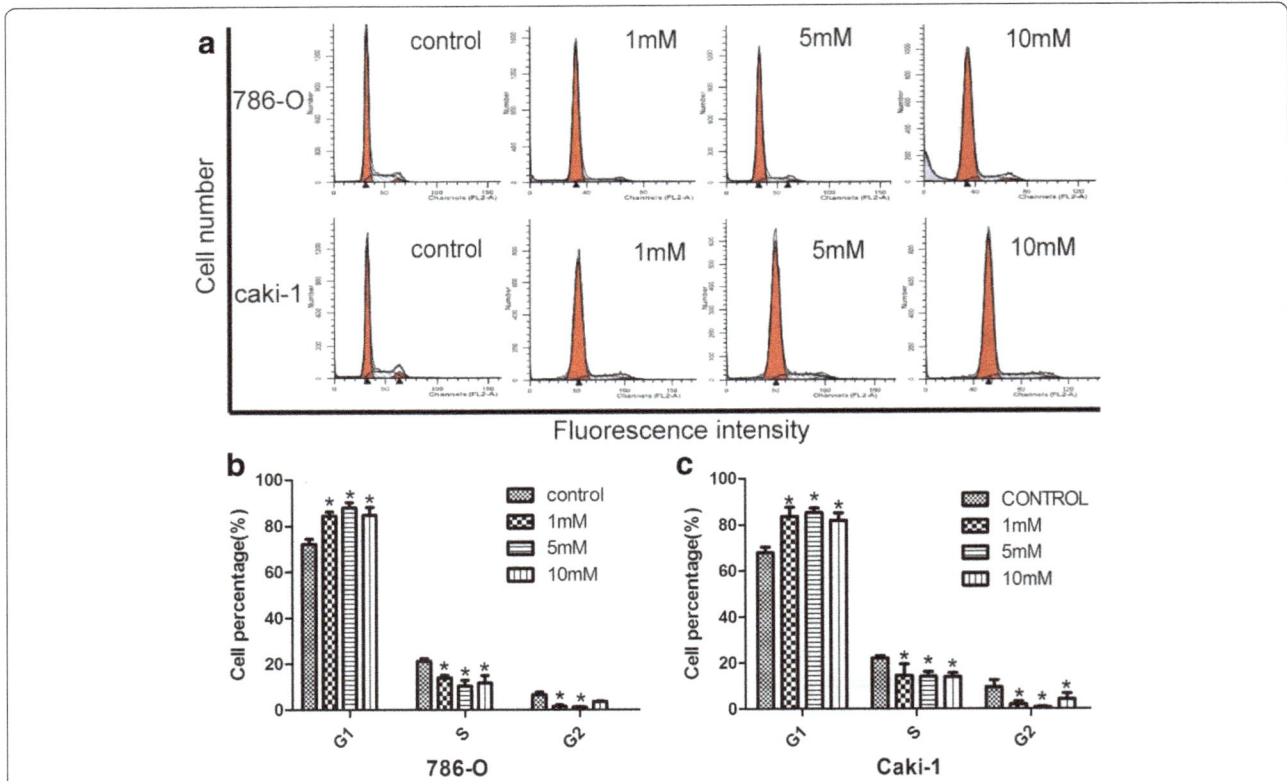

Fig. 4 Effects of Glucosamine on cell-cycle progression in human renal cancer cell lines (786-O and Caki-1). a Cell cycle distribution of 786-O and Caki-1 cells was examined after treatment with various concentrations of Glucosamine for 24 h. b, c Columns show the mean values of three experiments (± SD). *P < 0.05 compared with the control group (0 mM)

MTT assay was performed. Our data showed that Glucosamine inhibited the proliferation of RCC cells in a dose-dependent manner (Fig. 1). These results suggested that Glucosamine played an important anti-proliferative role in RCC cells.

Effects of Glucosamine on cell apoptosis

Previous studies have reported that Glucosamine induced apoptosis in various cell lines [25, 26]. Therefore, we investigated whether Glucosamine exerted anti-cancer role via inducing apoptosis in renal cancer cells lines. As shown in Fig. 2, the apoptosis rate of both cell lines was up-regulated by high concentration of Glucosamine (10 mM), but down-regulated by low concentrations of Glucosamine (1 mM and 5 mM), as compared with control group. These data suggested that low doses of Glucosamine-mediated proliferation inhibition of renal cancer cells was not due to apoptosis.

Members of caspases play vital role in the apoptotic process. The nuclear DNA repair enzyme poly (ADP-ribose) polymerase (PARP) is a target of caspase-3 and its cleavage is a biomarker for cell apoptosis [27, 28]. Thereby, we detected the expression of caspase-3, caspase-9 and

PARP in RCC cells by Western blot. Our results showed that the protein levels of caspase-3, caspase-9 and PARP were significantly down-regulated by Glucosamine as compared with the control in both 786-O and Caki-1 cells (Fig. 3). These results were in line with the results of Annexin V-FITC Apoptosis assay. All these results indicated that Glucosamine inhibited the proliferation of RCC cells was not by inducing apoptosis.

Glucosamine induces cell cycle arrest in RCC cells in a dose-dependent manner

Glucosamine could cause cell-cycle arrest in various types of cancer cell lines [29, 30]. To determine whether the anti-proliferation effect of Glucosamine was accompanied by the alteration in cell cycle process, we next investigated the cycle distribution of 786-O and caki-1 cells after Glucosamine treatment (0 mM, 1 mM, 5 mM, and 10 mM) for 24 h. As shown in Fig. 4, with the increasing doses of Glucosamine, G0/G1 cell population was gradually increased with the decrease of cells in S and G2/M phases. These results indicated that Glucosamine-mediated cell growth inhibition occurred at the G0/G1 to S transition phase.

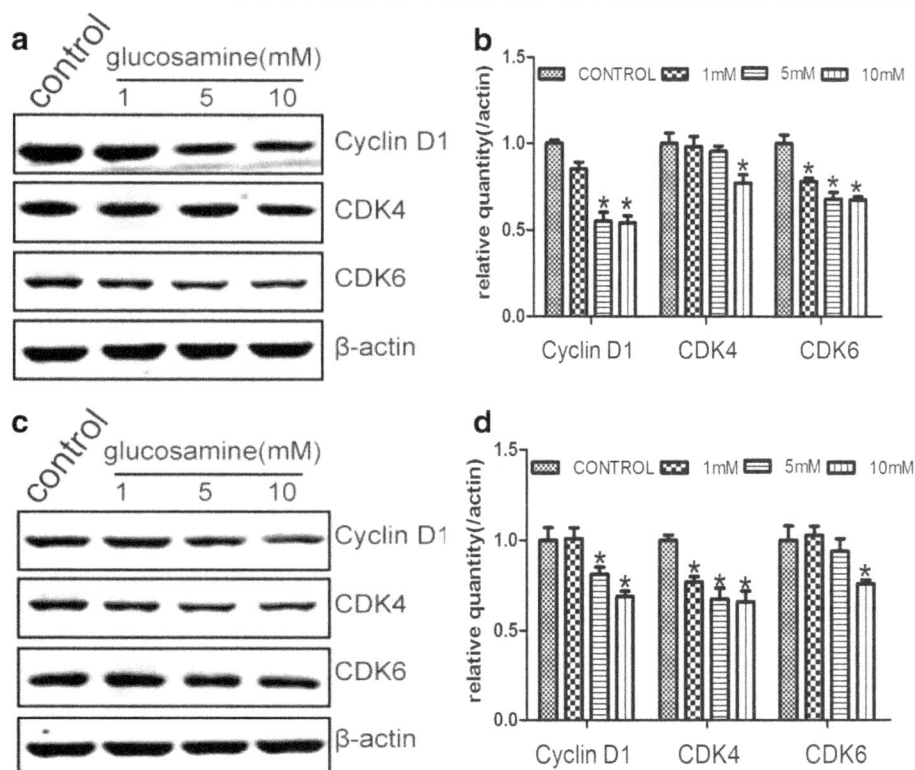

Fig. 5 The expression of Cyclin D1, CDK4 and CDK6 were down-regulated by Glucosamine. When 786-O (a, b) and Caki-1 (c, d) cells were treated with Glucosamine for 24 h, the expression of Cyclin D1, CDK4 and CDK6 were down-regulated. Cells were lysed with RIPA lysis buffer, and the lysates were then analyzed by Western blot. a, c Representative gels from 3 experiments are shown. b, d Densitometric analysis was performed for each protein band relative to β-actin in the same sample using Quantity one software. *P < 0.05 compared with the control group (0 mM)

Down-regulation of Cyclin D1 and CDK4/6 by glucosamine in RCC cells

Cyclin D1 was reported to be a key element in cell proliferation in many types of cancers [31]. Meanwhile, on account of CDK4 and CDK6 preferably associate with the D type cyclins during the G1 phase [32], the expression of Cyclin D1, CDK4 and CDK6 were examined. Western blot results demonstrated that Cyclin D1 expression significantly repressed by Glucosamine with the dose raising (Fig. 5). Simultaneously, CDK4 and CDK6 were also gradually suppressed by Glucosamine in a dose-dependent manner (Fig. 5).

Up-regulation of p53 and p21 by glucosamine in RCC cells

It is well known that the complexes of cyclins and CDKs, which is essential to the transition from G0/G1 to S phase, are inhibited by CDKIs [33]. p21 is one of the most important CDKI for CDK4/6. p53, a well-known tumor suppressor, can regulate cell cycle process by affecting the expression of p21 [17]. Thus, we examined the expression of p21 and p53 under the effect of Glucosamine. Glucosamine was found to gradually up-regulate the expression of p21 and p53 in protein levels (Fig. 6).

Discussion

Renal cell carcinoma is one of the deadliest urogenital malignancies. The morbidity of RCC is increasing annually and the causes are multifactorial [34]. Abnormal cell cycle progression, such as shortening of the G1-phase, is involved in tumorigenesis.

Glucosamine and its derivatives are obligatory structural components of many biologically important macromolecules, such as membrane glycoproteins and mucopolysaccharide [35]. Although the anticancer property of glucosamine has been reported more than 60 years ago [7], the molecular mechanism remained unclear. Recently, Glucosamine has been demonstrated to be an effective anticancer agent in prostate cancer, lung cancer, leukemia and colorectal cancer [2, 25, 36, 37]. However, its action in renal cell carcinoma has not been studied.

In the present study, we analyzed the anticancer role of Glucosamine in renal cancer cells. We demonstrated that Glucosamine functioned as an anti-proliferation drug in renal cancer 786-O and Caki-1 cells. Afterward, we tried to certify whether the apoptosis and cell cycle of RCC cells were influenced. Using Annexin V-FITC Apoptosis assay, we found the apoptosis of RCC cells was down-regulated

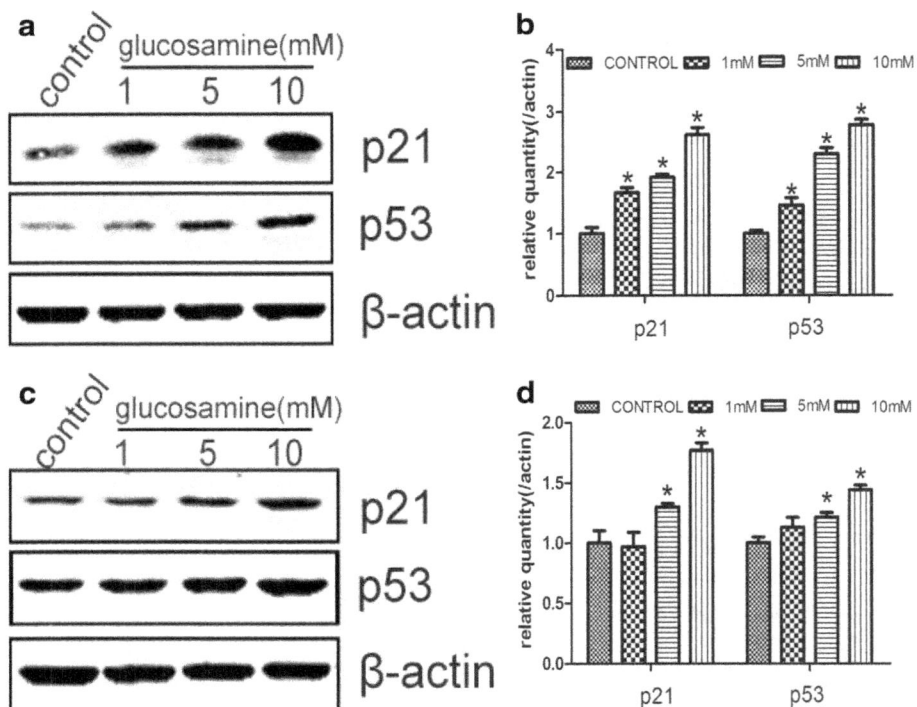

Fig. 6 Glucosamine affects the expression of p21 and p53 in 786-O and Caki-1 cells. The expression of p21 and p53 was tested by Western blot after 786-O and Caki-1 cells were treated with various concentrations of Glucosamine for 24 h. β-actin served as internal loading control. **a, c** Representative gels from 3 experiments are shown. **b, d** Densitometric analysis was performed for each protein band relative to β-actin in the same sample using Quantity one software. *P < 0.05 compared with the control group (0 mM)

significantly when treated with low dose of Glucosamine and was up-regulated only in a very high dose. Likewise, several apoptosis markers were down-regulated obviously, such as caspase-9, caspase-3 and PARP. Notably, Glucosamine induced G0/G1 arrest in the process of RCC cell cycle. Meanwhile, results of Western blot revealed significant down-regulation of Cyclin D1, CDK4, and CDK6 and up-regulation of p21 and p53 under treatment of Glucosamine, especially at the dose of 10 mM comparing with untreated samples. These results indicated that Glucosamine could exert its anticancer affect in RCC cells via causing cell cycle arrest and up-regulating cancer suppressor gene p21 and p53. However, the potential detailed mechanisms involved in the anti-tumor property of Glucosamine in RCC are required to be revealed in the future.

Our results implied that the antiproliferation role of Glucosamine in RCC cells was not related to apoptosis, and this result was consistent with the findings of Chang-Min Liang et al. [11]. They reported that Glucosamine did not induce apoptosis in the ARPE-19 cells, but inhibit epidermal growth factor-induced proliferation by causing cell cycle arrest. However, Zhe Wang et al. reported that Glucosamine sulfate induced apoptosis in chronic myelogenous leukemia K562 cells and this regulation was associated with translocation of cathepsin D and downregulation of Bcl-xL [25]. Otherwise, Ki-Hoon Song et al. showed that Glucosamine induced cell cycle arrest and apoptosis in NSCLC cells [26]. We assume that Glucosamine may play various roles in different types of cancers.

Conclusion

Current study found that, Glucosamine inhibited the proliferation of RCC cells mostly by causing cell cycle arrest at G0/G1 phase. Glucosamine treatment in RCC cells led to the down-regulation of Cyclin D1, CDK4 and CDK6, as well as the up-regulation of p21 and p53. Cumulatively, these findings indicate that Glucosamine might serve as a potential therapeutic in the future.

Abbreviations

CDK: Cyclin-dependent kinases; HBP: Hexosamine biosynthetic pathway; PARP: Poly (ADP-ribose) polymerase; RCC: Renal cell carcinoma

Acknowledgement
Not applicable.

Funding
National Natural Science Foundation of China (No. 01.02.12.054).

Authors' contributions
YXD and ZJH conceived and designed the experiments; WLS and CSJ performed the experiments; ZJF analyzed the data; LMN contributed reagents/materials/analysis tools; WLS and CSJ wrote the paper. We confirm that all authors read and approved the final manuscript.

Competing interests
The authors declare that they have no competing interests.

References

1. Al-Kurdi ZI, Chowdhry BZ, Leharne SA, Qinna NA, Al Omari MM, Badwan AA. Influence of glucosamine on the bioactivity of insulin delivered subcutaneously and in an oral nanodelivery system. Drug Des Devel Therapy. 2015;9:6167–76.
2. Hwang JA, Kim Y, Hong SH, Lee J, Cho YG, Han JY, Kim YH, Han J, Shim YM, Lee YS, et al. Epigenetic inactivation of heparan sulfate (glucosamine) 3-O-sulfotransferase 2 in lung cancer and its role in tumorigenesis. PLoS ONE. 2013;8(11):e79634.
3. Thomas SM, Coppelli FM, Wells A, Gooding WE, Song J, Kassis J, Drenning SD, Grandis JR. Epidermal growth factor receptor-stimulated activation of phospholipase Cgamma-1 promotes invasion of head and neck squamous cell carcinoma. Cancer Res. 2003;63(17):5629–35.
4. Al-Hamidi H, Edwards AA, Douroumis D, Asare-Addo K, Nayebi AM, Reyhani-Rad S, Mahmoudi J, Nokhodchi A. Effect of glucosamine HCl on dissolution and solid state behaviours of piroxicam upon milling. Colloids Surf B: Biointerfaces. 2013;103:189–99.
5. Liu BQ, Meng X, Li C, Gao YY, Li N, Niu XF, Guan Y, Wang HQ. Glucosamine induces cell death via proteasome inhibition in human ALVA41 prostate cancer cell. Exp Mol Med. 2011;43(9):487–93.
6. Reginster JY, Deroisy R, Rovati LC, Lee RL, Lejeune E, Bruyere O, Giacovelli G, Henrotin Y, Dacre JE, Gossett C. Long-term effects of glucosamine sulphate on osteoarthritis progression: a randomised, placebo-controlled clinical trial. Lancet. 2001;357(9252):251–6.
7. Quastel JH, Cantero A. Inhibition of tumour growth by D-glucosamine. Nature. 1953;171(4345):252–4.
8. Friedman SJ, Skehan P. Membrane-active drugs potentiate the killing of tumor cells by D-glucosamine. Proc Natl Acad Sci U S A. 1980;77(2):1172–6.
9. Chesnokov V, Sun C, Itakura K. Glucosamine suppresses proliferation of human prostate carcinoma DU145 cells through inhibition of STAT3 signaling. Cancer Cell Int. 2009;9(1):25.
10. Chesnokov V, Gong B, Sun C, Itakura K. Anti-cancer activity of glucosamine through inhibition of N-linked glycosylation. Cancer Cell Int. 2014;14:45.
11. Liang CM, Tai MC, Chang YH, Chen YH, Chen CL, Chien MW, Chen JT. Glucosamine inhibits epidermal growth factor-induced proliferation and cell-cycle progression in retinal pigment epithelial cells. Mol Vis. 2010;16:2559–71.
12. Mizuno H, Nakanishi Y, Ishii N, Sarai A, Kitada K. A signature-based method for indexing cell cycle phase distribution from microarray profiles. BMC Genomics. 2009;10:137.
13. Sherr CJ, Roberts JM. CDK inhibitors: positive and negative regulators of G1-phase progression. Genes Dev. 1999;13(12):1501–12.
14. Donnellan R, Chetty R. Cyclin D1 and human neoplasia. Mol Pathol. 1998;51(1):1–7.
15. Zuryn A, Litwiniec A, Safiejko-Mroczka B, Klimaszewska-Wisniewska A, Gagat M, Krajewski A, Gackowska L, Grzanka D. The effect of sulforaphane on the cell cycle, apoptosis and expression of cyclin D1 and p21 in the A549 non-small cell lung cancer cell line. Int J Oncol. 2016;48(6):2521–33.
16. Lima MS, Pereira RA, Costa RS, Tucci S, Dantas M, Muglia VF, Ravinal RC, Barros-Silva GE. The prognostic value of cyclin D1 in renal cell carcinoma. Int Urol Nephrol. 2014;46(5):905–13.
17. Liu PY, Chan JY, Lin HC, Wang SL, Liu ST, Ho CL, Chang LC, Huang SM. Modulation of the cyclin-dependent kinase inhibitor p21(WAF1/Cip1) gene by Zac1 through the antagonistic regulators p53 and histone deacetylase 1 in HeLa Cells. Mol Cancer Res. 2008;6(7):1204–14.
18. Waldman T, Kinzler KW, Vogelstein B. p21 is necessary for the p53-mediated G1 arrest in human cancer cells. Cancer Res. 1995;55(22):5187–90.
19. Siegel R, Naishadham D, Jemal A. Cancer statistics, 2013. CA Cancer J Clin. 2013;63(1):11–30.
20. Siegel RL, Miller KD, Jemal A. Cancer statistics, 2016. CA Cancer J Clin. 2016;66(1):7-30.
21. Znaor A, Lortet-Tieulent J, Laversanne M, Jemal A, Bray F. International variations and trends in renal cell carcinoma incidence and mortality. Eur Urol. 2015;67(3):519–30.
22. Cindolo L, Patard JJ, Chiodini P, Schips L, Ficarra V, Tostain J, de La Taille A, Altieri V, Lobel B, Zigeuner RE, et al. Comparison of predictive accuracy of four prognostic models for nonmetastatic renal cell carcinoma after nephrectomy: a multicenter European study. Cancer. 2005;104(7):1362–71.

23. Wang Q, Wang S, Sun SQ, Cheng ZH, Zhang Y, Chen G, Gu M, Yao HJ, Wang Z, Zhou J, et al. The effects of RNA interference mediated VEGF gene silencing on biological behavior of renal cell carcinoma and transplanted renal tumor in nude mice. Cancer Biomark. 2016;16(1):1–9.

24. Sternberg CN, Davis ID, Mardiak J, Szczylik C, Lee E, Wagstaff J, Barrios CH, Salman P, Gladkov OA, Kavina A, et al. Pazopanib in locally advanced or metastatic renal cell carcinoma: results of a randomized phase III trial. J Clin Oncol. 2010;28(6):1061–8.

25. Wang Z, Liang R, Huang GS, Piao Y, Zhang YQ, Wang AQ, Dong BX, Feng JL, Yang GR, Guo Y. Glucosamine sulfate-induced apoptosis in chronic myelogenous leukemia K562 cells is associated with translocation of cathepsin D and downregulation of Bcl-xL. Apoptosis. 2006;11(10):1851–60.

26. Song KH, Kang JH, Woo JK, Nam JS, Min HY, Lee HY, Kim SY, Oh SH. The novel IGF-IR/Akt-dependent anticancer activities of glucosamine. BMC Cancer. 2014;14:31.

27. Chereau D, Zou H, Spada AP, Wu JC. A nucleotide binding site in caspase-9 regulates apoptosome activation. Biochemistry. 2005;44(13):4971–6.

28. Chaitanya GV, Steven AJ, Babu PP. PARP-1 cleavage fragments: signatures of cell-death proteases in neurodegeneration. Cell Commun Signal. 2010;8:31.

29. Masson E, Wiernsperger N, Lagarde M, El Bawab S. Glucosamine induces cell-cycle arrest and hypertrophy of mesangial cells: implication of gangliosides. Biochem J. 2005;388(Pt 2):537–44.

30. Chuang KH, Lu CS, Kou YR, Wu YL. Cell cycle regulation by glucosamine in human pulmonary epithelial cells. Pulm Pharmacol Ther. 2013;26(2):195–204.

31. Kim JK, Diehl JA. Nuclear cyclin D1: an oncogenic driver in human cancer. J Cell Physiol. 2009;220(2):292–6.

32. Cordon-Cardo C. Mutations of cell cycle regulators. Biological and clinical implications for human neoplasia. Am J Pathol. 1995;147(3):545–60.

33. Zarkowska T, Mittnacht S. Differential phosphorylation of the retinoblastoma protein by G1/S cyclin-dependent kinases. J Biol Chem. 1997;272(19):12738–46.

34. Petejova N, Martinek A. Renal cell carcinoma: review of etiology, pathophysiology and risk factors. Biomed Pap Med Fac Univ Palacky Olomouc Czech. 2016;160(2):183–94.

35. Fujiwara T, Kubota K, Sato T, Matsuzawa T, Tada M, Iwata R, Itoh M, Hatazawa J, Sato K, Fukuda H, et al. N-[18 F] fluoroacetyl-D-glucosamine: a potential agent for cancer diagnosis. J Nucl Med. 1990;31(10):1654–8.

36. Ogunsina M, Pan H, Samadder P, Arthur G, Schweizer F. Structure activity relationships of N-linked and diglycosylated glucosamine-based antitumor glycerolipids. Mol. 2013;18(12):15288–304.

37. Kantor ED, Lampe JW, Peters U, Shen DD, Vaughan TL, White E. Use of glucosamine and chondroitin supplements and risk of colorectal cancer. Cancer Causes Control. 2013;24(6):1137–46.

7

Assembling and validating data from multiple sources to study care for Veterans with bladder cancer

Florian R. Schroeck[1,2,3,4*] , Brenda Sirovich[1,4], John D. Seigne[2,3], Douglas J. Robertson[1,4] and Philip P. Goodney[1,4]

Abstract

Background: Despite the high prevalence of bladder cancer, research on optimal bladder cancer care is limited. One way to advance observational research on care is to use linked data from multiple sources. Such big data research can provide real-world details of care and outcomes across a large number of patients. We assembled and validated such data including (1) administrative data from the Department of Veterans Affairs (VA), (2) Medicare claims, (3) data abstracted by tumor registrars, (4) data abstracted via chart review from the national electronic health record, and (5) full text pathology reports.

Methods: Based on these combined data, we used administrative data to identify patients with newly diagnosed bladder cancer who received care in the VA. To validate these data, we first compared the diagnosis date from the administrative data to that from the tumor registry. Second, we measured accuracy of identifying bladder cancer care in VA administrative data, using a random chart review ($n = 100$) as gold standard. Lastly, we compared the proportion of patients who received bladder cancer care among those who did versus did not have full text bladder pathology reports available, expecting that those with reports are significantly more likely to receive care in VA.

Results: Out of 26,675 patients, 11,323 (42%) had tumor registry data available. 90% of these patients had a difference of 90 days or less between the diagnosis dates from administrative and registry data. Among 100 patients selected for chart review, 59 received bladder cancer care in VA, 58 of which were correctly identified using administrative data (sensitivity 98%, specificity 90%). Receipt of bladder cancer care was substantially more common among those who did versus did not have bladder pathology available (96% vs. 43%, $p < 0.001$).

Conclusion: Merging administrative with electronic health record and pathology data offers new possibilities to validate the use of administrative data in bladder cancer research.

Keywords: Bladder cancer, Cystoscopy, Electronic health record, Validity

Background

Bladder cancer is the third and fourth most prevalent non-cutaneous cancer among men and women in the United States [1]. In spite of this high prevalence, there is fairly limited research on what entails optimal bladder cancer care [2], particularly for the majority of patients who are living with non-muscle invasive bladder cancer (NMIBC). This may be due to the fact that examining bladder cancer care using observational data often

represents a "moving target" [3]. Specifically, patients with bladder cancer tend to have multiple recurrences and after each recurrence their pathology and consequently their bladder cancer risk-classification can change [4, 5], impacting further treatment recommendations and follow-up [3].

One potential way to advance observational research on care for NMIBC is to use linked data from multiple sources to gain a more complete picture of the care patients receive and of the outcomes of that care. Sources may include administrative data from hospital electronic health records (EHR), claims data from Medicare, full text records (e.g. pathology reports) from the EHR, as

* Correspondence: florian.r.schroeck@dartmouth.edu
[1]White River Junction VA Medical Center, 215 N Main Street, White River Junction, VT 05009, USA
[2]Section of Urology, Dartmouth Hitchcock Medical Center, Lebanon, NH, USA
Full list of author information is available at the end of the article

well as data manually abstracted by chart review. Linking multiple sources into larger, combined datasets – sometimes called big data research [6] – provides the opportunity to capture procedures performed, details of pathology at time of diagnosis and at time of recurrence, and clinical details that can be abstracted from the patient chart, thus providing a more complete picture of patient care and outcomes. Moreover – as done here – these combined datasets allow for the validation of algorithms and results from the administrative data.

Here, we combine multiple data sources from the Department of Veterans Affairs (VA) Corporate Data Warehouse (CDW) to assemble a data set that can be used to study care for patients with bladder cancer. We describe an algorithm to identify patients with newly diagnosed bladder cancer who received bladder cancer care in VA and then examine its convergent, criterion, and concurrent validity. These validated data will provide the opportunity for future detailed research examining utilization and outcomes of surveillance care among patients with bladder cancer.

Methods
Data sources
We assembled and linked data from five distinct sources in order to provide a comprehensive picture of bladder cancer diagnosis, pathology, and care. This included (1) administrative data from the VA CDW (including both inpatient and outpatient encounter data), (2) Medicare claims data for the Veterans in our cohort, (3) data abstracted by tumor registrars at each individual VA facility which is then deposited into the CDW, (4) full text pathology reports from the Text Integration Utility files available in the CDW, and (5) data abstracted via chart review from the national electronic health record using the Compensation and Pension Records Interchange (CAPRI) and Veterans Health Information Systems and Technology Architecture (VistA) Web tools.

The VA Information Resource Center (VIReC) routinely obtains Medicare claims data for Veterans and matches these to VA data using established algorithms, based on social security number, gender, and date of birth [7, 8]. Medicare data for members of our cohort were then provided by VIReC. Medicare claims data, tumor registry data, and full text pathology data were linked using the scrambled social security number, a unique patient identifier created for research purposes by VIReC. Data abstracted via chart review were linked using the real social security number. The study was approved by the Dartmouth Committee for the Protection of Human Subjects (#28417) and by the Veteran's Institutional Review Board of Northern New England (#897920-1).

Algorithm to identify patients with newly diagnosed bladder cancer
We developed an algorithm based on administrative data to identify a cohort of Veterans with newly diagnosed bladder cancer. For this, we first identified any patient 66 years of age or older with a diagnosis code for bladder cancer (ICD9 codes 188.x, 233.7, 236.7, 239.4) within the VA CDW outpatient and inpatient files between 01/01/2005 and 12/31/2011. For the outpatient files, we required at least two diagnosis codes for bladder cancer at least 30 days apart to help exclude "rule-out" type diagnoses (e.g. a patient with a lesion seen on CT scan prompting a diagnosis code for bladder cancer but later cystoscopy failing to show a tumor within the bladder) [9]. We defined the first occurrence of a bladder cancer diagnosis date as the index date. Next, we excluded any patients with a preexisting diagnosis of bladder cancer (ICD9 188.x, 233.7, V10.51) within the VA CDW inpatient or outpatient data, or within the Medicare Provider Analysis and Review (MEDPAR), Medicare Outpatient, or Medicare Carrier files during the 365 days prior to the index date. Medicare data were queried, because approximately half of VA patients also receive care through Medicare [8]. This left us with a cohort of patients who had a diagnosis code for bladder cancer between 2005 and 2011 and did not have any preexisting bladder cancer diagnosis codes. However, a 365 day look back is arbitrary and may be too short for bladder cancer patients as some of them may only undergo follow-up once a year. Thus, we performed sensitivity analyses after excluding patients with a preexisting diagnosis of bladder cancer in the 730 days prior to the index date (n = 23,068). Results from these sensitivity analyses were not materially different in direction or effect size compared with those of our main analyses, so only the latter are presented.

Assessing the date of diagnosis – Convergent validity
Convergent validity is defined as the degree to which an operationalization is similar to (converges on) other operationalizations that it theoretically should be similar to [10]. In our study, we assessed convergent validity by comparing the diagnosis date from the claims algorithm (that is the index date after applying the 365 day look back as described above) to the diagnosis date from the tumor registry among the subset of patient who had tumor registry data available (Table 1). We calculated the proportion of patients who had the same diagnosis date in both sources and whose tumor registry date fell within a +/– 7 day, 30 day, or 90 day window around the algorithm-derived index date. In addition, we calculated the proportion of patients who did not have newly diagnosed bladder cancer, defined as a tumor registry

Table 1 For each type of validity, the question, the comparison, and the rationale for evaluation are shown

Question	Comparison	Rationale
Can we correctly identify the diagnosis date? (Convergent validity)	Diagnosis dates from claims algorithm vs those from tumor registry ($n = 11,323$)	Tumor registry data are deemed most reliable because registrars abstracted data directly from the chart. However, registry data are not available for all patients, necessitating development of a cohort based on administrative data.
Can we accurately identify bladder cancer care received within VA? (Criterion validity)	Bladder cancer care received in VA based on administrative data vs chart review (n = 100)	(1) Assure that algorithm does find all patients who did get bladder cancer care (sensitivity). (2) Assure that patients who were identified as receiving bladder cancer care with the algorithm actually did receive such care (positive predictive value).
If we apply the algorithm to the entire cohort, can we distinguish between groups that are conceptually more or less likely to receive bladder cancer care in VA? (Concurrent validity)	Bladder cancer care received in VA among patients with vs without full text bladder pathology reports available ($n = 26,675$)	Patients with full text bladder pathology reports are highly suspected to have received bladder cancer care in VA. Thus, the proportion receiving bladder cancer care in VA should be significantly higher among patients who have full text bladder pathology reports than among those who have not.

diagnosis date more than 90 days prior to the algorithm-derived date.

Assessing receipt of bladder cancer care in VA – Criterion validity

Criterion validity is defined as the performance of an operationalization against some criterion (gold standard) [10]. In our study, we assessed criterion validity by evaluating our ability to identify bladder cancer care in VA based on administrative data against a chart review of 100 randomly selected cases as the gold standard. We defined bladder cancer care as cystoscopy without or with biopsy or transurethral resection. Using established methods [11], we classified patients as receiving bladder cancer care in the VA if they had evidence for these procedures (see Additional file 1) within the VA administrative data between the index date and study end (12/31/2014). To better understand whether we can correctly identify bladder cancer care, we measured the accuracy of the administrative data to differentiate between patients who did versus those who did not receive bladder cancer care in VA (Table 1). For this, we randomly sampled 100 patients out of the entire cohort for a chart review. We used the national electronic health record to review all relevant clinical notes from 1 year prior to the index date to at least 2 years after the index date. Based on this review, we determined whether the patient did or did not receive bladder cancer care in VA. Using the chart review as the gold standard, we then calculated sensitivity, specificity, negative predictive value, positive predictive value, and accuracy of the claims-based algorithm to identify patients who received bladder cancer care in VA. We calculated confidence intervals (CIs) for these measures using a binomial distribution. Finally, we determined the reasons for not identifying bladder cancer care within VA administrative data, using Medicare enrollment and claims data as well as data from the chart review.

Assessing our ability to distinguish between groups that are conceptually more or less likely to receive bladder cancer care in VA – Concurrent validity

Concurrent validity examines the operationalization's ability to distinguish between groups that it should theoretically be able to distinguish between [10]. In our case, patients with full text bladder pathology reports were highly suspected to have received bladder cancer care in VA. Thus, our a priori expectation was that receipt of bladder cancer care in VA should be significantly more common among patients who have full text pathology reports than among those who have not (Table 1). As previously described, we identified full text pathology reports based on the report title indicating a pathology report and on presence of at least one of the three keywords "bladder", "urethra", or "ureter" within the full text [12]. We then used the chi-squared test to compare the proportion of patients receiving bladder cancer care among those who did versus who did not have pathology reports available.

Results

The final cohort consisted of 26,675 patients with newly diagnosed bladder cancer, after excluding patients with a pre-existing bladder cancer diagnosis in either VA administrative data or Medicare claims during the 365 days prior to the index date. Approximately two thirds of these patients ($n = 16,846$, 63%) received bladder cancer care in VA (Fig. 1).

Convergent validity and date of diagnosis

First, we evaluated whether we can correctly identify the diagnosis date from the administrative data. Thus, we

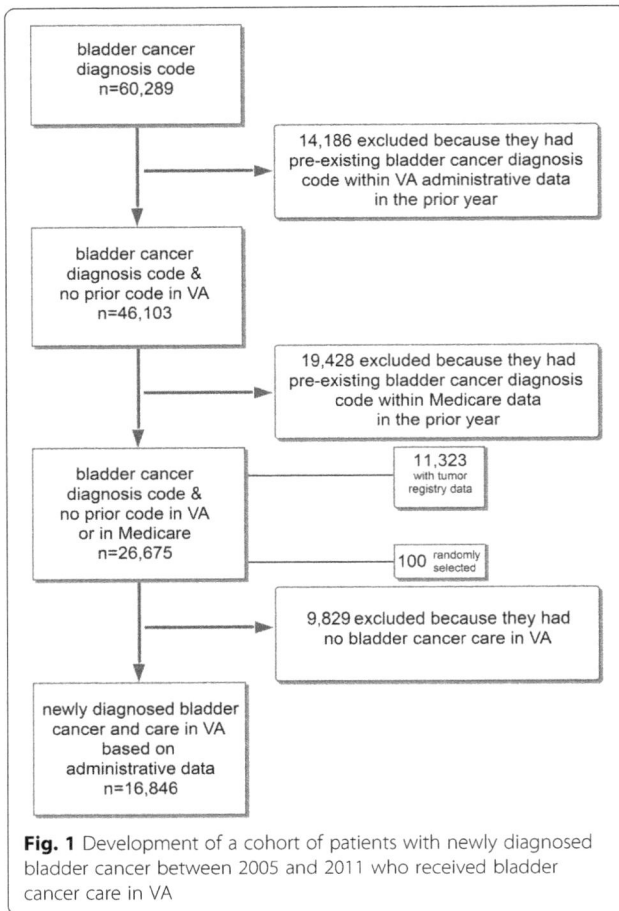

Fig. 1 Development of a cohort of patients with newly diagnosed bladder cancer between 2005 and 2011 who received bladder cancer care in VA

compared the diagnosis date obtained from the administrative data to the diagnosis date abstracted by the registrars among the subset of 11,323 patients (42%) with registry data available. About a quarter of patients (27%) had the same diagnosis date in both datasets. Ninety

percent had their tumor registry diagnosis date fall within a 90 day window around the date derived from the administrative data (Fig. 2). Only 2.9% did not have newly diagnosed bladder cancer, as their tumor registry date was more than 90 days prior to the date derived from the administrative data (Fig. 2).

Criterion validity and receipt of bladder cancer care in VA

Next, we assessed whether we can accurately identify patients who were newly diagnosed with bladder cancer and who received bladder cancer care in the VA based on administrative data. Using the chart review of 100 cases as the gold standard, we were able to differentiate patients who did versus who did not receive bladder cancer care in VA with an accuracy of 95% (95% CI 89% - 98%). All but one patient who had bladder cancer care based on chart review were identified by the use of administrative data (sensitivity 98%, 95% CI 91% - 100%, Table 2). Among the 62 patients who were identified as receiving bladder cancer care with administrative data, 58 actually did receive such care based on chart review (positive predictive value 94%, 95% CI 84% - 98%, Table 2).

Next, we evaluated reasons for not receiving bladder cancer care in VA. The most common reasons included receipt of care outside of the VA among patients who were enrolled in a Medicare HMO, a recent diagnosis of bladder cancer with the patient opting for palliative care only, and a remote history of bladder cancer without any recent recurrences or follow-up care (Additional file 2). We also evaluated the four patients who had no evidence for bladder cancer care in the chart review, but who did have administrative data suggesting such care (Table 2). These patients had unusual specific circumstances, including (1) a remote history of bladder cancer and cystectomy approximately 40 years ago with need for recurrent cystoscopic ureteral stent replacements, (2)

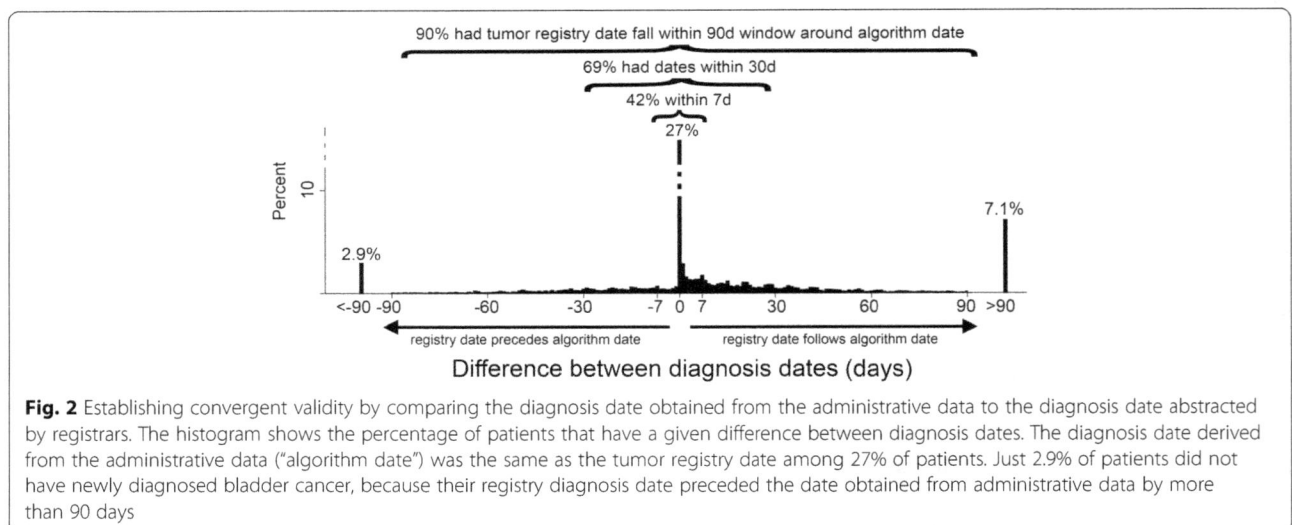

Fig. 2 Establishing convergent validity by comparing the diagnosis date obtained from the administrative data to the diagnosis date abstracted by registrars. The histogram shows the percentage of patients that have a given difference between diagnosis dates. The diagnosis date derived from the administrative data ("algorithm date") was the same as the tumor registry date among 27% of patients. Just 2.9% of patients did not have newly diagnosed bladder cancer, because their registry diagnosis date preceded the date obtained from administrative data by more than 90 days

Table 2 Accuracy of administrative data to identify bladder cancer care in VA among patients with newly diagnosed bladder cancer, based on chart review of 100 randomly selected cases (the gold standard). We were able differentiate between patients who did versus who did not receive bladder cancer care in VA with high accuracy (95%), with only 5 cases having discordant data between chart review and algorithm

Bladder cancer care in VA		Based on chart review (Gold standard)		Total
		Yes	No	
Based on administrative data	Yes	58	4	62
	No	1	37	38
Total		59	41	

a remote history of bladder cancer with subsequent need for cystoscopy with urethral dilation for a urethral stricture, (3) a patient whose prostate cancer diagnosis was miscoded as bladder cancer and who underwent a diagnostic cystoscopy after his prostate cancer treatment, and (4) a patient who had a benign ureteral mass excised and who had a subsequent cystoscopy for stent removal.

Assessing our ability to distinguish between groups that are conceptually more or less likely to receive bladder cancer care in VA – Concurrent validity

Finally, we assessed whether we can distinguish between groups of patients who should be more or less likely to receive bladder cancer care in VA. Examining the entire cohort, about two thirds of the cohort (16,846 patients, 63%) had bladder cancer care in VA (Fig. 1). We evaluated whether receipt of bladder cancer care was more common among those with full text pathology reports in the database as one would expect. Indeed, the proportion of patients receiving bladder cancer care in VA was significantly higher among those who had full text pathology reports available than among those who had not (96% vs. 43%, Table 3, $p < 0.001$).

Discussion

We combined data from multiple sources to validate the use of administrative data to examine bladder cancer care. Specifically, we provide evidence that we can accurately

identify patients with newly diagnosed bladder cancer who received care in the VA healthcare system. Comparison to tumor registry data showed that we can reliably identify an approximate diagnosis date for the vast majority of patients. We also established that we can accurately identify patients who received bladder cancer care in VA. Lastly, we were able to validate that patients who were highly likely to have received bladder cancer care in VA based on the presence of full text bladder pathology reports overwhelmingly also had evidence of that care in administrative data.

Our study leverages advantages conferred by additional data sources including full text pathology reports and chart review of the electronic health record. We were able to identify patients with newly diagnosed bladder cancer who received bladder cancer care in VA with a positive predictive value of 94%, very similar to the 93.8% positive predictive value reported by a study comparing administrative data from a primary care data base in the UK to a survey mailed to primary care physicians as the gold standard [13].

In addition to data obtained by chart review, we also used tumor registry data to validate the algorithm, similar to prior studies [14–17]. Comparing the diagnosis date obtained from the VA administrative data to the tumor registry diagnosis date, we found that about a quarter had the same date in both sources and for 90% the registry date fell within a 90 day window around the date obtained from the administrative data. These findings are very similar to those obtained in a prior study evaluating the accuracy of algorithms to identify newly diagnosed lung, colorectal, stomach, and breast cancers based on SEER-Medicare data (about a quarter had diagnosis dates on the same day and about 90% within a 60 day window) [17].

Our study has several limitations that warrant discussion. First, our approach and findings may not be generalizable to other big data sets from outside the VA. Nevertheless, our study highlights the unique opportunity to use big data on a national scale and may inspire other groups to use similar approaches in their data sets. Second, we were not able to examine the sensitivity of the algorithm to identify patients with bladder cancer. This would have required a national or regional sample

Table 3 Proportion of patients receiving bladder cancer care in VA based on administrative data, comparing those who did versus who did not have full text bladder pathology reports available. Applying the algorithm to the entire cohort, the proportion receiving bladder cancer care in VA is significantly higher among patients who have full text pathology reports in VA than among those who do not (96% vs 43%, p < 0.001, chi-squared test)

		Bladder cancer care in VA, Percent (N)		Total, Percent (N)
		Yes	No	
Full text pathology available, Percent (N)	Yes	96 (9893)	4 (432)	100 (10,325)
	No	43 (6953)	57 (9397)	100 (16,350)
Total, Percent (N)		63 (16,846)	37 (9829)	100 (26,675)

of patients with a confirmed bladder cancer diagnosis (regardless of their diagnosis codes) and then application of our algorithm to that cohort to examine whether these patients could be correctly identified. We did not have access to such a cohort, because our institutional review board approval is allowing us only access to patients with a bladder cancer diagnosis code. However, a previous study provided evidence of high sensitivity when identifying bladder cancer patients based on diagnosis codes [13]. Third, we acknowledge that only 42% of patients had tumor registry data available, which appears to be a low proportion. This is likely related to the fact that data is only abstracted among patients who receive their bladder cancer care within the VA. Among those who received their care in VA, the proportion with tumor registry data was substantially higher (9258 of 15,352 patients, 60%). Nevertheless, this relatively low proportion justifies the use of administrative data to assemble a cohort of bladder cancer patients for studies in which it is important to include the entire universe of patients receiving bladder cancer care.

In spite of these limitations, our study has important implications. We highlight the advantages of using big data, that is data from multiple sources merged into one comprehensive data set. This allowed us to validate the use of administrative data as done here and will allows us to develop a more comprehensive understanding of what does and does not matter when providing care for patients with bladder cancer in the future. Previously, the use of observational data to better understand care for patients with early stage bladder cancer has been hampered by the lack of important clinical details in most data sets. Care for early stage bladder cancer has been described as a "moving target" [3], because each patient's risk for recurrence and progression can change over time. For example, patients who are diagnosed with a low-risk early stage bladder cancer may have a recurrence of a high-risk cancer and vice versa [4, 5, 18]. Standard administrative and tumor registry data do not capture granular data on these recurrences and thus our ability to understand what entails high-quality care for these patients has remained limited. Our comprehensive data set includes administrative data from VA and Medicare, data abstracted by tumor registrars, and full text pathology reports. We expect that this data set validated herein will now make it possible to better understand how bladder cancer care is currently provided and how intensity of cancer care impacts outcomes such as tumor progression and recurrence.

Conclusions

We demonstrate how merging administrative data with data from the electronic health record, data abstracted by tumor registrars, and pathology data offers new possibilities to validate the use of administrative data. Our validated

cohort will now allow us to comprehensively evaluate care and outcomes for patients with bladder cancer.

Abbreviations
CAPRI: Compensation and pension records interchange; CDW: Corporate data warehouse; EHR: Electronic health record; MEDPAR: Medicare provider analysis and review; NMIBC: Non-muscle invasive bladder cancer; SEER: Surveillance, epidemiology, and end results; VA: Department of Veterans Affairs; VIReC: VA Information Resource Center; VistA: Veterans Health Information Systems and Technology Architecture

Acknowledgements
We acknowledge programming assistance from Stephen Oostema at the VA Salt Lake City Health Care System and University of Utah, Salt Lake City, UT.

Funding
FRS is supported by the Department of Veterans Affairs, Veterans Health Administration, VISN1 Career Development Award, by a pilot grant from the American Cancer Society (IRG-82-003-30), by a Conquer Cancer Foundation Career Development Award, and by the Dow-Crichlow Award of the Department of Surgery at the Dartmouth-Hitchcock Medical Center. PPG is supported by a grant from the Food and Drug Administration FDA (U01FD005478-01, Sedrakyan = PI).

Disclaimer
Opinions expressed in this manuscript are those of the authors and do not constitute official positions of the U.S. Federal Government or the Department of Veterans Affairs.

Authors' contributions
Conceptualization (FRS, PPG), Methodology (FRS, PPG), Analysis (FRS), Interpretation of data (FRS, BS, JDS, DJR, PPG), Resources (FRS, BS, PPG), Drafting of manuscript (FRS), Revision of manuscript for important intellectual content (BS, JDS, DJR, PPG), Visualization (FRS), Supervision (FRS, BS, PPG), Project Administration (FRS), Funding Acquisition (FRS, PPG). All authors have read and approved the final manuscript.

Competing interests
Florian R. Schroeck is Site PI (without any compensation) for the Phase III Trial of Vicinium (Viventia Biotech) and has received research funding from the U.S. Department of Veterans Affairs, Conquer Cancer Foundation, and American Cancer Society.
John D. Seigne is an owner of 100 shares of common stock of Johnson & Johnson. The remaining authors declare that they have no relevant financial interests.

Author details
¹White River Junction VA Medical Center, 215 N Main Street, White River Junction, VT 05009, USA. ²Section of Urology, Dartmouth Hitchcock Medical Center, Lebanon, NH, USA. ³Norris Cotton Cancer Center, Dartmouth Hitchcock Medical Center, Lebanon, NH, USA. ⁴The Dartmouth Institute for Health Policy and Clinical Practice, Geisel School of Medicine at Dartmouth College, Hanover, NH, USA.

References
1. Howlader N, Noone AM, Krapcho M, Garshell J, Miller D, Altekruse SF, et al. SEER cancer statistics review, 1975-2011. Bethesda: Natl Cancer Inst; 2014.
2. Carter AJ, Nguyen CN. A comparison of cancer burden and research spending reveals discrepancies in the distribution of research funding. BMC Public Health. 2012;12:526. doi: 10.1186/1471-2458-12-526.
3. Schroeck FR, Montie JE, Hollenbeck BK. Surveillance strategies for non-muscle invasive bladder cancer. AUA Update Ser. 2012;31:313–23.

4. Zieger K, Wolf H, Olsen PR, Hojgaard K. Long-term follow-up of noninvasive bladder tumours (stage Ta): recurrence and progression. BJU Int. 2000;85:824–8.
5. Leblanc B, Duclos AJ, Bénard F, Côté J, Valiquette L, Paquin JM, et al. Long-term followup of initial Ta grade 1 transitional cell carcinoma of the bladder. J Urol. 1999;162:1946–50.
6. Ward JS, Barker A. Undefined by data: a survey of big data definitions. ArXiv Prepr ArXiv13095821 2013.
7. VA Information Resource Center. Research findings from the VA medicare data merge initiative: veterans' enrollment, access and use of medicare and VA health services. US Dept Veterans Aff Health Serv Res Dev Serv 2003: Rpt No XVA-69001.
8. Hynes DM, Koelling K, Stroupe K, Arnold N, Mallin K, Sohn M-W, et al. Veterans' access to and use of medicare and veterans affairs health care. Med Care. 2007;45:214–23.
9. Klabunde CN, Potosky AL, Legler JM, Warren JL. Development of a comorbidity index using physician claims data. J Clin Epidemiol. 2000;53: 1258–67. doi: 10.1016/S0895-4356(00)00256-0.
10. Trochim WMK. Measurement validity types 2006. http://www. socialresearchmethods.net/kb/measval.php. Accessed 10 Oct 2016.
11. Hollenbeck BK, Ye Z, Dunn RL, Montie JE, Birkmeyer JD. Provider treatment intensity and outcomes for patients with early-stage bladder cancer. J Natl Cancer Inst. 2009;101:571–80. doi: 10.1093/jnci/djp039.
12. Schroeck FR, Pattison EA, Denhalter DW, Patterson OV, DuVall SL, Seigne JD, et al. Early stage bladder cancer – do pathology reports tell us what we need to know? Urology. 2016;98:58–63. doi: 10.1016/j.urology.2016.07.040.
13. Mamtani R, Haynes K, Boursi B, Scott FI, Goldberg DS, Keefe SM, et al. Validation of a coding algorithm to identify bladder cancer and distinguish stage in an electronic medical records database. Cancer Epidemiol Prev Biomark. 2015;24:303–7. doi: 10.1158/1055-9965.EPI-14-0677.
14. Cooper GS, Yuan Z, Stange KC, Dennis LK, Amini SB, Rimm AA. The sensitivity of medicare claims data for case ascertainment of six common cancers. Med Care. 1999;37:436–44.
15. Nattinger AB, Laud PW, Bajorunaite R, Sparapani RA, Freeman JL. An algorithm for the use of Medicare claims data to identify women with incident breast cancer. Health Serv Res. 2004;39:1733–50.
16. Baldi I, Vicari P, Di Cuonzo D, Zanetti R, Pagano E, Rosato R, et al. A high positive predictive value algorithm using hospital administrative data identified incident cancer cases. J Clin Epidemiol. 2008;61:373–9. doi: 10. 1016/j.jclinepi.2007.05.017.
17. Setoguchi S, Solomon DH, Glynn RJ, Cook EF, Levin R, Schneeweiss S. Agreement of diagnosis and its date for hematologic malignancies and solid tumors between medicare claims and cancer registry data. Cancer Causes Control. 2007;18:561–9. doi: 10.1007/s10552-007-0131-1.
18. Lebret T, Bohin D, Kassardjian Z, Herve JM, Molinie V, Barre P, et al. Recurrence, progression and success in stage Ta grade 3 bladder tumors treated with low dose bacillus Calmette-Guerin instillations. J Urol. 2000;163:63–7.

Alpha$_{1A}$-adrenoceptor antagonist improves underactive bladder associated with diabetic cystopathy via bladder blood flow in rats

Saori Yonekubo[*], Satoshi Tatemichi, Kazuyasu Maruyama and Mamoru Kobayashi

Abstract

Background: Patients with diabetes experience lower urinary tract symptoms. Cystopathy may evolve into underactive bladder (UAB), depending on the degree and duration of the symptoms. In the present study, we aimed to investigate the effects of silodosin, an alpha$_{1A}$-adrenoceptor (AR) antagonist, on UAB in a rat model of diabetes mellitus (DM).

Methods: Female Sprague-Dawley rats (6 weeks old) were administered streptozotocin (STZ) (50 mg/kg, i.v.) to establish a DM model. One week after STZ administration, vehicle or silodosin (0.3 or 1 mg/kg/day) was delivered subcutaneously through an osmotic pump. Nine weeks after STZ administration (8 weeks after drug treatment), a catheter was implanted into the bladder under urethane anesthesia. After the measurement of emptied bladder blood flow (BBF), saline was continuously infused into the bladder and intravesical pressure and micturition volume were measured. In another experiment, the bladder was isolated and nerve markers were quantified.

Results: A cystometrogram showed that bladder capacity (BC), residual volume (RV), and bladder extension (BC/ bladder weight) increased by 7.43, 10.47, and 3.59 times, respectively, in vehicle rats in comparison with normal rats. These findings suggested the occurrence of UAB-like symptoms in this model. Silodosin (1 mg/kg/day) inhibited the increase in BC and RV by 49.0% and 46.8%, respectively, and caused a decrease in BBF of approximately 25.5% (when the difference between normal and vehicle was set as 100%) in STZ rats. The nerve marker expression levels tended to be decreased in the bladders of STZ rats and these effects were ameliorated by silodosin.

Conclusions: The STZ rats showed increased bladder extension and RV, symptoms that were suggestive of UAB, and these symptoms were ameliorated by silodosin. These results suggested that the alpha$_{1A}$-AR antagonist would be useful for the prevention or treatment of UAB.

Keywords: Alpha-adrenergic receptor, Blood flow, Diabetes, Underactive bladder

Background

More than 371 million people worldwide suffered from diabetes in 2012 [1]. Various complications are associated with diabetes. Over 50% of diabetic patients have diabetic cystopathy, such as overactive bladder (OAB) syndrome and incontinence [2, 3]. In diabetic patients with lower urinary tract symptoms (LUTS), OAB may evolve into underactive bladder (UAB), or detrusor underactivity (DUA), depending on the degree and duration of the symptoms. Diabetic UAB is characterized by an impaired sensation of bladder fullness, increased bladder capacity (BC), decreased bladder contractility, and increased post voiding residual volume (RV) [4, 5]. When urinary symptoms in patients become severe, they may develop into incontinence, ischuria, and/or hydronephrosis. OAB became a common disease, whereas UAB has not been studied in detail [4].

Diabetes mellitus (DM), bladder outlet obstruction (BOO), and aging are considered factors contributing to

---

* Correspondence: saori_yonekubo@pharm.kissei.co.jp
Central Research Laboratories, Kissei Pharmaceutical Co., Ltd, 4365-1 Kashiwabara, Hotaka, Azumino-City, Nagano-Pref 399-8304, Japan

the development of UAB symptoms. Rat models of DM, BOO, aging, and pelvic nerve transection have been reported previously [4, 6]. Changes in parameters suggesting the functional decline of the bladder have been observed in all models. DM rats have DUA, hypoesthesia, and a large RV. Bladder nerves and vessels have been reported to show decreased density in DM rat models [7–9]. Diabetes is known to induce functional changes related to neuropathy, and blood flow is thought to be closely related to the nerves. However, there have been few detailed reports regarding the nerve changes associated with bladder blood flow (BBF) in DM models.

The pharmacological treatment options for UAB syndrome are limited. This condition can be improved with the use of agents that increase detrusor contractile activity and/or decrease outlet resistance. Current standard pharmacotherapy includes the use of muscarinic receptor agonists, such as bethanechol, to stimulate detrusor muscarinic receptors, or cholinesterase inhibitors, such as distigmine, to reduce the degradation of acetylcholine [10]. Alpha$_1$-Adrenoceptor (AR) antagonists have also been reported to be an used for treatment for UAB [11–13]. The mechanism of action of alpha$_1$-AR antagonists involves a cancellation of confinement through the inhibition of alpha$_{1A}$-ARs distributed mainly over the urethra (prostatic part) [14]. Urapidil is used for relaxing the urethra and reducing resistance to urine flow and is the only alpha$_1$-AR antagonist that can be used in women [11]. However, hypotension develops concomitantly with urethral relaxation because urapidil has a lower selectivity for alpha$_{1A}$-ARs [15, 16] than for alpha$_{1B}$-ARs, which are mainly involved in blood pressure regulation [17]. Recent studies showed that chronic treatment with tamsulosin (alpha$_{1A/1D}$–AR antagonist) prevented a decrease in BBF and controlled the increase in urinary frequency in rats [18, 19]. Furthermore, chronic treatment with silodosin (alpha$_{1A}$-AR antagonist) reportedly improved bladder dysfunction by restoring the BBF in a rat model of atherosclerosis-induced bladder ischemia without BOO [20, 21]. These results suggest that alpha$_1$-AR antagonists can not only relax urethral obstruction, which is their primary action (prostatic effect), but also improve BBF (bladder effect). Therefore, it is considered that alpha$_1$-AR antagonists may improve BBF and ameliorate bladder dysfunction in addition to inducing urethral relaxation.

In this study, we investigated the effects of silodosin on the changes in bladder function in a streptozotocin (STZ)-induced DM rat model.

Methods
Animals
Female Sprague–Dawley rats (Charles River, Yokohama, Japan) were housed under a 12-h/12-h light cycle (lights on, 08:00–20:00 h) under controlled conditions and fed a laboratory chow diet and water ad libitum. All animal experiments were performed in accordance with the guidelines approved by the Laboratory Animal Committee of Kissei Pharmaceutical Co., Ltd., which conform to the current Japanese law.

Induction of diabetes
In this study, diabetes was induced as reported previously [22]. Briefly, rats were injected with STZ dissolved in 0.03 mol/L citrate buffer at pH 4.5, which was used at a dose of 50 mg/kg (i.v.). Age-matched non-diabetic rats were injected with vehicle alone. After 1 week, non-fasting serum glucose levels were measured using Antsense III (Horiba, Kyoto, Japan), and rats with values above 300 mg/dL were considered diabetic. Rats were assigned based on body weight (BW) and blood glucose level. The rats that did not meet the experimental criterion were euthanized using the method of inhalation of carbon dioxide (CO_2).

Drug treatment
Drug treatment was performed using a procedure similar to that described previously [20]. When the blood glucose level was measured the following day, an osmotic pump (2ML4; Alzet, Cupertino, CA) was inserted under the dorsal skin. The silodosin group was subcutaneously administered the drug at each constant infusion rate for 8 weeks via the osmotic pump. Steady-state free plasma concentrations of silodosin were estimated using constant infusion equations, total clearance, and the percentage of silodosin binding to rat plasma proteins. Concentrations at the constant infusion rates of each dose were calculated as 1.13×10^{-9} mol/L (silodosin, 0.3 mg/kg/day) and 3.78×10^{-9} mol/L (silodosin, 1.0 mg/kg/day) [20]. Similarly, the sham treatment and DM groups were subcutaneously infused with Hartmann's solution as the vehicle via the osmotic pump for 8 weeks.

BBF
Measurements were performed using a procedure similar to that described previously [20]. Nine weeks after the induction of diabetes, the rats were anesthetized by the subcutaneous administration of urethane (1.0 g/kg). A midline abdominal incision was made to expose the anterior bladder. An 18-gauge catheter was implanted in the bladder through the dome and the bladder was emptied. BBF was determined using an Omegazone laser speckle blood flow imager (Omegawave, Tokyo, Japan), which shows blood flow as high-resolution 2-dimensional color images.

Cystometrogram (CMG)
After the BBF study, cystometric measurements were performed. Briefly, the rat was placed in the supine

position, and a bladder catheter was connected via a tube to a KDS-100 infusion pump (Muromachi Kikai, Tokyo, Japan) for continuous saline infusion into the bladder and a DT-4812 pressure transducer (Nihon Becton Dickinson, Tokyo, Japan) for bladder pressure recording. Micturition volume (MV) was measured using a GF-300 digital balance (A&D, Tokyo, Japan) located below the plastic cage. During cystometric evaluation, saline was infused to achieve a voiding interval of about 20 min (infusion rate, Normal rats: $1 \sim 3$ mL/h, DM rats: $6 \sim 24$ mL/h). Bladder pressure and MV were recorded continuously on a Rectigraph-8 K (NEC San-ei, Tokyo, Japan). The cystometric parameters obtained were intravesical pressure (IVP), MV, and RV. Rats used for CMG measurement were euthanized by exsanguination of the abdominal aorta.

Real-time RT-PCR

Nine weeks after the induction of diabetes, total RNA in the bladder was extracted using an RNeasy® Fibrous Tissue Mini Kit (Qiagen, Hilden, Germany). For this experiment, we used different rats from those used for the blood flow measurement and CMG. Rats used for PCR and immunohistochemistry studies were euthanized by exsanguination of the abdominal aorta using isoflurane anesthesia. The mRNA expression levels corresponding to target genes were determined by real-time quantitative RT-PCR with an Applied Biosystems 7500 Fast (Life Technologies Japan, Tokyo, Japan) using a PrimeScript™ RT reagent kit (Takara, Shiga, Japan) and SYBR® Premix Ex Taq™ (Takara). The levels of β-actin, neurofilament-M (NF-M), and peripherin mRNA expression were quantified by the reverse-transcription of total bladder RNA using primers purchased from Takara. After extraction of total bladder RNA as described above, first-strand cDNA was synthesized from 0.4 mg of the total RNA using a GeneAmp PCR System 9700 (Life Technologies Japan) for RT-PCR. The total bladder RNA from normal rats was used to determine the standard curve. After correction for β-actin mRNA levels, the expression levels of the test genes were normalized to those in normal rats.

Immunohistochemistry

The bladders were immersed in Mildform® (Wako, Osaka, Japan), embedded in paraffin, and cut into 5-μm-thick sections. Briefly, the sections were deparaffinized and then heated in a microwave oven for 30 min for antigen retrieval. After cooling and washing the sections with water, nonspecific binding of immunoglobulin was prevented using a protein block reagent (Agilent Technologies, Denmark, Denmark) for 10 min. After overnight incubation at 4 °C with anti-NF-M (AB1987, dilution 1:200; Merck KGaA, Darmstadt, Germany) or anti-peripherin (AB1530, dilution 1:100; Merck KGaA)

antibody, the sections were rinsed with phosphate-buffered saline 3 times for 5 min each. The sections were then treated with Alexa Fluor® 488 goat anti-rabbit IgG (A11034, dilution 1:500; Life Technologies Japan) for 2 h at room temperature. After rinsing with phosphate-buffered saline 3 times for 5 min each, propidium iodide was added to stain the nuclei, followed by mounting with Fluoromount/Plus™ (Diagnostic BioSystems, Pleasanton, CA).

Photomicrographs (10×) of labeled bladder sections were taken using a DP72 digital camera (Olympus, Tokyo, Japan) attached to an Olympus IX71 microscope. The whole area of the bladder was photographed and tiled with high accuracy using the cellSens digital imaging software (Olympus), and WinROOF image processing, image measurement, image analysis, and data processing software (Mitani, Fukui, Japan) were used to measure the total area of the photographed bladder and immunopositive bundles.

Drug

The test drug silodosin (KMD-3213; Kissei Pharmaceutical Co. Ltd., Matsumoto, Japan) was dissolved and diluted in Hartmann's solution of the following composition (w/v%): 0.60 NaCl, 0.03 KCl, 0.02 CaCl$_2$, and 0.31 lactic acid, containing hydrobromide at a 2-fold equivalent of silodosin.

Data analysis

Data are presented as means ± S.E.M. Statistical analyses were performed using SAS version 8.20 (SAS Institute, Cary, NC). Data were analyzed among the 3 groups as follows. When equality of variances was indicated by Bartlett's test, statistical analysis was performed using one-way analysis of variance (ANOVA) followed by parametric Dunnett's multiple comparison test. When equality of variances was not indicated by Bartlett's test, statistical analysis was performed using nonparametric Dunnett's multiple comparison test. Comparisons between two groups were performed as follows. When equality of variances was indicated by an F-test, statistical analysis was performed using the Student's t-test; when equality of variances was not indicated, statistical analysis was performed using the Aspin–Welch t-test. A value of $P < 0.05$ was considered statistically significant.

Results

General physical characteristics

Blood glucose levels, BWs, and bladder weights (BlaWs) are shown in Table 1. The blood glucose levels of DM rats (541.0 ± 25.3 mg/dL) were about 3-fold higher than those of normal rats (161.4 ± 7.6 mg/dL). Silodosin did not affect blood glucose levels. The BlaW of DM rats (0.220 ± 0.010 g) were approximately double that of normal rats (0.107 ± 0.005 g).

Table 1 Chronic effects of silodosin on blood glucose, BW, and BlaW in STZ-induced DM rats

Group	Blood glucose (mg/dL)	BW (g)	BlaW (g)
Normal	161.4 ± 7.6	278.5 ± 10.7	0.107 ± 0.005
DM-Vehicle	541.0 ± 25.3[†††]	260.4 ± 4.6	0.220 ± 0.010[†††]
DM-Silodosin 0.3 mg/kg/day	521.4 ± 15.2[†††]	262.5 ± 4.2	0.223 ± 0.014[†††]
DM-Silodosin 1.0 mg/kg/day	474.6 ± 27.5[†††]	271.8 ± 8.1	0.210 ± 0.014[†††]

Data are presented as means ± S.E.M ($n = 10$–13). [†††]$P < 0.001$ versus normal rats. BW, body weight; BlaW, bladder weight; DM, diabetes mellitus

CMG study

Cystometry performed in anesthetized DM rats indicated that BC and RV significantly increased 9 weeks after STZ injection, as compared to normal rats. In contrast, IVP did not differ between the DM rats and normal rats. In addition, the baseline pressure and threshold pressure did not differ between the DM rats and normal rats (data not shown). Silodosin significantly decreased BC and RV (Fig. 1A and B). In addition, the bladder extension (BC/BlaW ratio) increased in DM rats, indicating that the bladder had become thin (i.e., bladder hyperextension). Silodosin decreased the ratio almost to that observed in normal rats (Fig. 1C). Silodosin had no effect on IVP (Fig. 1D).

BBF measurement

A significant decrease in BBF in the empty bladder was observed in DM rats compared with normal rats. Silodosin at a dose of 1.0 mg/kg/day significantly suppressed the diabetes-induced decrease in BBF in the empty bladder (Fig. 2).

Evaluation of nerve markers

We evaluated the expression of the neuron-specific markers NF-M (an intermediate filament that provides support for neuronal structure) and peripherin (a sensory neuron-specific marker) [23] by RT-PCR and immunohistochemistry. The mRNA expressions trended to decrease in DM rats and suppressed in silodosin-treated rats (Fig. 3A and B). Immunohistochemical analysis

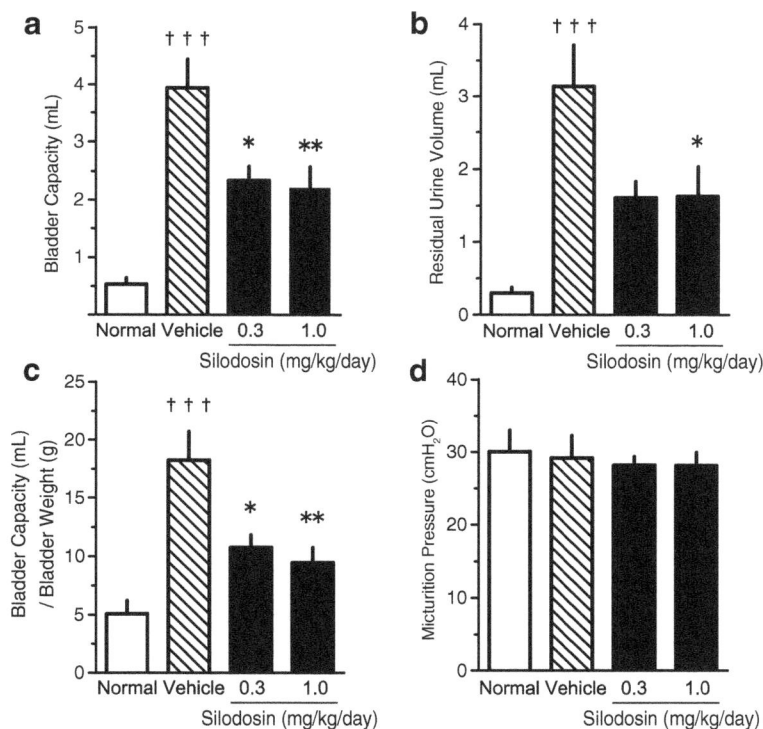

Fig. 1 Effects of silodosin (0.3 and 1.0 mg/kg/day, s.c.) on bladder capacity (BC) (**a**), residual volume (RV) (**b**), BC/bladder weight (BlaW) (**c**), and intravesical pressure (IVP) (**d**) in rats on cystometrography. Data are presented as means ± S.E.M. ($n = 10$–13). †††$P < 0.001$ versus normal rats (Student's t-test or Aspin–Welch t-test). *$P < 0.05$, **$P < 0.01$ versus diabetes mellitus (DM)-Vehicle rats (Dunnett's test)

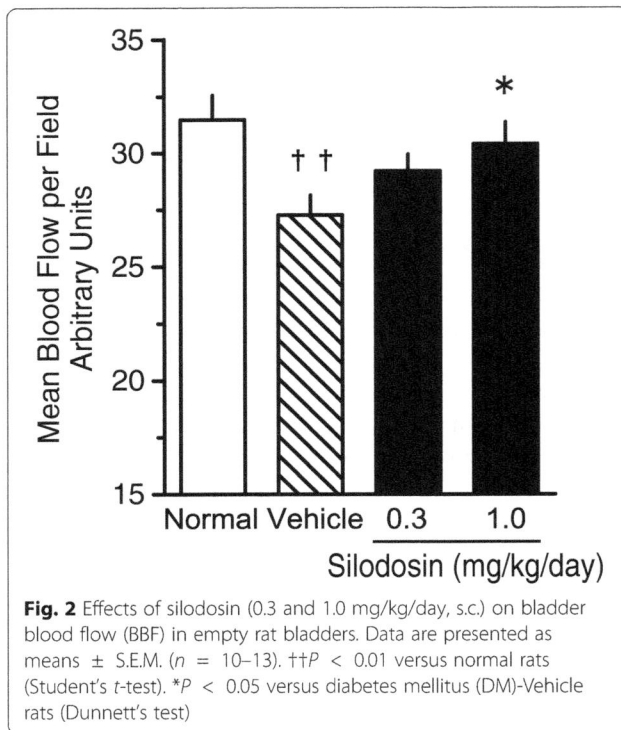

Fig. 2 Effects of silodosin (0.3 and 1.0 mg/kg/day, s.c.) on bladder blood flow (BBF) in empty rat bladders. Data are presented as means ± S.E.M. ($n = 10–13$). ††$P < 0.01$ versus normal rats (Student's t-test). *$P < 0.05$ versus diabetes mellitus (DM)-Vehicle rats (Dunnett's test)

this decrease was suppressed by silodosin. Similar improvement in NF-M was observed on immunohistochemical analysis.

Discussion

In this study, we examined the changes in bladder function and the effects of silodosin in STZ-induced DM rats. Nine weeks after STZ induction, urinary dysfunction was observed on a CMG. Increases in BC and RV were observed in the DM group, and the BC/BlaW ratio was high. Furthermore, BBF was decreased and both gene and protein expression levels of NF-M and peripherin, which are neuronal markers, were decreased in bladder tissue in the DM group. These results suggest that a decrease in BBF and bladder hyperextension with sensory disorder, i.e., UAB-like symptoms, occurred in the DM group. The alpha$_{1A}$-AR antagonist silodosin showed inhibitory effects against all of these changes in the DM group. Silodosin shows preventive or curative effects against UAB-like symptoms in DM, and these effects may be caused by the improvement in the sensory disorder by preventing the decrease in BBF.

Autonomic nervous system disorders due to peripheral neuropathy, which is one of the 3 major complications of DM, are known to be responsible for urination disorders. LUTS have been reported in various DM rat models. The STZ-induced DM rats showed pathological progress from bladder irritation symptoms (compensatory response), such as frequent urination, to UAB symptoms (decompensatory response), such as increases in BC and RV [5, 7, 24]. In the CMG study, no change in IVP was observed in the DM group 9 weeks after STZ treatment, but increases in BC and RV were

indicated that peripherin was distributed in the smooth muscular layer (low-power field) (Fig. 4A and B), and a weaker signal was observed at high magnification (Fig. 4C). These signals were weaker in full bladders in DM rats than in those in normal rats (Fig. 5). The signals in the silodosin group were similar to those in the normal group. Quantified signals are shown in Fig. 6. Signals for peripherin were significantly decreased in DM rats, and

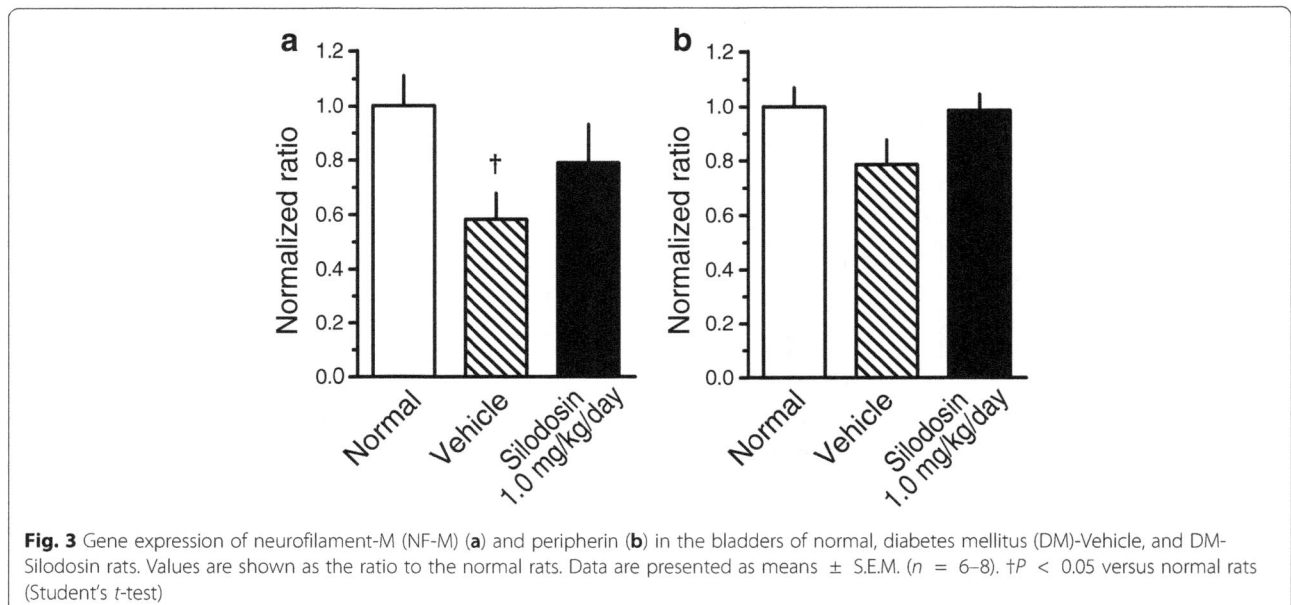

Fig. 3 Gene expression of neurofilament-M (NF-M) (**a**) and peripherin (**b**) in the bladders of normal, diabetes mellitus (DM)-Vehicle, and DM-Silodosin rats. Values are shown as the ratio to the normal rats. Data are presented as means ± S.E.M. ($n = 6–8$). †$P < 0.05$ versus normal rats (Student's t-test)

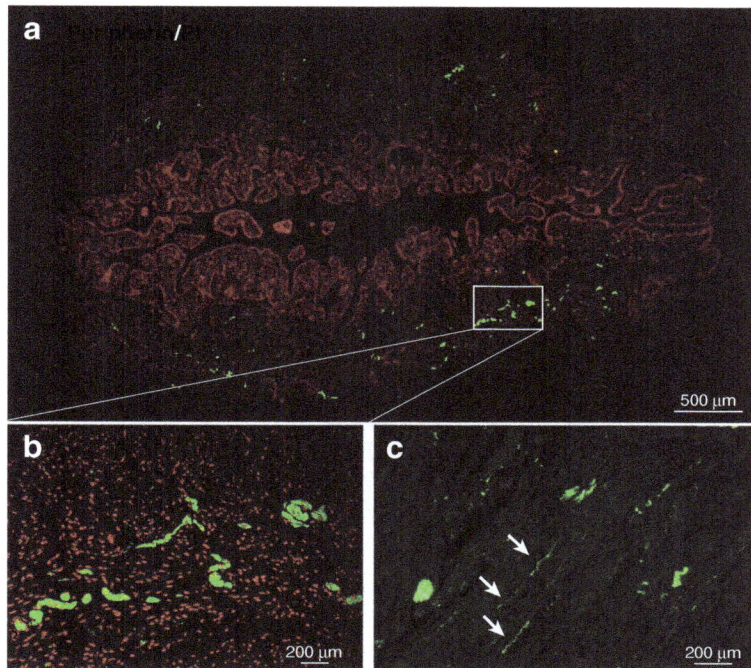

Fig. 4 Representative immunofluorescence staining of peripherin-immunoreactive nerves (green) and propidium iodide-positive nuclei (red) in vertical sections of the bladder. **a** Whole bladder. **b** and **c**, Extended image. A few axons branched off from the plexus. A weaker b signal was observed under increased magnification

observed. We did not identify the reason IVP did not change, but we think that a longer treatment period may be required to observe the differences. In the present experiment, UAB-like symptoms were examined by the evaluation of RV and bladder hyperextension, although changes in IVP were not observed.

We used the BC/BlaW ratio as a new index to evaluate bladder extension in this study. The BC/BlaW ratio was

high in the DM group compared with the normal group. Increases in BC and RV were also observed in the BOO rat model. However, there was little difference in the BC/BlaW ratio between the normal and BOO rats [25, 26]. As powerful contractions due to urethral obstruction are noted in the BOO rat model, the bladder smooth muscles probably became thick [27]. On the other hand, bladder sensation of DM rats decrease, and BC increase that is

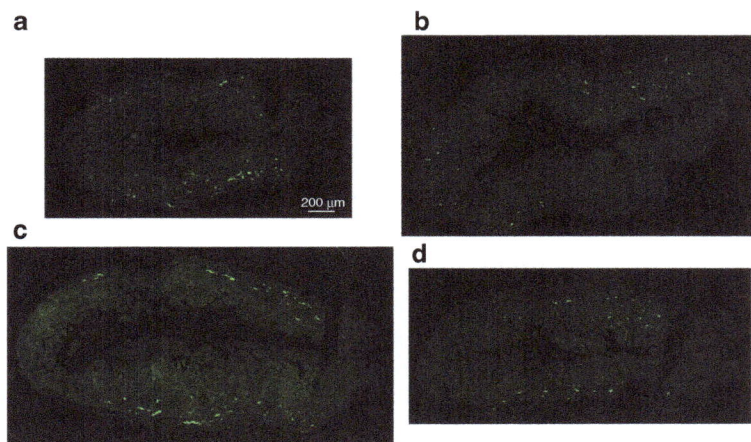

Fig. 5 Peripherin expression in the vertical section of the whole bladder. Photomicrographs of labeled bladder sections were captured using a DP72 digital camera (Olympus, Tokyo, Japan) attached to an Olympus IX71 microscope. **a** Normal bladder. **b** Streptozotocin (STZ)-induced diabetes mellitus (DM)-Vehicle bladder. **c** and **d**, STZ-induced DM-chronic s.c. infusion of silodosin 0.3 and 1.0 mg/kg/day bladder, respectively

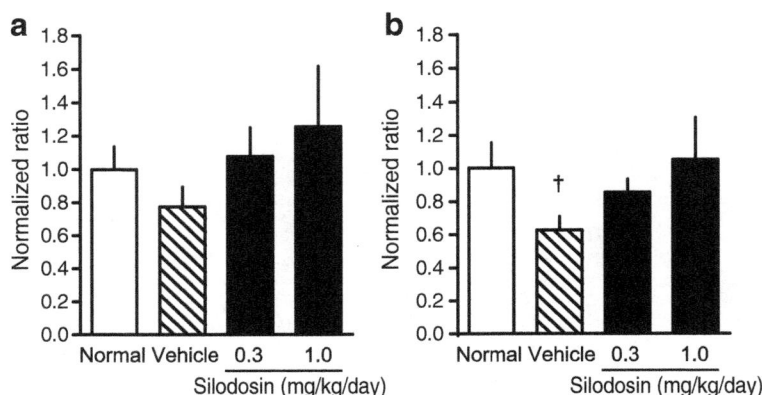

Fig. 6 Immunohistochemical analysis of the effects of silodosin on neurofilament-M (NF-M) (**a**) and peripherin (**b**) in the bladder. The whole bladder was photographed and tiled with high accuracy using cellSens software. WinROOF was used to measure the total area of the photographed bladder and immunopositive bundles. Values are shown as the ratio to the normal rats. Data are presented as means ± S.E.M. (n = 7–8). †P < 0.05 versus normal rats (Student's t-test)

bladder smooth muscles became thin. Therefore, it is possible that the BC/BlaW ratio would be a useful index to quantitatively evaluate bladder extension accompanied with diminished bladder sensation.

As noted above, diminished bladder sensation is a symptom of peripheral neuropathy. The vascular supply in peripheral nerves is sparse and blood flow is likely to be compromised and lack autoregulation. The system causes peripheral nerves to be vulnerable to ischemia [28]. Therefore, it is suggested that peripheral neuropathy is closely related to decreased blood flow. In this study, BBF and the levels of neuronal markers, NF-M and peripherin, were measured in the bladder. NF-M and peripherin are intermediate filaments expressed in nerve cells, and peripherin is used as a specific marker of sensory neurons [23]. Therefore, measurement of peripherin expression in the bladder would be a useful index for evaluating bladder sensation. In this study, BBF decreased after 9 weeks of STZ treatment in DM rats. Although it was reported that blood vessel density decreased in DM rat bladders after 20 weeks of STZ treatment [8], ischemia was considered to have occurred after 9 weeks of STZ treatment because a decrease in BBF was observed at this time. Therefore, bladder nerve density was thought to have decreased, resulting in diminished bladder sensation.

We examined the effects of the alpha$_{1A}$-AR antagonist silodosin on these changes in DM rats. Urinary function improved after chronic injection of silodosin for 8 weeks. In addition, silodosin inhibited the decrease in BBF and improved the decrease in the number of peripherin-positive sensory nerves in addition to NF-M-positive nerves.

The mechanism underlying the improvement in bladder dysfunction did not involve a decrease in blood glucose levels, as silodosin did not affect the blood glucose levels. Generally, poor contractility, detrusor sphincter dyssynergia, and decline of bladder sensation are considered to be the causes of RV increase and bladder hyperextension. At these concentrations, silodosin specifically inhibited alpha$_{1A}$-AR but not alpha$_{1B}$-AR or alpha$_{1D}$-AR [29]. Silodosin shows urethral relaxation effect. But it was reported that urethral resistance is weaker in female than in male rats [30]. The BBF decrease is closely related to peripheral neuropathy, and alpha$_1$-ARs are expressed in the bladder arteries. Furthermore, it has been reported that alpha$_1$-AR antagonists increase BBF [18–20]. It may be possible that silodosin improved the decreased bladder sensation due to inhibition of ischemia by ameliorating the decrease in BBF in this DM rat model.

In the present study, silodosin treatment was initiated in the early stages of DM. Therefore, further studies are required to examine the curative effect of silodosin administered after DM progression. Furthermore, in this study, we did not perform comparisons with other alpha$_1$-AR antagonists. A more detailed investigation is required to clarify the mechanism underlying the involvement of alpha$_1$-AR subtypes in UAB by the comparison with other alpha$_1$-AR antagonists with different alpha$_1$-AR subtype selectivity.

Conclusions

In conclusion, the alpha$_{1A}$-AR antagonist silodosin showed a protective effect against impaired bladder function indicated by UAB-like symptoms characterized by increased RV and bladder hyperextension in STZ-induced DM rats.

Abbreviations
AR: Adrenoceptor; BBF: Bladder blood flow; BC: Bladder capacity; BlaW: Bladder weight; BOO: Bladder outlet obstruction; BW: Body weight; CMG: Cystometrogram; DM: Diabetes mellitus; DUA: Detrusor underactivity; IVP: Intravesical pressure; LUTS: Lower urinary tract symptoms; MV: Micturition volume; NF-M: Neurofilament-M; OAB: Overactive bladder; RV: Residual volume; STZ: Streptozotocin; UAB: Underactive bladder

Acknowledgements
Not applicable

Funding
This study and writing assistance for this manuscript were funded by Kissei Pharmaceutical Co., Ltd. All authors are employees of Kissei Pharmaceutical Co., Ltd.

Authors' contributions
All authors have read and approved the final manuscript, and author contributions are in accordance with ICMJE guidelines. Conception, design, and acquisition of data: SY and ST. Analysis and interpretation of data: SY, ST, KM, MK.

Competing interests
This study was funded by Kissei Pharmaceutical Co., Ltd. SY, ST, KM and MK are current employees of Kissei. This does not alter the authors' adherence to all the BMC Urology policies on sharing data and materials, as detailed online in the guide for authors.

References
1. Bhatia J, Gamad N, Bharti S, Arya DS. Canagliflozin-current status in the treatment of type 2 diabetes mellitus with focus on clinical trial data. World J Diabetes. 2014;5:399–406.
2. Ellenberg M. Development of urinary bladder dysfunction in diabetes mellitus. Ann Intern Med. 1980;92:321–3.
3. Brown JS, Wessells H, Chancellor MB, Howards SS, Stamm WE, Stapleton AE, Steers WD, Van Den Eeden SK, McVary KT. Urologic complications of diabetes. Diabetes Care. 2005;28:177–85.
4. Miyazato M, Yoshimura N, Chancellor MB. The other bladder syndrome: underactive. bladder. Rev Urol. 2013;15:11–22.
5. Chancellor MB. The overactive bladder progression to underactive bladder hypothesis. Int Urol Nephrol. 2014;46(Suppl 1):23–7.
6. Tyagi P, Smith PP, Kuchel GA, de Groat WC, Birder LA, Chermansky CJ, Adam RM, Tse V, Chancellor MB, Yoshimura N. Pathophysiology and animal modeling of underactive bladder. Int Urol Nephrol. 2014; 46(Suppl 1):S11–21.
7. Sasaki K, Chancellor MB, Phelan MW, Yokoyama T, Fraser MO, Seki S, Kubo K, Kumon H, Groat WC, Yoshimura N. Diabetic cystopathy correlates with a long-term decrease in nerve growth factor levels in the bladder and lumbosacral dorsal root ganglia. J Urol. 2002;168:1259–64.
8. Liu G, Li M, Vasanji A, Daneshgari F. Temporal diabetes and diuresis-induced alteration of nerves and vasculature of the urinary bladder in the rat. BJU Int. 2011;107:1988–93.
9. Daneshgari F, Huang X, Liu G, Bena J, Saffore L, Powell CT. Temporal differences in bladder dysfunction caused by diabetes, diuresis, and treated diabetes in mice. Am J Physiol Regul Integr Comp Physiol. 2006;290:1728–35.
10. Andersson KE. Bladder underactivity. Eur Urol. 2014;65:399–401.
11. Yamanishi T, Yasuda K, Homma Y, Kawabe K, Morita T. A multicenter placebo-controlled, double-blind trial of urapidil, an alpha-blocker, on neurogenic bladder dysfunction. Eur Urol. 1999;35:45–51.
12. Sakakibara R, Hattori T, Uchiyama T, Suenaga T, Takahashi H, Yamanishi T, et al. Are alpha blockers involved in lower urinary tract dysfunction in multiple system atrophy? A comparison of prazosin and moxisylyte. J Auton Nerv Syst. 2000;79:191–5.
13. Schulte-Baukloh H, Michael T, Miller K, Knispel HH. Alfuzosin in the treatment of high leak-point pressure in children with neurogenic bladder. BJU Int. 2002;90:716–20.
14. Michel MC, Vrydag W. Alpha1-, alpha2- and beta-adrenoceptors in the urinary bladder, urethra and prostate. Br J Pharmacol. 2006;147(Suppl 2): S88–S119.
15. Ohtake A, Sato S, Sasamata M, Miyata K. Effects of tamsulosin on resting urethral pressure and arterial blood pressure in anaesthetized female dogs. J Pharm Pharmacol. 2006;58:345–50.
16. Sato S, Hatanaka T, Yuyama H, Ukai M, Noguchi Y, Ohtake A, Taguchi K, Sasamata M, Miyata K. Tamsulosin potently and selectively antagonizes human recombinant α(1A/1D)-adrenoceptors: slow dissociation from the α(1A)-adrenoceptor may account for selectivity for α(1A)-adrenoceptor over α(1B)-adrenoceptor subtype. Biol Pharm Bull. 2012;35:72–7.
17. Cavalli A, Lattion AL, Hummler E, et al. Decreased blood pressure response in mice deficient of the α1b-adrenergic receptor. Proc Natl Acad Sci U S A. 1997;94:11589–94.
18. Okutsu H, Matsumoto S, Ohtake A, Suzuki M, Sato S, Sasamata M, Uemura H. Effect of tamsulosin on bladder blood flow and bladder function in a rat model of bladder over distention/emptying induced bladder overactivity. J Urol. 2011;186:2470–7.
19. Okutsu H, Matsumoto S, Hanai T, Noguchi Y, Fujiyasu N, Ohtake A, Suzuki M, Sato S, Sasamata M, Uemura H, Kurita T. Effects of tamsulosin on bladder blood flow and bladder function in rats with bladder outlet obstruction. Urology. 2010;75:235–40.
20. Goi Y, Tomiyama Y, Nomiya M, Sagawa K, Aikawa K, Yamaguchi O. Effects of silodosin, a selective α1A-adrenoceptor antagonist, on bladder blood flow and bladder function in a rat model of atherosclerosis induced chronic bladder ischemia without bladder outlet obstruction. J Urol. 2013;190:1116–22.
21. Inoue S, Saito M, Tsounapi P, Dimitriadis F, Ohmasa F, Kinoshita Y, Satoh K, Takenaka A. Effect of silodosin on detrusor overactivity in the male spontaneously hypertensive rat. BJU Int. 2012;110:E118–24.
22. Kiguchi S, Imamura T, Ichikawa K, Kojima M. Oxcarbazepine antinociception in animals with inflammatory pain or painful diabetic neuropathy. Clin Exp Pharmacol Physiol. 2004;31:57–64.
23. Mizuseki K, Sakamoto T, Watanabe K, Muguruma K, Ikeya M, Nishiyama A, Arakawa A, Suemori H, Nakatsuji N, Kawasaki H, Murakami F, Sasai Y. Generation of neural crest-derived peripheral neurons and floor plate cells from mouse and primate embryonic stem cells. Proc Natl Acad Sci U S A. 2003;100:5828–33.
24. Daneshgari F, Liu G, Imrey PB. Time dependent changes in diabetic cystopathy in rats include compensated and decompensated bladder function. J Urol. 2006;176:380–6.
25. Schroder A, Colli E, Maggi M, Andersson KE. Effects of a vitamin D(3) analogue in a rat model of bladder outlet obstruction. BJU Int. 2006;98:637–42.
26. Zeng J, Xie K, Jiang C, Mo J, Lindstrom S. Bladder mechanoreceptor changes after artificial bladder outlet obstruction in the anesthetized rat. Neurourol Urodyn. 2012;31:178–84.
27. McConnell JD. Epidemiology, etiology, pathophysiology, and diagnosis of benign prostatic hyperplasia. In: Walsh PC, Retik AB, Vaughan Jr. ED, and Wein AJ eds. Campbell's Urology, 7th ed. W. B. Saunders Co., Philadelphia; 1998. p. 1429–1477.
28. Yagihashi S, Mizukami H, Sugimoto K. Mechanism of diabetic neuropathy: where are we now and where to go? J Diabetes Investig. 2011;24(2):18–32.
29. Tatemichi S, Kobayashi K, Maezawa A, Kobayashi M, Yamazaki Y, Shibata N. Alpha1-adrenoceptor subtype selectivity and organ specificity of silodosin (KMD-3213). Yakugaku Zasshi. 2006;126:209–16.
30. Akiyama K, Hora M, Tatemichi S, Masuda N, Nakamura S, Yamagishi R, Kitazawa M. KMD-3213, an uroselective and long-acting alpha (1a)-adrenoceptor antagonist, tested in a novel rat model. J Pharmacol Exp Ther. 1999;291:81–91.

A low psoas muscle volume correlates with a longer hospitalization after radical cystectomy

Yoko Saitoh-Maeda[1], Takashi Kawahara[1,2]* iD, Yasuhide Miyoshi[1], Sohgo Tsutsumi[1], Daiji Takamoto[1], Kota Shimokihara[1], Yuutaro Hayashi[1], Taku Mochizuki[1], Mari Ohtaka[1], Manami Nakamura[1], Yusuke Hattori[1], Jun-ichi Teranishi[1], Yasushi Yumura[1], Kimito Osaka[2], Hiroki Ito[2], Kazuhide Makiyama[2], Noboru Nakaigawa[2], Masahiro Yao[2] and Hiroji Uemura[1]

Abstract

Background: Recently, sarcopenia has been reported as a new predictor for patient outcomes or likelihood of post-operative complications. The purpose of this study was to evaluate the association of the psoas muscle volume with the length of hospitalization among patients undergoing radical cystectomy.

Methods: A total of 63 (80.8%) male patients and 15 (19.2%) female patients who underwent radical cystectomy for their bladder cancer in our institution from 2000 to 2015 were analyzed. The psoas muscle index (PMI) was calculated by normalizing the psoas muscle area calculated using axial computed tomography at the level of the umbilicus (cm^2) by the square of the body height (m^2). Longer hospitalization was defined as hospitalization exceeding 30 days after surgery.

Results: The median PMIs (mean ± standard deviation) were 391 (394 ± 92.1) and 271 (278 ± 92.6) cm^2/m^2 in men and women, respectively. Thus, the PMIs of male patients were significantly larger than those of females ($p < 0.001$). Based on the differences in gender, we analyzed 63 male patients for a further analysis. In male patients, those hospitalized longer showed a significantly smaller PMI than those normally discharged (377 ± 93.1 vs. 425 ± 83.4; $p = 0.04$). Similarly, male patients with a small PMI (<400) had a significantly worse overall survival ($p = 0.02$) than those with a large PMI (≥400).

Conclusions: The presence of sarcopenia was found to be associated with significantly longer hospitalization after radical cystectomy in male patients. Furthermore, in men, a PMI <400 may suggest a significantly worse prognosis.

Keywords: Bladder cancer, Radical cystectomy, Sarcopenia, Psoas muscle

Background

For locally advanced bladder cancer, radical cystectomy is still the gold standard therapy [1, 2]. However, despite its effectiveness, the perioperative complication rate is reported to be around 30%, and the 30- and 90-day post-operative mortality rates are 3.2% and 5.2%,

respectively [1–3]. The indication for radical cystectomy is usually considered based on the patient's age, complications, and performance status [4, 5]. Recently, sarcopenia was reported as a new predictor for the prognosis or risk of post-operative complications [1, 6, 7].

Sarcopenia is the age-related loss of skeletal muscle mass [8]. Previous studies have defined the sum of the muscle masses of the four limbs as the appendicular skeletal mass in order to calculate the psoas muscle index (PMI) [9, 10]. A correlation between sarcopenia and oncologic outcomes has been reported in malignant melanoma, breast cancer, and hepatocellular carcinoma

* Correspondence: takashi_tk2001@yahoo.co.jp
[1]Departments of Urology and Renal Transplantation, Yokohama City University Medical Center, 4-57 Urafune-cho, Minami-ku, Yokohama, Kanagawa 2320024, Japan
[2]Department of Urology, Yokohama City University Graduate School of Medicine, Yokohama, Japan

[11–14]. In patients with bladder cancer, several studies have suggested that sarcopenia correlates with a worse prognosis than in those without sarcopenia [1, 7]. However, whether or not the PMI easily determined using the one-side psoas volume in non-contrast computed tomography (CT) precisely predicts post-operative complications as well as the long-term oncologic outcomes in patients undergoing radical cystectomy remains controversial.

We therefore explored the value of sarcopenia in bladder cancer patients who underwent radical cystectomy.

Methods

Patients

A total of 78 patients (63 males and 15 females) underwent radical cystectomy for bladder cancer at Yokohama City University Medical Center (Yokohama, Japan) from 2000 to 2015. All of the patients were Japanese. The institutional review board of Yokohama City University Medical Center approved this study [D1507018]. The patients were followed up every three months for two years after cystectomy and every six months thereafter using CT.

Clinical assessments

The volume and area of the psoas muscle were calculated using axial CT at the level of the umbilicus before radical cystectomy. The PMI (cm^2/m^2) was calculated by normalizing the psoas muscle area (cm^2) by the square of the body height (m^2).

Longer hospitalization was defined as hospitalization exceeding 30 days after surgery. Based on observed differences in gender, we analyzed the 63 male patients in a further analysis. The overall survival (OS) was compared between the high- (≥400) and low- (<400) PMI groups. The patients' perioperative complications were assessed and scored according to the modified Clavien grading system.

Statistical analysis

The patients' characteristics and preoperative factors were analyzed using the Mann-Whitney U and chi-squared tests. The Kaplan-Meier product limit estimator was used to estimate the OS. The survival duration was defined as the time between radical cystectomy and death. The log-rank test was performed for comparison. A p value of <0.05 was considered to be statistically significant.

Results

Patients' characteristics

The median/mean (± standard deviation (SD)) follow-up times in male and female patients after radical cystectomy were 24.8/36.6 (± 30.9) and 25.4/31.5 (± 24.6) months, respectively The median/mean (± SD) durations of post-operative hospitalization were 36/39.7 (± 17.4) days in male patients and 37.0/42.1 (± 15.3) days in female patients.

Length of hospitalization vs. psoas muscle volume

The median/mean (± SD) psoas areas of the 63 male and 15 female patients were 1078/1085 (± 254) and 632/634 (± 239) cm^2, respectively, and the PMIs were 391/393 (± 92.1) and 271/278 (± 92.6) cm^2/m^2, respectively. Thus, male patients had a significantly higher PMI than female patients ($p < 0.001$, Fig. 1). Among the male patients, those hospitalized longer showed a significantly smaller psoas muscle volume than those normally discharged (Fig. 2). A similar trend was noted among female patients (longer hospitalized group: 763/1045 ± 826 cm^2/m^2 vs. control group: 774/670 ± 373 cm^2/m^2), but the difference was not statistically significant ($p = 0.405$), possibly due to the small number of female subjects.

Histopathological features

Histopathological features in male patients, including tumor grade, pathological T stage, lymph node metastasis, and the presence of concurrent carcinoma in situ (CIS), are summarized in Table 1. The frequencies of clinical T and N stage showed no marked differences between the high- and low-PMI groups. In the male, older patients tended to have a lower PMI than the younger patients; however, the difference did not reach statistical significance. The correlation coefficient (R2) was 0.022.

Correlation of PMI with the OS

The OS was compared in male patients with high versus low PMI. Kaplan-Meier and log-rank tests revealed that the patients with a high PMI had a significantly better OS than those with a low PMI ($p = 0.023$, Fig. 3). The mean survivals were 2889 days

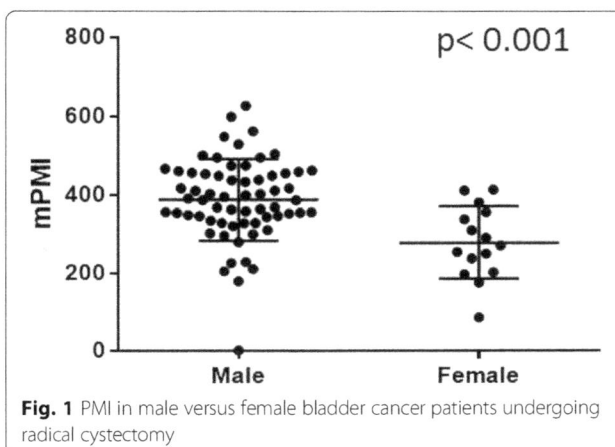

Fig. 1 PMI in male versus female bladder cancer patients undergoing radical cystectomy

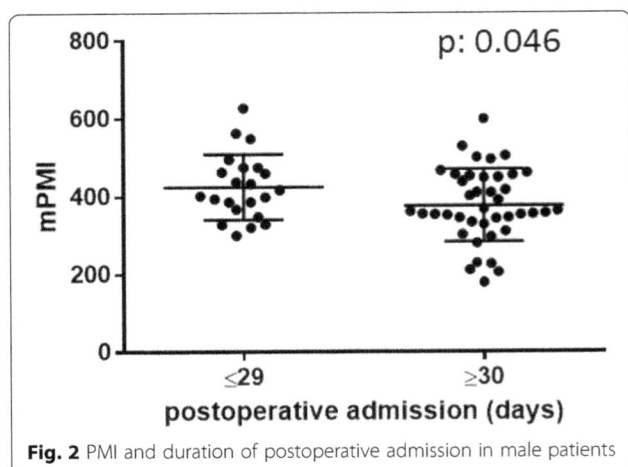

Fig. 2 PMI and duration of postoperative admission in male patients

in the high-PMI group and 2009 days in the low-PMI group.

Perioperative complications

In male patients, the low-PMI group showed a significantly higher rate of complications than the high-PMI group (82.9% vs 31.8%, $p < 0.001$). Furthermore, the patients in the low-PMI group experienced severe complications (Clavien grade $\geq$ 3, 19.5%) (Table 2).

Discussion

Sarcopenia is defined as a low volume of skeletal muscle. Sarcopenic patients show a worse swallowing function and nutritional condition than those without sarcopenia [15]. One study reported that sarcopenic patients had a lower activity of daily life than those without sarcopenia at $\geq$65 years of age [16]. Recently, sarcopenia has been reported as a predictive factor for postoperative complications and the survival in several cancers. For instance, in patients

Table 1 Patient characteristics and psoas muscle volume in male patients

	Total (male only) ($n = 63$)	PMI < 400 ($n = 34$)	PMI $\geq$ 400 ($n = 29$)	P value
Age				
< 65 years	30 (47.6%)	12 (35.3%)	18 (62.1%)	0.062
$\geq$ 65 years	33 (52.4%)	22 (64.7%)	11 (37.9%)	
Pathological Tumor Grade				
1	1 (1.2%)	0 (0%)	1 (38.5%)	0.477
2	25 (39.7%)	13 (41.0%)	12 (46.1%)	
3	32 (50%)	19 (59.4%)	13 (50%)	
Pathological T Stage				
$\leq$ pT2	46 (74.2%)	21 (63.6%)	25 (93.1%)	0.047
$\geq$ pT3	14 (25.8%)	12 (37.4%)	2 (6.9%)	
Lymph Node Metastasis				
pN0	56 (88.9%)	30 (88.2%)	26 (89.7%)	0.097
pN+	7 (11.1%)	4 (11.8%)	3 (10.3%)	
Concurrent CIS				
Yes	12 (19.0%)	5 (14.7%)	7 (24.1%)	0.521
No	51 (81.0%)	29 (85.3%)	22 (75.9%)	
Prognosis				
Death	10 (15.9%)	8 (23.5%)	2 (6.9%)	0.258
Alive	53 (84.1%)	26 (76.5%)	27 (93.1%)	
Body Height				
Median, Mean $\pm$ SD	166, 166 $\pm$ 5.84	166, 165 $\pm$ 6.32	167, 167 $\pm$ 5.31	0.595
Psoas area (cm2)				
Median, Mean $\pm$ SD	1078, 1085 $\pm$ 255	920, 896 $\pm$ 152	1297,1307 $\pm$ 149	<0.001
Psoas Muscle Index (cm2/m2)				
Median, Mean $\pm$ SD	391, 393 $\pm$ 92.1	347,327 $\pm$ 57.3	347, 472 $\pm$ 56.7	<0.001

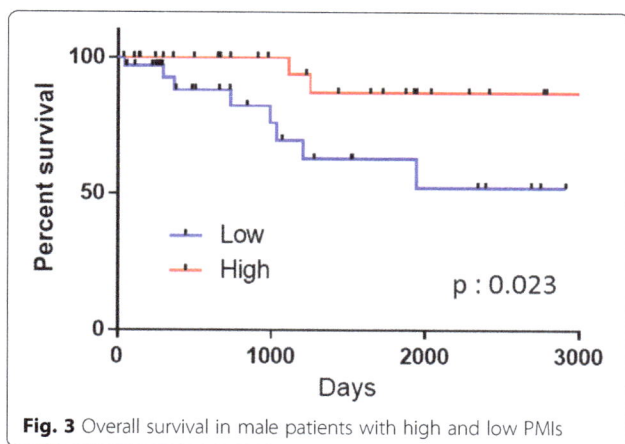

Fig. 3 Overall survival in male patients with high and low PMIs

with stage 2 or 3 gastric cancer undergoing gastrectomy, sarcopenia was found to be correlated with higher rates of postoperative complications and a poorer overall and disease-free survival than in those without sarcopenia [17]. Another study found that male sarcopenia patients who underwent pancreatectomy showed a poorer overall survival than those without sarcopenia [18].

Although the detailed mechanism underlying the association between sarcopenia and post-operative complications remains unknown, body frailty is suspected to be involved, as body failure or reduced body durability results in longer admission duration [19]. Sarcopenia develops due to body frailty with aging or in the presence of malignant disease.

The present study showed that, in male patients, those with a lower psoas muscle volume who underwent radical cystectomy had a longer hospitalization than those with a normal volume. In bladder cancer, there have been several studies regarding sarcopenia in patients undergoing radical cystectomy. Psutka et al. reported that, compared with non-sarcopenic patients, sarcopenic patients showed a significantly lower cancer-specific 5-year survival (49% vs 72%; $p = 0.003$) and OS (39% vs. 70%; $p = 0.003$) [1]. Wan et al. showed that sarcopenia increased the risk of severe complications after radical cystectomy [20]. Smith et al. reported that sarcopenic female patients had an increased risk of post-operative complications compared with non-sarcopenic patients [21]. Consistent

with these data, our results showed that a lower preoperative psoas muscle volume was associated with a prolonged hospitalization after radical cystectomy, suggesting that the psoas muscle volume might be a reliable factor for predicting a long hospitalization, presumably due to postoperative complications.

Most patients who undergo radical cystectomy for muscle-invasive bladder cancer are relatively old. Accordingly, predicting postoperative complications is important before performing radical cystectomy in such vulnerable patients. Thus far, combination therapy, including transurethral resection, systemic chemotherapy, and radiation therapy, have been thought to be the most effective bladder-preserving therapies, with a 5-year survival rate of around 50% to 60% [2, 22]. In patients over 70 years of age, intra-arterial systemic chemotherapy combined with radiation has been shown to be associated with a more favorable prognosis than radical cystectomy. Similarly, if radical cystectomy is contraindicated due to advanced age, sarcopenic patients may also be good candidates for bladder preservation.

According to the previous studies on the association of sarcopenia with the prognosis or postoperative complications, dual-energy X-ray absorptiometry and bioelectrical impedance analysis have been used to detect muscle volume. We used standard axial CT at the level of the umbilicus. A low psoas muscle volume detected by CT in this manner was associated with a longer post-operative admission due to postoperative complications. Our method is easy to perform, and in most patients undergoing radical cystectomy, no additional procedures for measuring the psoas muscle volume are required.

Conclusion

In the present study, we showed that sarcopenia is a predictor of longer hospitalization, and sarcopenic patients had a significantly worse OS than those without sarcopenia among male patients. The present findings support sarcopenia as a meaningful factor influencing the choice of therapy for locally advanced bladder cancer.

Abbreviations
OS: Overall survival; PMI: Psoas muscle index; SD: Standard deviation

Acknowledgements
We would like to thank R. Shimizu, Y. Nakamkura, and T. Yamaki for their technical assistance.

Funding
Grants from KAKENHI grants (16 K20152) from the Ministry of Education, Culture, Sports, Science and Technology of Japan.

Table 2 Postoperative complications (male patients only)

Clavien Grading Score	PMI < 400	PMI ≥ 400	p value
0	7 (17.1%)	15 (68.2%)	<0.001
1	24 (58.5%)	6 (27.3%)	
2	2 (4.9%)	1 (4.5%)	
≥3	8 (19.5%)	0 (0.0%)	

Authors' contributions

Conceived and designed the experiments: YS-M, TK, HU. Analyzed data: YS-M, TK, HI. Performed the experiments: YM ST DT KS YHay TM MO MN YHat JT YY KO KM NN MY HU. Wrote the paper: YS-M, TK. All authors read and approved the final manuscript.

Competing interests

The authors declare that they have no competing interests.

References

1. Psutka SP, Carrasco A, Schmit GD, Moynagh MR, Boorjian SA, Frank I, Stewart SB, Thapa P, Tarrell RF, Cheville JC, et al. Sarcopenia in patients with bladder cancer undergoing radical cystectomy: impact on cancer-specific and all-cause mortality. Cancer. 2014;120(18):2910–8.
2. Efstathiou JA, Spiegel DY, Shipley WU, Heney NM, Kaufman DS, Niemierko A, Coen JJ, Skowronski RY, Paly JJ, McGovern FJ, et al. Long-term outcomes of selective bladder preservation by combined-modality therapy for invasive bladder cancer: the MGH experience. Eur Urol. 2012;61(4):705–11.
3. Kawahara T, Furuya K, Nakamura M, Sakamaki K, Osaka K, Ito H, Ito Y, Izumi K, Ohtake S, Miyoshi Y, et al. Neutrophil-to-lymphocyte ratio is a prognostic marker in bladder cancer patients after radical cystectomy. BMC Cancer. 2016;16:185.
4. Hautmann RE, de Petriconi RC, Pfeiffer C, Volkmer BG. Radical cystectomy for urothelial carcinoma of the bladder without neoadjuvant or adjuvant therapy: long-term results in 1100 patients. Eur Urol. 2012;61(5):1039–47.
5. Zahran MH, El-Hefnawy AS, Zidan EM, El-Bilsha MA, Taha DE, Ali-El-Dein B. Health-related quality of life after radical cystectomy and neobladder reconstruction in women: impact of voiding and continence status. Int J Urol. 2014;21(9):887–92.
6. Sejima T, Morizane S, Yao A, Isoyama T, Saito M, Amisaki T, Koumi T, Takenaka A. Prognostic impact of preoperative hematological disorders and a risk stratification model in bladder cancer patients treated with radical cystectomy. Int J Urol. 2014;21(1):52–7.
7. Ahmadi H, Montie JE, Weizer AZ, Morgan T, Montgomery JS, Lee CT. Patient Psoas muscle mass as a predictor of complications and survival after radical Cystectomy. Curr Urol Rep. 2015;16(11):79.
8. Cruz-Jentoft AJ, Baeyens JP, Bauer JM, Boirie Y, Cederholm T, Landi F, Martin FC, Michel JP, Rolland Y, Schneider SM, et al. Sarcopenia: European consensus on definition and diagnosis: report of the European working group on sarcopenia in older people. Age Ageing. 2010;39(4):412–23.
9. Kwon HJ, Ha YC, Park HM. The reference value of skeletal muscle mass index for defining the sarcopenia of women in Korea. J Bone Metab. 2015;22(2):71–5.
10. Baumgartner RN, Koehler KM, Gallagher D, Romero L, Heymsfield SB, Ross RR, Garry PJ, Lindeman RD. Epidemiology of sarcopenia among the elderly in New Mexico. Am J Epidemiol. 1998;147(8):755–63.
11. Mir O, Coriat R, Blanchet B, Durand JP, Boudou-Rouquette P, Michels J, Ropert S, Vidal M, Pol S, Chaussade S, et al. Sarcopenia predicts early dose-limiting toxicities and pharmacokinetics of sorafenib in patients with hepatocellular carcinoma. PLoS One. 2012;7(5):e37563.
12. Del Fabbro E, Parsons H, Warneke CL, Pulivarthi K, Litton JK, Dev R, Palla SL, Brewster A, Bruera E. The relationship between body composition and response to neoadjuvant chemotherapy in women with operable breast cancer. Oncologist. 2012;17(10):1240–5.
13. Sabel MS, Lee J, Cai S, Englesbe MJ, Holcombe S, Wang S. Sarcopenia as a prognostic factor among patients with stage III melanoma. Ann Surg Oncol. 2011;18(13):3579–85.
14. Demark-Wahnefried W, Kenyon AJ, Eberle P, Skye A, Kraus WE. Preventing sarcopenic obesity among breast cancer patients who receive adjuvant chemotherapy: results of a feasibility study. Clin Exerc Physiol. 2002;4(1):44–9.
15. Shiozu H, Higashijima M, Koga T. Association of sarcopenia with swallowing problems, related to nutrition and activities of daily living of elderly individuals. J Phys Ther Sci. 2015;27(2):393–6.
16. Tanimoto Y, Watanabe M, Sun W, Tanimoto K, Shishikura K, Sugiura Y, Kusabiraki T, Kono K. Association of sarcopenia with functional decline in community-dwelling elderly subjects in Japan. Geriatr Gerontol Int. 2013;13(4):958–63.
17. Zhuang CL, Huang DD, Pang WY, Zhou CJ, Wang SL, Lou N, Ma LL, Yu Z, Shen X. Sarcopenia is an independent predictor of severe postoperative complications and long-term survival after radical Gastrectomy for gastric cancer: analysis from a large-scale cohort. Medicine (Baltimore). 2016;95(13):e3164.
18. Onesti JK, Wright GP, Kenning SE, Tierney MT, Davis AT, Doherty MG, Chung MH. Sarcopenia and survival in patients undergoing pancreatic resection. Pancreatology. 2016;16(2):284–9.
19. Makary MA, Segev DL, Pronovost PJ, Syin D, Bandeen-Roche K, Patel P, Takenaga R, Devgan L, Holzmueller CG, Tian J, et al. Frailty as a predictor of surgical outcomes in older patients. J Am Coll Surg. 2010;210(6):901–8.
20. Wan F, Zhu Y, Gu C, Yao X, Shen Y, Dai B, Zhang S, Zhang H, Cheng J, Ye D. Lower skeletal muscle index and early complications in patients undergoing radical cystectomy for bladder cancer. World J Surg Oncol. 2014;12:14.
21. Smith AB, Deal AM, Yu H, Boyd B, Matthews J, Wallen EM, Pruthi RS, Woods ME, Muss H, Nielsen ME. Sarcopenia as a predictor of complications and survival following radical cystectomy. J Urol. 2014;191(6):1714–20.
22. Koga F, Kihara K. Selective bladder preservation with curative intent for muscle-invasive bladder cancer: a contemporary review. Int J Urol. 2012;19(5):388–401.

The neutrophil-to-lymphocyte ratio (NLR) predicts adrenocortical carcinoma and is correlated with the prognosis

Taku Mochizuki[1], Takashi Kawahara[1,2]* (iD), Daiji Takamoto[1], Kazuhide Makiyama[2], Yusuke Hattori[1], Jun-ichi Teranishi[1], Yasuhide Miyoshi[1], Yasushi Yumura[1], Masahiro Yao[2] and Hiroji Uemura[1]

Abstract

Background: The neutrophil-to-lymphocyte ratio (NLR) is reported as a biomarker for some solid malignant diseases. Thus far, however, no reports of the relationship between the NLR and adrenal tumors have been published. We analyzed the utility of the preoperative NLR as a biomarker for predicting the prognosis or diagnosis of malignant disease.

Methods: A total of 59 patients with adrenal tumors (13 cases of malignant disease and 46 with benign disease) were analyzed in this study from February 2004 to June 2015 at our institute. The NLR was obtained just before adrenalectomy. The diagnosis of adrenal tumor was confirmed by a pathological examination of surgical specimens.

Results: The NLR in malignant adrenal tumor specimens was significantly higher than in non-malignant specimens ($p = 0.028$). Adrenocortical carcinoma (ACC) showed the highest NLR among all adrenal tumors. In ACC, the higher NLR group (NLR ≥ 5) showed a significantly poorer overall survival than the lower NLR group (NLR < 5) ($p = 0.032$).

Conclusions: In adrenal tumors, a higher NLR indicates a higher incidence of malignancy. The NLR might be a new biomarker for predicting the prognosis of adrenal tumor patients.

Keywords: Biomarker, Neutrophil-to-lymphocyte ratio, Adrenal tumor, Adrenocortical carcinoma

Background

Adrenocortical carcinoma (ACC) is a very rare disease with an incidence of 0.5 to 2.0 patients/100,000,000 patients/year and has one of the poorest prognoses among all solid malignancies [1, 2]. A large number of patients are diagnosed at an advanced stage. About 70% of ACCs are reported to be diagnosed as extra-adrenal lesions [3]. However, despite this poor prognosis, some patients have achieved a long disease-free survival [4]. There were no confirmed risk to predict a poorer prognosis. Several candidate prognostic factors of ACC have been reported, including the tumor size, rate of Ki-67 positivity, completeness of resection of the surgical margin, and the clinical stage [5].

A number of studies have revealed that the neutrophil-to-lymphocyte ratio (NLR) is an independent prognostic factor in various solid malignancies, including prostatic carcinoma and renal cell carcinoma [6, 7]. The NLR has also been suggested to be not only a predictor of the systemic inflammatory response in critical care patients but also a prognostic factor for certain solid malignancies [8–10]. The NLR can be easily calculated from routine complete blood counts (CBCs) in peripheral blood.

The aims of this study were to compare the NLR in ACC patients with those in patients with other non-malignant adrenal tumors and to evaluate the NLR as a prognostic marker in ACC patients.

Methods

Patients

A total of 59 consecutive cases, including 33 adrenocortical adenoma, 13 pheochromocytoma, 9 adrenocortical

* Correspondence: takashi_tk2001@yahoo.co.jp
[1]Departments of Urology and Renal Transplantation, Yokohama City University Medical Center, 4-57 Urafune-cho, Minami-ku, Yokohama, Kanagawa, 2320024, Japan
[2]Department of Urology, Yokohama City University, Graduate School of Medicine, Yokohama, Japan

Table 1 Each adrenal tumor's characteristics

	adrenocortical adenoma	pheochromocytoma	adrenocortical carcinoma	malignant lymphoma
n	33	13	9	4
Sex (male: female)	10: 23	6: 7	1: 8	3: 1
Age (median)	50	57	64	70
Maximum tumor diameter (mm) (mean)	22	40	100	91
NLR (median)	2.84	2.03	6.02	3.30

cancer, and 4 malignant lymphoma, at our institute from February 2004 to June 2015 were analyzed in this study.

Clinical and laboratory assessments

The NLR was calculated using the neutrophil and lymphocyte counts obtained via CBCs just before adrenalectomy as part of the routine preoperative workup of patients. We set the cut-off point of 5.0 as the threshold defining an elevated NLR, in accordance with a previous report [11]. None of the patients demonstrated systemic inflammation or blood disease at the time of the blood examinations.

Statistical analyses

The patients' characteristics were analyzed using the Mann-Whitney U and chi-squared tests. The cut-off NLR was determined based on the results of a receiver operative curve (ROC) analysis and a multivariate analysis was performed to investigate the factors associated with malignancy in adrenal tumors. Spearman's correlation coefficients were calculated to investigate the correlation between the NLR and tumor size. The Kaplan-Meier product limit estimator was used to estimate the overall survival. A log-rank test was performed for comparison. The statistical analyses were performed using the Graph Pad Prism software program (Graph Pad Software, La Jolla, CA, USA). P values of <0.05 were considered to indicate statistical significance.

Results

Patients

We examined a total of 59 cases of adrenal tumor, including 33 cases of adrenal carcinoid (mean size, 22 mm; median (mean ± standard deviation) NLR, 2.84 (3.41 ± 1.89)), 13 cases of pheochromocytoma (mean size, 40 mm; NLR, 2.03 (2.47 ± 1.54)), nine cases of ACC (mean size, 100 mm; NLR, 6.02 (5.04 ± 3.09)), and four cases of malignant lymphoma (mean size, 91 mm; NLR, 3.30 (3.82 ± 2.18)) [Table 1]. Regarding the ACC cases, 8 (88.9%) were female and one (11.1%) was male. One of the four patients showed endocrine activity and capsule invasion. The median age was 64 years old, and the median follow-up period was 17 months. The ACC patients' backgrounds, including the tumor volume and clinical stage, are shown in Table 2.

NLR values and patient outcomes

Malignant adrenal tumors showed a significantly higher NLR (mean ± standard deviation, standard error of the mean: 4.76 ± 2.93, 0.81) than non-malignant adrenal tumors (3.01 ± 1.78, 0.27; p = 0.016). The NLR in ACC showed the highest NLR [Figs. 1 and 2]. The cut-off NLR for predicting malignant disease was 3.15 (area under ROC: 0.668) [Fig.3]. A multivariate analysis showed that the NLR was an independent predictor (GR 8.990, p: 0.037) (Table 3). The tumor size was weakly correlated with the NLR (r^2: 0.08, p: 0.034). In ACC subjects, the higher NLR group (≥ 5) showed a significantly poorer overall survival than the lower

Table 2 Adrenocortical carcinoma patients' characteristics

No	Age	Sex	Maximum diameter (mm)	Endocrine activity	Capsule invasion	Clinical stage	Chemotherapy	Outcome	Observation period (months)
1	85	F	96	−	NA	StageIV	−	dead	1
2	19	F	125	+	+	StageIII	+	dead	5
3	64	F	72	−	NA	StageIV	+	dead	42
4	62	M	100	−	+	StageIV	+	dead	9
5	64	F	105	−	NA	StageIV	+	dead	2
6	66	F	70	−	+	StageIV	+	dead	30
7	42	F	108	−	−	StageIV	+	dead	17
8	34	F	125	−	−	StageIV	−	dead	17
9	72	F	18	−	+	StageI	−	alive	27

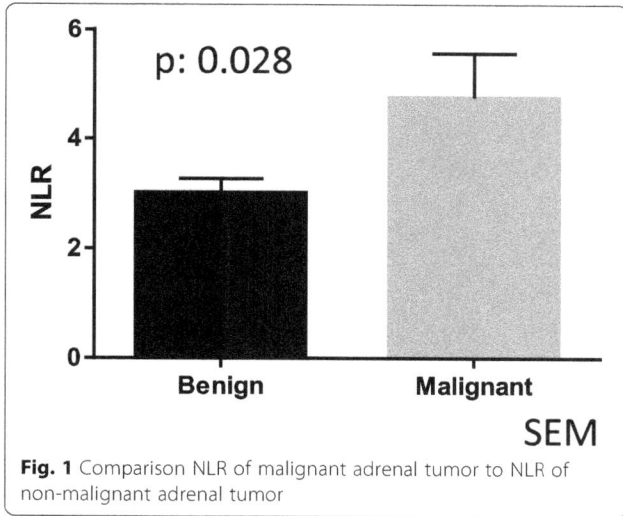

Fig. 1 Comparison NLR of malignant adrenal tumor to NLR of non-malignant adrenal tumor

NLR group (< 5) with a median survival of 174 vs. 917 days ($p = 0.032$) [Fig. 4].

Discussion

Recently, NLR had been shown to be an independent prognostic risk factor for certain solid malignancies [6–10]. Only one study comparing the NLR and the prognosis of ACC has been reported—by Bagante et al. [11]. They found that an NLR > 5.0 was associated with a poorer disease-specific survival and progression-free survival in ACC. No other reports have investigated the effectiveness of NLR in detecting the malignancy of an adrenal tumor. In the present study, we found that a higher NLR in adrenal tumors was associated with a higher incidence

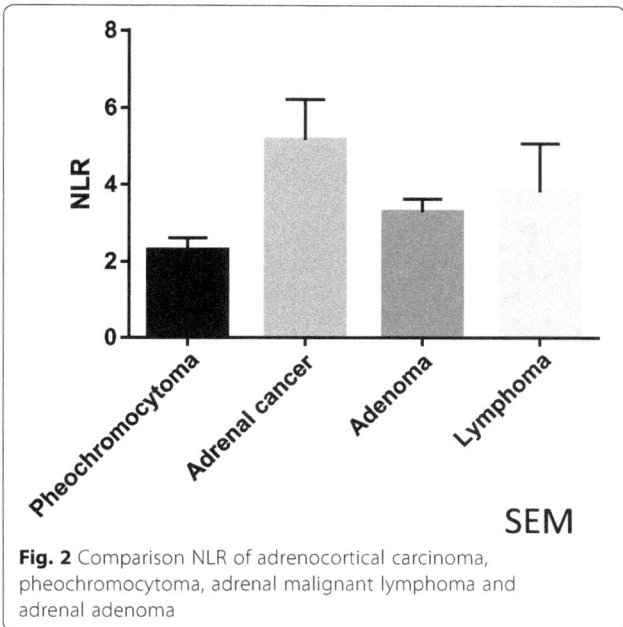

Fig. 2 Comparison NLR of adrenocortical carcinoma, pheochromocytoma, adrenal malignant lymphoma and adrenal adenoma

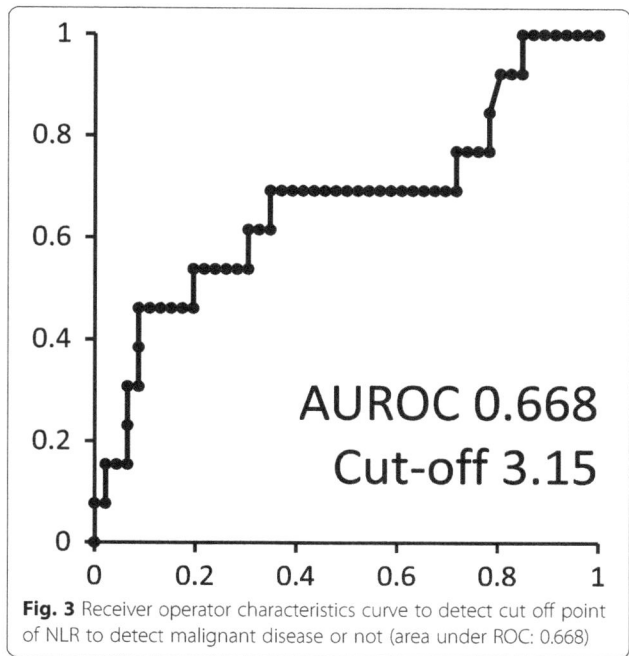

Fig. 3 Receiver operator characteristics curve to detect cut off point of NLR to detect malignant disease or not (area under ROC: 0.668)

of malignancy. These findings might contribute to the prediction of malignant disease for differentiating incidentaloma.

Among incidental adrenal tumors, ACC is difficult to diagnose using preoperative imaging findings. A tumor size >4 cm is a well-known imaging finding for differentiating malignant tumors, with a sensitivity of 81% [5]. A previous report showed that 16% of adrenal tumors with diameters of <5 cm were ACCs [12].

Due to the marked increase in the rate of imaging analyses being performed at medical check-ups, small ACC would be increased. So, differentiated diagnosis except tumor size would be needed.

Irregular margins are usually seen in ACC, but some benign adrenal tumors also showed irregular margins [13]. Computed tomography (CT) shows a finding of a low Hounsfield unit value (< 10) with 98% specificity. Chemical-shift imaging with magnetic resonance imaging (MRI) has also been reported to be useful for detecting adrenal adenomas [14]. However, the specific imaging findings indicative of ACC remain unclear. The NLR can be easily calculated during a daily clinical examination. The combination of imaging findings on CT and/or MRI

Table 3 The results of the multivariate analysis

	P value	HR	95% CI
Gender (male)	0.332	0.353	0.043–2.892
Age (≥57)	0.099	5.720	0.719–45.504
NLR (≥3.15)	0.037	8.990	1.142–70.547
Size (≥40 mm)	<0.001	112.400	7.39–1710.5

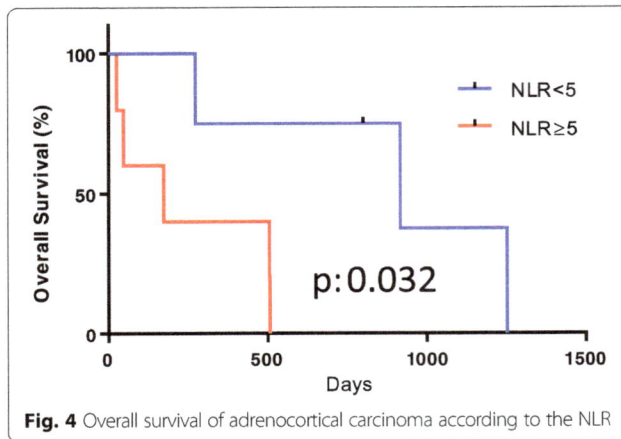

Fig. 4 Overall survival of adrenocortical carcinoma according to the NLR

Further study is needed to confirm the usefulness of NLR in ACC to confirm the sensitivity and specificity.

Conclusion

Malignant adrenal tumors showed a higher NLR than non-malignant ones. In addition, the ACC patients with a higher NLR showed a significantly poorer survival than those with lower values.

Funding

Grants from KAKENHI grants (16 K20152) from the Ministry of Education, Culture, Sports, Science and Technology of Japan.

Authors' contributions

Conceived and designed the experiments: TM, TK. Analyzed data: TM, TK. Performed the experiments: TM, TK, DT, KM, YH, JT, YY, YM, MY, HU. Wrote the paper: TM, TK. All authors have read and approved of the final manuscript.

Competing interests

The authors declare that they have no competing interests.

and the NLR may support the preoperative diagnosis of adrenal tumor.

Previous reports have shown that an NLR > 5.0 indicates a poor prognosis in pancreas cancer and liver metastatic rectal cancer [15, 16]. Our previous study showed that an NLR > 2.4 was associated with a high risk of prostate cancer in patients with a PSA of 4–10 ng/mL [17]. However, due to the small number of patients, that study could not detect an adequate NLR cut-off point. In the present study, we found that an NLR cut-off point of 5.0 was adequate for predicting the prognosis of ACC. The cut-off NLR of 5.0 was the same as a previous report and was the median value in this study. The cut-off NLR of 5.0 was relatively high in comparison to other studies, which indicated the aggressive nature of ACC in comparison to other types of cancer. Further studies are needed to validate the clinical utility of this parameter.

In this study, the multivariate analysis revealed that the tumor size and NLR were found to be independent predictors of malignant disease. The combination of the NLR and imaging findings might support the preoperative diagnosis and detection of malignant adrenal tumors, including ACC and malignant lymphoma, as well as benign adrenal tumors, helping in the planning of an adequate surgical approach.

This study showed that an NLR of 5.0 was a candidate cut-off point for predicting the prognosis in ACC. In localized ACC, the surgical margin was confirmed to be the most important prognostic factor. The 5-year overall survival in completely surgically resected patients ranges from 40 to 50%, while the median overall survival in unresectable case is <1 year [6]. In cases preoperatively predicted to have a poor outcome, a preoperative surgical plan with extended resection might be suggested in order to obtain a negative surgical margin.

This study was limited by its small sample size and retrospective nature, both due to the rarity of ACC.

References

1. Wajchenberg BL, Albergaria Pereira MA, Medonca BB, Latronico AC, Campos Carneiro P, Alves VA, et al. Adrenocortical carcinoma: clinical and laboratory observations. Cancer. 2000;88(4):711–36.
2. Kebebew E, Reiff E, Duh QY, Clark OH, McMillan A. Extent of disease at presentation and outcome for adrenocortical carcinoma: have we made progress? World J Surg. 2006;30(5):872–8.
3. Phan AT. Adrenal cortical carcinoma–review of current knowledge and treatment practices. Hematol Oncol Clin North Am. 2007;21(3):489–507. viii-ix
4. Tran TB, Postlewait LM, Maithel SK, Prescott JD, Wang TS, Glenn J, et al. Actual 10-year survivors following resection of adrenocortical carcinoma. J Surg Oncol. 2016;114(8):971–6.
5. Lebastchi AH, Kunstman JW, Carling T. Adrenocortical carcinoma: current therapeutic state-of-the-art. J Oncol. 2012;2012:234726.
6. Ohno Y, Nakashima J, Ohori M, Hatano T, Tachibana M. Pretreatment neutrophil-to-lymphocyte ratio as an independent predictor of recurrence in patients with nonmetastatic renal cell carcinoma. J Urol. 2010;184(3):873–8.
7. Kawahara T, Yokomizo Y, Ito Y, Ito H, Ishiguro H, Teranishi J, et al. Pretreatment neutrophil-to-lymphocyte ratio predicts the prognosis in patients with metastatic prostate cancer. BMC Cancer. 2016;16:111.
8. Walsh SR, Cook EJ, Goulder F, Justin TA, Keeling NJ. Neutrophil-lymphocyte ratio as a prognostic factor in colorectal cancer. J Surg Oncol. 2005;91(3):181–4.
9. Azab B, Bhatt VR, Phookan J, Murukutla S, Kohn N, Terjanian T, et al. Usefulness of the neutrophil-to-lymphocyte ratio in predicting short- and long-term mortality in breast cancer patients. Ann Surg Oncol. 2012;19(1):217–24.
10. Yamanaka T, Matsumoto S, Teramukai S, Ishiwata R, Nagai Y, Fukushima M. The baseline ratio of neutrophils to lymphocytes is associated with patient prognosis in advanced gastric cancer. Oncology. 2007;73(3–4):215–20.
11. Bagante F, Tran TB, Postlewait LM, Maithel SK, Wang TS, Evans DB, et al. Neutrophil-lymphocyte and platelet-lymphocyte ratio as predictors of disease specific survival after resection of adrenocortical carcinoma. J Surg Oncol. 2015;112(2):164–72.
12. Fishman EK, Deutch BM, Hartman DS, Goldman SM, Zerhouni EA, Siegelman SS. Primary adrenocortical carcinoma: CT evaluation with clinical correlation. AJR Am J Roentgenol. 1987;148(3):531–5.
13. Benitah N, Yeh BM, Qayyum A, Williams G, Breiman RS, Coakley FV. Minor morphologic abnormalities of adrenal glands at CT: prognostic importance in patients with lung cancer. Radiology. 2005;235(2):517–22.
14. Blake MA, Cronin CG, Boland GW. Adrenal imaging. AJR Am J Roentgenol. 2010;194(6):1450–60.
15. Kou T, Kanai M, Yamamoto M, Xue P, Mori Y, Kudo Y, et al. Prognostic model for survival based on readily available pretreatment factors in patients with advanced pancreatic cancer receiving palliative

Real life persistence rate with antimuscarinic treatment in patients with idiopathic or neurogenic overactive bladder: a prospective cohort study with solifenacin

Marloes J. Tijnagel*, Jeroen R. Scheepe and Bertil F. M. Blok

Abstract

Background: Several studies have shown that the antimuscarinic treatment of overactive bladder is characterized by low long-term persistence rates. We have investigated the persistence of solifenacin in real life by means of telephonic interviews in a prospective cohort. We included both patients with idiopathic overactive bladder as well as neurogenic overactive bladder.

Methods: From June 2009 until July 2012 patients with idiopathic or neurogenic overactive bladder who were newly prescribed solifenacin were included. In total 123 subjects were followed prospectively during one year by means of four telephonic interviews, which included questions about medication use and adverse events.

Results: After one year 40% of all patients included was still using solifenacin, 50% discontinued and 10% was lost to follow-up. In the neurogenic group 58% was still using solifenacin versus 32% in the idiopathic group after one year ($p < 0,05$). The main reasons to stop solifenacin were lack of efficacy, side effects and a combination of both.

Conclusions: This prospective cohort study showed a real life continuation rate of 40% after 12 months. This continuation rate is higher than found in most other studies.
The use of regular telephonic evaluation might have improved medication persistence. The findings of this study also suggest that patients with neurogenic overactive bladder have a better persistence with this method of evaluation compared to patients with idiopathic overactive bladder.

Keywords: Muscarinic antagonists, Overactive bladder, Urge urinary incontinence, Adverse effects, Medication adherence

Background

Antimuscarinics are the first-line therapy in the treatment of overactive bladder (OAB). This applies to idiopathic OAB (iOAB) as well as neurogenic OAB (nOAB). The use of antimuscarinics in patients with iOAB is characterized by very low persistence rates. Results from short-term studies show discontinuation rates ranging from 4 to 31% [1]. The long-term persistence to antimuscarinics in OAB is not well investigated. A systematic review conducted by Veenboer et al. found that persistence beyond 1 year rarely exceeded 10% of the patients [2]. These data might even represent an overestimation of the persistence because reviews of medical claims data show much higher discontinuation rates (up to 83% within the first 30 days) [1]. Furthermore, patients who have collected the prescribed medications might not use them because of other reasons, like fear for adverse effects.

* Correspondence: mtijn@hotmail.com
Department of Urology, Erasmus University Medical Center, P.O. Box 2040
3000 CA Rotterdam, The Netherlands

Regarding the use of antimuscarinics in the treatment of nOAB much less studies have been performed compared to iOAB. Patients with nOAB are a heterogeneous group with different underlying neurologic conditions, such as multiple sclerosis, spinal cord injury, Parkinson disease, cerebral palsy and meningomyelocele [3]. Patients often suffer from incontinence, urgency, frequency or impaired bladder emptying. It has been shown that the use of antimuscarinics in this group is associated with better patient-reported cure/improvement compared to placebo. However, there is a higher incidence of adverse events [4].

This prospective study was carried out to investigate the persistence rate in real life among patients with idiopathic or neurogenic OAB who were prescribed solifenacin. We followed them during one year by means of telephonic interviews.

Furthermore, we wanted to investigate the reasons why patients stopped taking their medications. Third, we wanted to investigate if we could find any differences between patients with idiopathic OAB versus neurogenic OAB.

Methods

This study was undertaken at the urology department of the Erasmus University Medical Center, Rotterdam, The Netherlands. The ethics committee of the hospital approved the study protocol. The inclusion was carried out from June 2009 until July 2012. After giving informed consent, patients older than 18 years and newly prescribed solifenacin because of complaints of idiopathic or neurogenic OAB, were included. Solifenacin, under the trade name Vesicare, is a urinary antispasmodic of the anticholinergic class. It is produced by Astellas Pharma BV. It is available in 5 and 10 mg. The starting dose was chosen by the doctor who prescribed the solifenacin but could be adjusted during the study period. Because this observational study investigated the persistence rate in real life in patients who had been prescribed solifenacin by their own doctor, they had to collect the solifenacin themselves at a pharmacy of choice.

Patients who had used anticholinergic drugs less than 7 days before they started solifenacin were excluded. Participants were allowed to continue possible other urologic medications, for example alfa-blockers, but not other anticholinergic drugs.

Telephonic surveys were taken at 1, 3, 6 and 12 months after starting solifenacin. The patients were asked whether they were continuing the medication. They were also interviewed about possible side effects and if they had discontinued the therapy, what had been reasons for stopping.

Statistical analysis was performed using SPSS statistical software. The Chi-square test was used to evaluate the differences between groups.

Results

During the study period a total number of 123 patients were included in this study. Twelve patients were lost to follow-up. Table 1 displays the demographic characteristics. Eighty-three patients received solifenacin because of idiopathic OAB and 40 patients because of neurogenic OAB. Among this group 17 patients had a spinal cord injury, 10 multiple sclerosis. The rest was diagnosed with other conditions as you can find in Fig. 1.

After one year 40% of all patients included were still using solifenacin, 50% discontinued and 10% was lost to follow-up. Table 2 shows the persistence rate after one year in patients with idiopathic OAB and neurogenic OAB. Persistence in the neurogenic group was 58% versus 32% in the idiopathic group ($p < 0,05$).

The main reasons to stop taking solifenacin were lack of efficacy (39%), side effects (30%) and a combination of both (13%).

Of the total group of 111 interviewed patients 64 patients (58%) experienced side effects within one year. Most common side effects were dry mouth, constipation, blurred vision, dry eyes and abdominal pain.

Discussion

Antimuscarinic drugs have been available for many years for the treatment of OAB.

OAB is a chronic condition and long-term effective treatment might be of importance for the quality of life. Unfortunately, adherence and persistence to antimuscarinics are poor. OAB medication is known to have the lowest persistence in comparison to other chronic oral medication like cardiovascular, antidiabetic and osteoporosis treatments [5].

Table 1 Demographics

Characteristic	Patients included
Age: years	
Mean (S.D.)	61.7 (15.4)
Range	20.1 – 90.2
Gender: no (%)	
Men	70 (57%)
Women	53 (43%)
Starting dose : no (%)	
10 mg/day	12 (9.8)
5 mg/day	106 (86.2)
5 mg/2 days	3 (2.4)
2.5 mg/2 days	1 (0.8)
unknown	1 (0.8)
Condition: no (%)	
Idiopathic OAB	83 (67.5)
Neurogenic OAB	40 (32.5)

S.D. Standard deviation

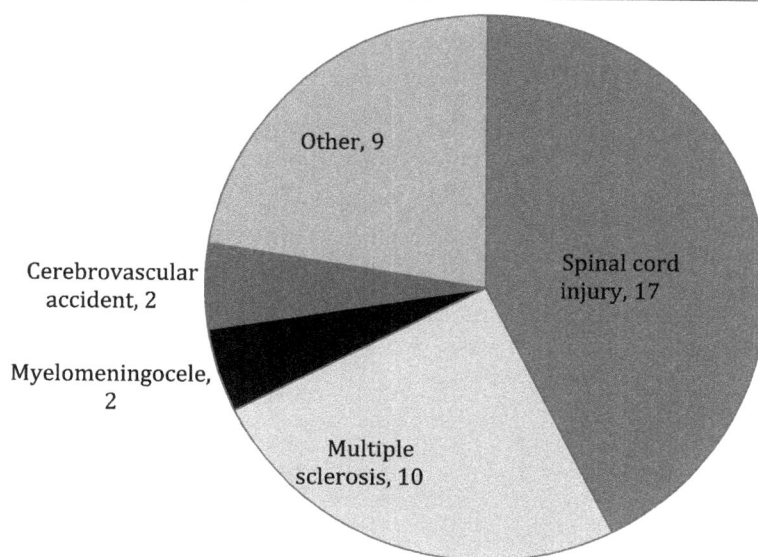

Fig. 1 Patient distribution neurogenic OAB

Regarding the use of benign prostate hyperplasia (BPH) medication, a large population-based cohort study using an administrative prescription database showed that the persistence was 29% after one year [6].

Doses of solifenacin succinate (5 mg and 10 mg) once daily (OD) have proven to be effective [7–9]. Haab et al. showed that 81% of the patients completed 40 weeks of open-label treatment with only 4,7% discontinuation because of adverse events [10]. Clinical and prescription database studies demonstrated much lower continuation rates varying from 9 to 35%. [11–15].

In our study we found a continuation rate of 40% after 12 months. This continuation rate is higher than found in most other studies. We think that this difference might be explained by the fact that the patients received telephonic interviews regularly. This is somewhat in line with other studies, which suggest that compliance to OAB therapy improves with patient education about OAB en its treatment [16, 17].

Furthermore, an additional difference in our study was the possibility of adjusting the medication dose during the study period. Patients who complained about side effects could receive a lower dose, whereas people who had little effect could receive a higher dose. This possible adjustment might have contributed to a higher persistence. This observation might encourage other caregivers

to evaluate regularly patients who receive antimuscarinic medication for OAB.

A possible tool for the future is the use of Short Message Service (SMS) to improve utilization of and adherence to anticholinergic medication. It is a simple and inexpensive strategy, which has proven to help patients taking their medications on time [18]. Furthermore, it has been used to increase medication adherence to a variety of medication classes on a short term [19–22]. This tool could educate people with OAB and help them to improve persistence with antimuscarinic medication on the long term.

A large screening survey performed in the USA to identify patient-reported reasons for discontinuing overactive bladder medication found that the most mentioned reasons were: "didn't work as expected"," switched to new medication", "learned to get by without medication" and "I had side effects" [23].

These reported reasons are similar to our study were the main reasons to stop taking the medications were lack of efficacy (39%), side effects (30%) and a combination of both (13%). A possible confounder of our study is that Dutch patients usually have to pay a part of the medication costs themselves when the product is still patented. No one reported these costs as a reason to stop, but we did not ask explicitly.

As mentioned before, antimuscarinic treatment in patients with neurogenic OAB has not been thoroughly evaluated. Treatment for neurogenic OAB is important in order to provide more bladder control, decrease urinary incontinence and, therefore, decrease the risk of decubitus ulcers, prevent UTI's and ultimately to preserve renal function [24]. Antimuscarinics are advised to use

Table 2 Persistence rate solifenacin after one year

	Patients still using	Patients discontinued	Lost to FU
All patients	50 (40.7%)	61 (49.6%)	12 (9.7%)
Neurogenic OAB	23 (57.5%)	13 (32.5%)	4 (10%)
Idiopathic OAB	27 (32.5%)	48 (57.8%)	8 (9.7%)

as a first line medical treatment, but data on persistence in nOAB are lacking [25]. A study on the epidemiology and healthcare utilization of neurogenic bladder patients performed in the US found that 71, 5% was using one of more OAB drugs during the study period of one year. Only 29% of the patients continued that therapy. Another 38% of the patients stopped and did not restart, 34% stopped and restarted [24]. This suggests that neurogenic bladder patients are not adequately managed. In our study 32% of the patients with neurogenic OAB discontinued versus 58% of the patients with idiopathic OAB, which was a significant difference. This suggests that patients with neurogenic OAB have a better persistence compared to patients with idiopathic OAB.

Conclusions

This prospective cohort study showed a real life continuation rate of solifenacin of 40% after 12 months. This continuation rate is higher than found in most other studies.

The use of regular telephonic evaluation might have improved medication persistence. This observation should be further investigated. The findings of this study also suggest that patients with neurogenic overactive bladder have a better persistence with this method of evaluation compared to patients with idiopathic overactive bladder.

Abbreviations
OAB: Overactive bladder; iOAB: Idiopathic overactive bladder; nOAB: Neurogenic overactive bladder; UTI: Urinary tract infection; BPH: Benign prostatic hyperplasia; SMS: Short message service

Acknowledgements
Not applicable.

Funding
The study was supported by a grant from Astellas. With this grant a research nurse who performed the interviews was funded.
Astellas Pharma BV had no role in the design of the study and collection, analysis, and interpretation of data and in writing the manuscript.

Authors' contributions
All authors made substantial contributions to conception and design, of acquisition of data. MT analyzed and interpreted the patient data. JS and BB have been involved in revising it critically. All authors read and approved the final manuscript.

Competing interests
Astellas Pharma BV (who financially supported this study) manufactures solifenacin. The persistence rate of this drug was observed during this study.

References

1. Sexton CC, Notte SM, Dmochowki RR, Cardozo L, Subramanian D, Coyne KS. Persistence and adherence in the treatment of overactive bladder syndrome with anticholinergic therapy: a systematic review of literature. Int J Clin Pract. 2011;65(5):567–85.
2. Veenboer PW, Bosch JL. Long-term adherence to antimuscarinic therapy in everyday practice: a systematic review. J Urol. 2014;191(4):1003–8.
3. Chancellor MB, Anderson RU, Boone TB. Pharmacotherapy for neurogenic detrusor overactivity. Am J Phys Med Rehabil. 2006;85(6):536–45.
4. Madhuvrata P, Singh M, Hasafa Z, Abdel-Fattah M. Anticholinergic drugs for adult neurogenic detrusor overactivity: a systematic review and meta-analysis. Eur Urol. 2012;62(5):816–30.
5. Yeaw J, Benner JS, Walt JG, Sian S, Smith DB. Comparing adherence and persistence across 6 chronic medication classes. J Manag Care Pham. 2009; 15(9):728–40.
6. Cindolo L, Pirozzi L, Fanizza C, et al. Drug adherence and clinical outcomes for patients under pharmacological therapy for lower urinary tract symptoms related to benign prostatic hyperplasia: population-based cohort study. Eur Urol. 2015;68(3):418–25.
7. Chapple CR, Martinez-Garcia R, Selvaggi L, et al. A comparison of the efficacy and tolerability of solifenacin succinate and extended realease tolterodine at treating overactive bladder syndrome: results of the STAR trial. Eur Urol. 2005;48(3):464–70.
8. Luo D, Liu L, Han P, Wei Q, Shen H. Solifenacin for overactive bladder: a systematic review and meta-analysis. Int Urogynecol J. 2012;23(8):983–91.
9. Cardozo L, Hessdorfer E, Milani R, et al. Solifenacin in the treatment of urgency and other symptoms of overactive bladder: results from a randomnized, double-blind, placebo-controlled, rising-dose trial. BJU Int. 2008;102(9):1120–7.
10. Haab F, Cardozo L, Chapple C, Ridder AM. Long-term open-label Solifenacin treatment associated with persistence with therapy in patients with overactive bladder syndrome. Eur Urol. 2005;47(3):376–38.
11. Yokoyama T, Koide T, Hara R, Fukumoto K, Miyaji Y, Nagai A. Long-term safety and efficacy of two different antimuscarinics, imidafenacin and solifenacin, for treatment of overactive bladder: a prospective randomized controlled study. Urol Int. 2013;90(2):161–7.
12. Brostrom S, Hallas J. Persistence of antimuscarinic drug use. Eur J Clin Pharmacol. 2009;65(3):309–14.
13. Gopal M, Haynes K, Bellamy SL, Arya LA. Discontinuation rates of anticholinergic medications used for the treatment of lower urinary tract symptoms. Obstet Gynecol. 2008;112(6):1311–8.
14. Wagg A, Compion G, Fahey A, Siddiqiu E. Persistence with prescribed antimuscarinic therapy for overactive bladder: a UK experience. BJU Int. 2012;11:1767–74.
15. Sicras-Mainar A, Rejas J, Navarro-Artieda R, et al. Antimuscarinic persistence patterns in newly treated patients with overactive bladder: a retrospective comparative analysis. Int Urolgynecol J. 2014;25(4):485–92.
16. Brubaker L, Fanning K, Goldberg EL, et al. Predictors of discontinuing overactive bladder medications. BJU Int. 2010;105(9):1283–90.
17. Wyman JF, Burgio KL, Newman DK. Practical aspects of lifestyle modifications and behavioral interventions in the treatment of overactive bladder and urinary incontinence. Int J Clin Prac. 2009;63:1177–91.
18. Huang HL, Li YCJ, Chou YC, et al. Effects of and satisfaction with short message service reminders for patient medication adherence: a randomized controlled study. BMC Med Inform Decis Mak. 2013;13:127.
19. Strandbygaard U, Thomsen SF, Backer V. A daily SMS reminder increases adherence to asthma treatment: a three-month follow-up study. Respir Med. 2010;104(2):166–71.
20. Vervloet M, Van Dijk L, De Bakker DH, et al. Short- and long-term effects of real-time medication monitoring with short message service (SMS) reminders for missed doses on the refill adherence of people with Type 2 diabetes: Evidence from a randomized controlled trial. Diabet Med. 2014; 31(7):821–8.
21. Da Costa TM, Barbosa BJP, Gomes e costa DA, et al. Results of a randomized controlled trial to assess the effects of a mobile SMS-based intervention on treatment adherence in HIV/AIDS-infected Brazilian women and impressions and satisfaction with respect to incoming messages. Int J Med Inform. 2012; 81(4):257 69.
22. Wang K, Wang C, Xi L, et al. A randomized controlled trial to asses adherence to allergic rhinitis treatment following a daily short message service (SMS) via the mobile phone. Int Arch Allergy Immunol. 2014;163:51–8.

12

Ureteral reconstruction using a tapered non-vascularized bladder graft

Lujia Zou[†], Shanhua Mao[†], Shenghua Liu, Limin Zhang, Tian Yang, Yun Hu, Qiang Ding and Haowen Jiang[*]

Abstract

Background: Reconstruction of ureteral defects and strictures remains problematic for urologists. We aimed to investigate the possibility of a tapered non-vascularized bladder graft as a novel substitute for ureteral reconstruction.

Methods: This experimental study was conducted on nine beagles. Under general anesthesia, a full-thickness graft with 5–6 cm in length was disassociated from the anterior upper wall of the bladder, and tapered into 1/3 to 1/2 thickness, remaining the urothelial surface. After removal of 5 cm of right-sided mid-ureter, the tapered bladder graft was tubularized along the long axis and then respectively anastomosed to the upper and lower stumps of the ureter. A retrograde urography through a cystostomy was performed 8 weeks after the ureteral reconstruction. The animals were euthanized, and histopathologic examinations of the neoureters were performed.

Results: There were no severe complications during postoperative follow-up. The urography indicated patent urine excretion and no fistula or stenosis. Histopathologic examinations of the neoureters showed open lumen with urothelial lining. Nutrient vessels were observed in healthy submucosa, lamina muscularis and peripheral connective tissue.

Conclusions: Our study implied that ureteral reconstruction by a tapered non-vascularized bladder graft was anatomically possible in our animal model. Further studies are expected to confirm long-term and functional outcomes.

Keywords: Animal model, Bladder graft, Non-vascularized, Reconstruction, Ureter

Background

Ureteral injuries usually arise from traumatic or iatrogenic causes [1]. In most cases, an end-to-end anastomosis without additional material can be applied for management of a short-segment ureteral defect or stricture. Furthermore, several classical surgical reconstructive methods have been well recognized, including ureteroplasty using a bladder muscle flap (Boari flap), ileal ureteral substitution, and renal autotransplantation [2].

However, these traditional methods have limitations in practical application. The Boari flap can reconstruct a limited length of distal or mid-ureter [3]. The ileal substitution has a variety of postoperative complications due to the characteristics of intestinal mucosa, including reabsorption of ammonium [4–6] and mucus secretion that may subsequently induce urinary tract infection and lithogenesis [5, 6]. Renal autotransplantation calls for a complicated procedure and is associated with possible infection and loss of renal function [1]. The Monti and Mitrofanoff techniques have been successfully developed to decrease postoperative intestinal complications, while intestinal involvement may still be related to leakage and ileus [7–9]. Concerning reconstructive materials, a

* Correspondence: huashanurologyhwj@163.com
[†]Equal contributors
Department of Urology, Huashan Hospital, Fudan University, No.12 Wulumuqi Middle Road, Shanghai 200040, People's Republic of China

bladder flap (or graft) with urothelial lining, which is similar to the ureter, seems ideal for ureteral replacement. We hypothesized that it may be possible to use a non-vascularized bladder graft for reconstruction of upper or mid-ureter. The primary concern was whether the bladder graft was able to survive without a vessel pedicle.

The main objective of our study was to investigate the possibility of a novel method using a tapered non-vascularized bladder graft to reconstruct the ureter in a canine animal model.

Methods

This experimental study was conducted on 9 healthy male beagles (approximately 1-year-old), which were obtained from School of Agriculture, Shanghai Jiao Tong University. The mean weight of the beagles at operation time was 10.6 kg (range 8.4–12.2 kg). The dogs were housed individually in the stainless-steel cages in a controlled environment. Filtered water and a standard animal diet were available ad libitum. The study was carried out at the laboratory animal unit in School of Pharmacy, Fudan University during March to August, 2015.

The right ureter was chosen for the experimental procedures, while the left side was reserved as control. The surgical field was prepared and sterilized with povidone-iodine. Then a prophylactic dose of cefazolin was applied intramuscularly. The procedure was performed under general endotracheal anesthesia. The anesthesia was induced through intravenous administration of propofol (4 mg/kg), lidocaine (1 mg/kg), and diazepam (0.3 mg/kg) and maintained with isoflurane in 100% oxygen. The laparotomy was conducted through a full-length midline abdominal incision. Abdominal viscera were inspected to exclude any possible abnormalities, particularly of the urinary system.

A rectangular region was marked by four loose ligations at each vertex on the anterior upper wall of the filling bladder, the volume of which was approximately 30-40 mL. The region was designed with 5–6 cm in length and 1 cm in width. After full thickness resection, the bladder graft was temporarily preserved in normal saline and gently squeezed until it turned pale.

Through the cystostomy, a 4.7-Fr ureteral stent was retrogradely inserted into the right ureter from the ureteral orifice. The right ureter was mobilized from the retroperitoneal tissue, and then approximately 5 cm was removed from the middle part. The non-vascularized bladder graft was tapered carefully by an ophthalmic scissor into 1/3 to 1/2 thickness (2–3 mm), keeping the urothelial surface intact. Thereafter, the tapered bladder graft was tubularized along the long axis, with the stent inside. The two ends of the graft tube were respectively anastomosed to the upper and lower stumps of the

ureter by four sutures. (Figs. 1 and 2) After the anastomoses were checked in case of hemorrhage and urine leakage, the abdominal fascia was closed by 3–4 sutures. The surgical wound was then closed layer by layer.

All animals received cefazolin and flurbiprofen for the next 3 days and cefazolin for an additional 4 days. Specific signs were monitored twice a day, including temperature, respiratory rate, pulse, appetite, activity, defecation and urination. The surgical wound was observed and sterilized at the time of monitoring. Liquid diet was started a few hours after the procedure, and it was advanced to regular diet the next day. The ureteral stent was maintained for the postoperative 6 weeks and removed through a brief cystostomy. 8 weeks after the reconstructive procedure, a retrograde urography by a 5-Fr tube was performed through another cystostomy to assess the possibility of leakage or stenosis.

The animals were then euthanized by intravenous injection of potassium chloride under general anesthesia. After thorough exploration of the abdominal cavity and surgical field, the right-sided kidney, ureter (together with peripheral connective tissue) and part of the bladder were resected and fixed with formalin immediately. The specimens were embedded with paraffin and stained with hematoxylin & eosin. Two experienced genitourinary pathologists separately finished the microscopic examination.

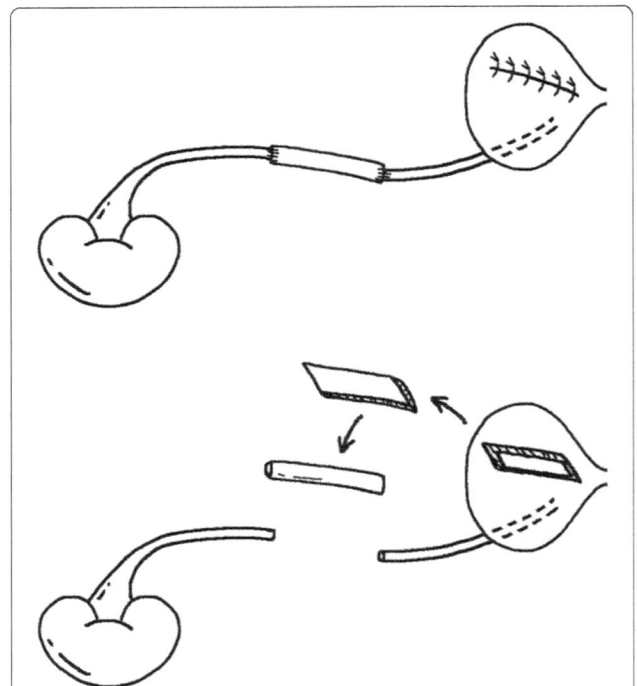

Fig. 1 The schematic diagram of the procedure

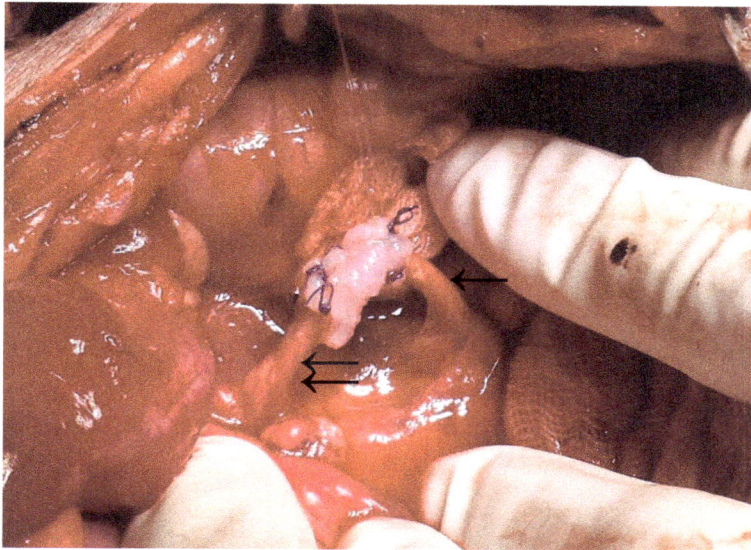

Fig. 2 A picture of the operation. Single arrow: upper ureter. Double arrow: lower ureter

Results

At the end point of the experiment, all the 9 dogs tolerated the procedure and survived. All had regular eating and activities. A subcutaneous abscess at the abdominal incision occurred to one dog, and was solved by a surgical debridement. There were otherwise no obvious signs of complications including severe gross hematuria, peritoneal infection or urine leakage. The ureteral stents in 7 animals were in place till the removal, and had been delivered out of the urinary tract in the other two. No obvious alteration of micturition rhythm was observed.

Through the abdominal exploration after the euthanasia, there was no hematoma, infection or urine leakage in the abdominal cavity. The reconstructive segments of the right ureters were intensely wrapped by fibrous adhesion. Mild hydronephrosis was observed in the right kidneys and upper ureters. Through the second cystostomy, urine was observed continuously outflowing from the orifices of the right ureters.

During the retrograde urography, the lumen of the neo-ureters easily accepted the 5-Fr tubes. The urography indicated normal ureteral caliber and patent urine excretion, without obvious fistula or stenosis. Grade of hydronephrosis assessed through the urography was accordant with the gross examination (Fig. 3).

The microscopic examination of the reconstructive ureteral segments showed that the open lumen was almost completely covered with pseudostratified urothelial lining. The urothelial cells formed the arrangement of 5–7 rows, similar to that of an empty bladder. In the denuding area, the basement membrane of urothelium was also complete. The submucosa and lamina muscularis were alive and healthy with abundant nutrient vessels.

Meantime, infiltration of inflammatory cells was observed in the submucosa. The smooth muscle fibers had disordered trends near the periureteral connective tissue, without serosa between the two layers. Nutrient vessels were also noticed in the periureteral connective tissue (Fig. 4).

Discussion

Ureteral injuries usually require surgical management, except for ureteral contusion and perforation. A short segment of ureteral defect can be repaired by end-to-

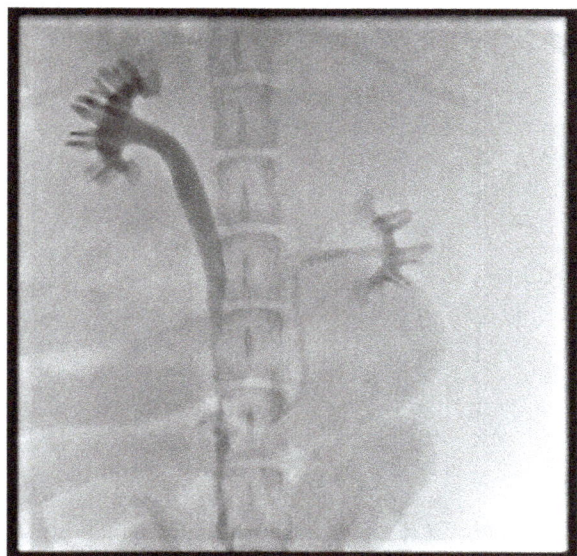

Fig. 3 The urography showing patent urine excretion and no fistula or stenosis (the left side as control)

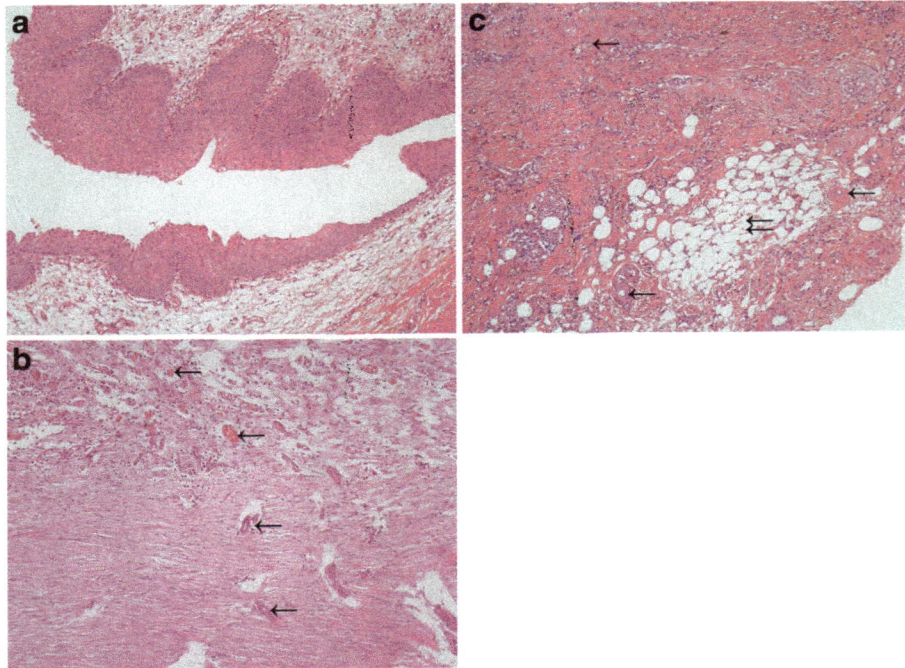

Fig. 4 Histological examination of reconstructive ureter (H.E.). **a** Longitudinal section view showing open lumen with complete urothelial lining in the neo-ureter. (×10) **b** The healthy submucosa and lamina muscularis with nutrient vessels. (×10) Single arrow: nutrient vessels in submucosa and lamina muscularis. **c** The disordered smooth muscle fibers, without a serosa between the lamina muscularis and connective tissue; nutrient vessels in the periureteral connective tissue. (×10) Single arrow: The nutrient vessels of the reconstructive ureter. Double arrow: the periureteral connective tissue

end anastomosis, while a long-segment defect usually calls for advanced procedures and additional materials to reconstruct the continuity of injured ureter [1, 10]. Tissue lined with urothelium may be the ideal material for ureteral reconstruction [1]. The reasons are associated with the characteristics of urothelial lining, including no reabsorption of ingredients of urine and no mucus secretion that may cause infection and lithogenesis. In brief, the urothelial lining can maintain the normal physiological functions of the ureter. The technique of a Boari flap is a classical example [3].

By contrast, intestinal or ileal substitution was regarded as the most accepted procedure for long-segment ureteral reconstruction so far. The advantages include adequate substitutive material and available blood supply for long-segment reconstruction [11]. However, it also involves numerous postoperative complications [12]. The absorptive and secretory functions of intestinal mucosa may lead to urine leakage, infection, anastomotic stenosis, lithogenesis, electrolyte and/or acid-base imbalance, and even renal function loss. The oversized caliber may exacerbate hydronephrosis and consequently accelerate impairment of renal function [4–6, 12]. Interference to the gastrointestinal tract can also bring about postoperative problems [12]. The development of the Monti and Mitrofanoff techniques is an

important improvement of intestinal substitution. Some previous studies claimed that the techniques were effective for ureteral replacement with sustained promising long-term results and consequent absence of metabolic complications [7, 8]. On the other hand, some studies reported the postoperative intestinal complications such as ileus and leakage, which called for second operations sometimes [8, 13].

Novel methods using different materials for ureteral reconstruction have been developed, mostly avoiding involvement of intestinal mucosa. An intestinal seromuscular tunnel [1] and a seromuscular tapered ileal tube [10] were reported to form neo-ureter with complete urothelial lining of the inner surface. Previous studies demonstrated that it was feasible to rebuild normal urothelial lining of the reconstructive segment [14, 15]. Moreover, an intestinal seromuscular segment with autograft of bladder mucosa was also proved applicable for ureteral reconstruction [16]. However, demucosalized intestinal segments may be complicated by shrinkage and regrowth of original gastrointestinal epithelium [17]. The efficacy of modified methods using intestinal segments demand further investigation. An autologous graft of granulation tissue capsule was also mentioned as a new material for ureteral substitution [12].

Recently, a spiral bladder muscle flap with vascular pedicles was designed to reconstruct full-length ureteral defects in 6 patients [2]. This procedure can avoid complex preoperative preparation and metabolic complications caused by intestinal substitution. It was claimed that the procedure can retain peristaltic function of bladder smooth muscle and consequently prevent dilation, fluid accumulation and lithogenensis. However, the authors also noted that kidney descent and fixation and a psoas hitch should be performed simultaneously to improve the success rate. Furthermore, preservation of superior vesical arteries required extremely subtle surgical techniques, which may lead to increased postoperative complications and limited popularization.

Considering its good compliance for the experimental surgery and resistance to infection, we selected beagles to establish the animal model. In our study, the gross examination and the urography identified that the neo-ureters were patent, only with mild hydronephrosis, which probably resulted from urine reflux due to the ureteral stent. The microscopic examination proved that the tapered bladder grafts were survivable without a vessel pedicle. Partial loss of urothelial lining, which was quite slight and local, may result from the retrograde catheterization and instillation of the contrast agent. The intact basement membrane allowed the healing of urothelium and thus avoided ureteral stenosis. Based on our histologic findings, we supposed that the nutrient vessels from periureteral connective tissue were sufficient to nourish the graft. Theoretically, the tapering procedure can reduce the volume of the graft tissue, and consequently decrease the nutrient demand. Meanwhile, it can create a raw surface of smooth muscle, cause inflammatory exudation and thus increase nutrient vessels and attachment between the graft and peripheral connective tissue. Our preliminary experience implied that a tapered non-vascularized bladder graft was a novel possible substitute material for ureteral reconstruction.

Another concern arose from the different capacity of bladder between the animal model and human beings. According to the previous studies, a 10-kg-heavy dog has a bladder capacity of approximately 40–70 ml [18, 19], while an adult human being has 300–500 ml. Comparatively, the beagles and human beings have a similar bladder capacity with respect to their own weight. Alteration of micturition rhythm was not observed in the animals, which indicated that the bladder capacity was not apparently influenced by the procedure. There was no concern about the application of our procedure for ureteral reconstruction in human beings.

The potential clinical application of this procedure is reconstruction of defect and stricture in upper and mid-ureter, for which a psoas hitch or a Boari flap is unsuitable. The bladder has sufficient substituted material for required length of the neo-ureter. However, the primary limitations of our study were a small sample size and a short-term follow-up. Therefore, the efficacy and safety of this procedure must be confirmed by a larger sample size and longer postoperative follow-up assessments.

Conclusion

Reconstruction of ureteral defect and stricture maintains a troublesome problem for urologists. Additional to the traditional intestinal substitution, a number of new procedures and materials have been developed for ureteral reconstruction. Our findings showed that it was anatomically possible to use a tapered non-vascularized bladder graft for ureteral reconstruction in the experimental animal model. In consideration of the limitations of our study, further investigations with a larger sample size are expected to evaluate the long-term functional efficacy and safety.

Acknowledgements
There were no particular people or institutions to be acknowledged during this study.

Funding
This study was funded by the National Natural Science Foundation of China, No.81400705 and the National Basic Research Program of China (973 Program), No.2015CB943003.

Authors' contributions
HJ and QD conceived and designed the study. Surgical operation was conducted by SM, LZo, SL, LZh and HJ. Histological examination was done by TY and YH. LZo drafted and wrote the manuscript, and HJ provided critical review. All authors read and approved the final manuscript.

Competing interests
The authors declare that they have no competing interests.

References
1. Hodjati H, Paidar JK, Kumar PV, Johari HG. Intestinal seromuscular tunneling: a novel method for ureteral replacement-an experimental design. Int Urol Nephrol. 2015;47(8):1351–5.
2. Li Y, Li C, Yang S, Song C, Liao W, Xiong Y. Reconstructing full-length ureteral defects using a spiral bladder muscle flap with vascular pedicles. Urology. 2014;83(5):1199–204.
3. Stein R, Rubenwolf P, Ziesel C, Kamal MM, Thuroff JW. Psoas hitch and Boari flap ureteroneocystostomy. BJU Int. 2013;112(1):137–55.
4. Jednak R, Schimke CM, Barroso UJ, Barthold JS, Gonzalez R. Further experience with seromuscular colocystoplasty lined with urothelium. J Urol. 2000;164(6):2045–9.
5. Jednak R, Schimke CM, Ludwikowski B, Gonzalez R. Seromuscular colocystoplasty. BJU Int. 2001;88(7):752–6.
6. Kaefer M, Tobin MS, Hendren WH, Bauer SB, Peters CA, Atala A, Colodny AH, Mandell J, Retik AB. Continent urinary diversion: the Children's hospital experience. J Urol. 1997;157(4):1394–9.
7. Ali-el-Dein B, Ghoneim MA. Bridging long ureteral defects using the Yang-Monti principle. J Urol. 2003;169(3):1074–7.
8. Castellan M, Gosalbez R. Ureteral replacement using the Yang-Monti principle: long-term follow-up. Urology. 2006;67(3):476–9.
9. Bakari AA, Gadam IA, Aliyu S, Suleiman I, Ahidjo AA, Pindiga UH. Use of mitrofanoff and yang-monti techniques as ureteric substitution for severe schistosomal bilateral ureteric stricture: a case report and review of the literature. Niger J Surg. 2012;18(1):30–3.

10. Ibrahim ME, Ezzat MM, Ezzat WM. The use of seromuscular tapered ileal tube in ureteral replacement: an experimental model. Int Urol Nephrol. 2010;42(3):697–701.

11. Shokeir AA, Ghoneim MA. Further experience with the modified ileal ureter. J Urol. 1995;154(1):45–8.

12. Zhang J, GL G, Liu GH, Jiang JT, Xia SJ, Sun J, Zhu YJ, Zhu J. Ureteral reconstruction using autologous tubular grafts for the management of ureteral strictures and defects: an experimental study. Urol Int. 2012;88(1):60–5.

13. Maigaard T, Kirkeby HJ. Yang-Monti ileal ureter reconstruction. Scandinavian journal of urology. 2015;49(4):313–8.

14. Kuzaka B, Szymanska K, Borkowski A, Krus S. Restoration of the continuity of dog ureter after resection of its 5 cm middle segment. Br J Urol. 1996;77(3):342–6.

15. Kaefer M, Hendren WH, Bauer SB, Goldenblatt P, Peters CA, Atala A, Retik AB. Reservoir calculi: a comparison of reservoirs constructed from stomach and other enteric segments. J Urol. 1998;160(6 Pt 1):2187–90.

16. Zou J, Huang X, Su X, Lv D, Liao Y, Gong B, Qiu M. Experimental study on reconstruction of ureter by intestinal sero-muscular segment with autograft of bladder mucosa. Zhongguo xiu fu chong jian wai ke za zhi = Zhongguo xiufu chongjian waike zazhi = Chinese journal of reparative and reconstructive surgery. 2010;24(5):594–8.

17. Heaney JA, Althausen AF, Parkhurst EC. Ileal conduit undiversion: experience with tunneled vesical implantation of tapered conduit. J Urol. 1980;124(3):329–33.

18. Geisse AL, Lowry JE, Schaeffer DJ, Smith CW. Sonographic evaluation of urinary bladder wall thickness in normal dogs. Vet Radiol Ultrasound. 1997;38(2):132–7.

19. Atalan G, Barr FJ, Holt PE. Estimation of bladder volume using ultrasonographic determination of cross-sectional areas and linear measurements. Vet Radiol Ultrasound. 1998;39(5):446–50.

13

Heterogeneity in high-risk prostate cancer treated with high-dose radiation therapy and androgen deprivation therapy

Daniel N. Cagney[1*], Mary Dunne[1,2], Carmel O'Shea[1,2], Marie Finn[1,2], Emma Noone[1,2], Martina Sheehan[1,2], Lesley McDonagh[1,2], Lydia O'Sullivan[1,2], Pierre Thirion[1] and John Armstrong[1,2]

Abstract

Background: Our aim was to assess the heterogeneity of high-risk (HR) prostate cancer managed with high-dose external beam radiotherapy (EBRT) with androgen deprivation therapy (ADT).

Methods: We identified 547 patients who were treated with modern EBRT from 1997 to 2013, of whom 98% received ADT. We analyzed biochemical relapse-free survival (bRFS) and distant metastases-free survival (DMFS).

Results: Median EBRT dose was 74 Gy, and median ADT duration was 8 months. At 5 years, the DMFS was 85%. On multivariate analysis, significant predictors of shorter bRFS were biopsy Gleason score (bGS) of 8 to 10, higher prostate-specific antigen (PSA) level, shorter duration of ADT and lower radiation dose while predictors of shorter DMFS were bGS of 8 to 10, higher PSA level, and lower radiation dose. We identified an unfavorable high-risk (UHR) group of with 2–3 HR factors based on 2015 National Comprehensive Cancer Network (NCCN) criteria and a favorable high-risk (FHR) group, with 1 HR feature. Comparing very-HR prostate cancer, UHR & FHR, 5 year bRFS rates were 58.2%, 66.2%, and 69.2%, and 5 year DMFS rates were 78.4%, 81.2%, and 88.0%.

Conclusion: Patients with multiple HR factors have worse outcome than patients with 1 HR factor. Future studies should account for this heterogeneity in HR prostate cancer.

Background

Risk stratifying newly diagnosed prostate cancer aids physicians and patients to choose an optimal management approach. The most widely used classification system for prostate cancer was developed in 1998 [1] and this has been adapted by the National Comprehensive Cancer Network (NCCN) [2]. High-risk prostate cancer is defined by the 2015 NCCN guidelines as biopsy Gleason Score (bGS) of 8 to 10, or prostate-specific antigen (PSA) concentration of >20 ng/ml, or clinical stage T3a [2]. Patients with multiple intermediate risk factors (for example, a bGS of 7 and PSA of 10–20 ng/ml) may also be considered for management similar to patients with high-risk disease [2, 3]. This risk stratification scheme was originally based on biochemical outcomes of patients treated with standard

doses of external beam radiation therapy (EBRT) in the order of 70 Gy or less [1].

A current standard of care for the management of high-risk disease is radiation dose escalation combined with androgen deprivation therapy (ADT). This combination has shown improvement in rates of biochemical failure and distant metastases compared to standard dose radiation alone [4–8]. It remains unclear whether the original high-risk definition based on biochemical outcomes remains applicable to patients treated in this manner for more clinically relevant endpoints of distant metastases and prostate cancer-specific mortality.

Although most high-risk prostate cancer patients fare well after curative therapy, a subgroup of patients still succumbs to their disease despite aggressive treatment. Therefore, there is a need to revisit our classification system and attempt to better stratify patients within this heterogeneous disease. The aim of our study was to sub-stratify high-risk prostate cancer patients treated

* Correspondence: danielcagney@yahoo.com
[1]Department of Radiation Oncology, St. Luke's Radiation Oncology Network, Highfield Road Rathgar, Dublin, Ireland
Full list of author information is available at the end of the article

with high-dose, image-guided, conformal radiation therapy and androgen deprivation into prognostic subgroups using combinations of accepted risk factors.

Methods

Using prospectively gathered data from our six prostate cancer clinical trials (ICORG 97–01, ICORG 02–01, ICORG 05–04, ICORG 06–15, ICORG 06–16, ICORG 08–17,) we identified 547 patients who were treated with definitive EBRT (≥70Gy) at the St Luke's Radiation Oncology Network from 1997 to 2013.

Routine workup included history and physical examination and digital rectal examination. Patients with distant or nodal metastatic disease as identified on bone scans or CT scans of the abdomen and pelvis were excluded. All patients were treated with either high-dose three-dimensional conformal radiotherapy or intensity-modulated RT (IMRT). Radiotherapy was delivered in accordance with trial protocol (e.g. for 05–03 and 06–15 it was as per institutional policy; for 06–16 and 08–17 the clinical target volume included the prostate and seminal vesicles, and for 97–01 and 02–01 the clinical target volume included the prostate and seminal vesicles, and the planning target volume encompassed the clinical target volume with a margin of 1 cm). The pelvic lymph nodes were not electively irradiated. No patient received a brachytherapy boost. All radiation treatment was delivered with image guidance per trial protocol.

Androgen deprivation therapy (ADT) was used in 98% of patients, with a luteinizing hormone-releasing hormone agonist given before and/or concurrently with and after EBRT. The use of an additional oral non-steroidal anti-androgen and the total duration of ADT were either prescribed by the trial protocol or left to the discretion of the treating physician. Patients were routinely followed with serum PSA testing at least every 6 months, and metastatic workup was initiated only if clinically indicated.

Statistical analyses

Biochemical failure was calculated using the nadir PSA plus 2 ng/ml definition [9]. The percentage of biopsy cores positive for prostate cancer and the pre-treatment PSA velocity were not available for all patients and were not included in this analysis. BRFS (time to any event including biochemical relapse, irrespective of cause, except for any second primary cancers) and DMFS (time to lymph node/ bone/ distant soft tissue metastasis or death from any cause) were defined as the time from the start of RT to date of event or the date of last follow-up if there was no event.

The Kaplan-Meier method was used to estimate bRFS and DMFS [10]. The Cox proportional hazards model] was used to assess the impact of potential explanatory variables on survival times [11]. These included clinical stage (T1b- T2a, T2b-T2c and T3a), PSA (continuous), bGS (≤6, 7, 8–10), duration of ADT (continuous and stratified by ≤6 months vs. >6 months), and radiation dose (continuous). The log-rank test was used to compare differences in survival. All statistical tests were two-sided and assessed for significance at the 0.05 level. Statistical analyses were carried out using IBM® SPSS® statistical software version 22.

Four subgroups were defined: (1) two to three NCCN Intermediate risk factors (n = 104); (2) one NCCN High risk factor (n = 225); (3) two to three NCCN High risk factors (n = 92); (4) NCCN very high risk factor (n = 126). Subgroups (2 and 3) were then split into two dichotomous groups based on 5-year DMFS rates, either above or below the median DMFS rate for all patients, to define a favourable high-risk (FHR) cohort and an unfavourable high-risk (UHR) cohort of high-risk prostate cancer. These groups were then compared to the very high-risk group for bRFS and DMFS.

Results

For the 547 patients, the median age was 68 years old (range, 46–83 years old), the median baseline PSA was 14.5 ng/ml (range, 0.6–263 ng/ ml), and 27% of patients had a bGS of 8 to 10. The median EBRT dose to the planning target volume was 74 Gy (range, 70–81 Gy) in 2Gy/ fraction biologically equivalent doses, and IMRT was used with 21% of all patients. Overall, 98% of men received ADT for a median duration of 8 months and a mean duration of 15 months (range, 2–72 months).

The median follow-up was 62.3 months (range, 0–183.7 months). For the entire study cohort, the 2-year bRFS rate was 87%, the 2-year and 5-year DMFS rates were 95% and 85%.

On univariate analysis for all patients, using Cox proportional hazards regression, statistically significant predictors of longer bRFS were T stage (T1b-T2a and T2b-T2c versus T3b-T4), PSA level at randomisation, duration of ADT, and radiation dose (Table 1). T3a stage did not predict for longer bRFS than T-stages T3b–T4. BGS (<7, 7, 8–10) was not a statistically significant predictor of bRFS but was retained in the multivariate model because of its clinical significance. A bGS <7 and =7 (vs. 8–10; $p < .0005$ and $p = .010$ respectively), PSA level ($p < .0005$), duration of ADT (continuous; $p = .017$), and radiation dose ($p < .0005$) were significant predictors for longer bRFS on multivariate analysis. T-stage did not remain significant in the presence of the other variables ($p = .112$).

On univariate analysis, statistically significant predictors of longer DMFS were low PSA level, and higher radiation dose (Table 1). Shorter duration of ADT, T-stage (grouped), and bGS (grouped) were not statistically

Table 1 Univariate and multivariate analysis of risk factors for bRFS and DMFS

Risk factor	Reference category	Univariate analysis			Multivariate analysis		
		HR	95% CI	p	HR	95% CI	p
bRFS							
T-stage	T3b-T4			0.047			0.112
T1b-T2a		0.64	0.43–0.94	0.025	0.653	0.44–0.98	0.038
T2b-T2c		0.60	0.39–0.91	0.016	0.672	0.43–1.04	0.075
T3a		0.76	0.53–1.09	0.134	0.91	0.63–1.30	0.608
PSA		1.01	1.01–1.02	<.0005	1.015	1.01–1.02	<0.0005
Gleason score	GS > 7			0.148			<0.0005
< 7		0.68	0.46–1.00	0.053	0.349	0.23–0.53	<0.0005
= 7		0.83	0.58–1.19	0.307	0.604	0.41–0.89	0.010
ADT duration (continuous)		0.97	0.96–0.99	0.001	0.979	0.96–1.00	0.017
Radiation dose		0.83	0.77–0.89	<0.0005	0.859	0.79–0.93	<0.0005
DMFS							
T-stage	T3b-T4			0.204			0.272
T1b-T2a		0.62	0.37–1.02	0.061	0.634	0.38–1.06	0.081
T2b-T2c		0.65	0.38–1.11	0.117	0.695	0.40–1.22	0.204
T3a		0.84	0.54–1.29	0.424	0.916	0.59–1.42	0.694
PSA		1.01	1.00–1.02	0.004	1.009	1.00–1.01	0.011
Gleason score	GS > 7			0.137			0.013
< 7		0.61	0.37–0.99	0.047	0.482	0.29–0.79	0.004
= 7		0.77	0.49–1.21	0.254	0.730	0.46–1.17	0.189
ADT duration (continuous)		0.99	0.97–1.01	0.366			
Radiation dose		0.86	0.78–0.95	0.004	0.853	0.77–0.95	0.003

Abbreviations: *bRFS* biochemical relapse-free survival, *CI* confidence interval, *DMFS* distant metastases-free survival

significant predictors of DMFS, but T-stage (grouped) and bGS (grouped) were retained in the multivariate model because of their clinical significance. A bGS <7 (vs. 8–10; p = .004), low PSA level (p = .011), and higher radiation dose (p = .003) were significant predictors for longer DMFS on multivariate analysis. T-stage (p = .272) was not a significant predictor of DMFS.

Kaplan-Meier curves were generated, and 5-year DMFS rates were calculated for each of the four subgroups (Fig. 1, Table 2). These patients were then split into two dichotomous groups (1) FHR: 1 high risk factor (n = 225); and (2) UHR (n = 92): 2–3 high risk factors. The patient and treatment characteristics of these high-risk cohorts are listed in Table 3. The median duration of ADT use was 8 and 13.5 respectively. The estimated 2-year rates of bRFS were 91.6% and 78.8%, respectively for FHR and UHR. The 5 year bRFS rates were 69.2%, 66.2% and 58.2%, respectively, for FHR, UHR and very-high risk groups. The 2-year rates of DMFS were 96.5% and 93.0%, respectively, for FHR and UHR (Table 4). The 5-year rates of DMFS were 88.0% and 81.2% respectively, for FHR and UHR. The estimated 10-year rates of DMFS were 66.7% and 54.5%

respectively, for FHR and UHR. These results are graphically shown in Fig. 2. The estimated 5 and 10-year rates of DMFS for the very high-risk group were 78.4% and 57.4% respectively. On Cox proportional hazards regression analysis, There was a trend to shorter distant metastasis free survival for UHR than for FHR patients (p = 0.097). The median DMFS was not yet reached for the FHR group compared to 10.9 years for the UHR group. (Fig. 2) On Cox proportional hazards regression analysis, there was a trend towards a higher risk of biochemical relapse and distant metastasis for UHR than for FHR patients (Table 5). The estimated hazards or risks of biochemical relapse and distant metastasis increases by 1.4 and 1.5 times, respectively, for those with UHR compared to those with FHR.

Discussion
Numerous definitions of high-risk prostate cancer exist [1, 12–16]. Lack of clarity and consensus on a single precise definition represents a potential barrier for patient-specific counselling and comparative assessment of different treatment modalities.

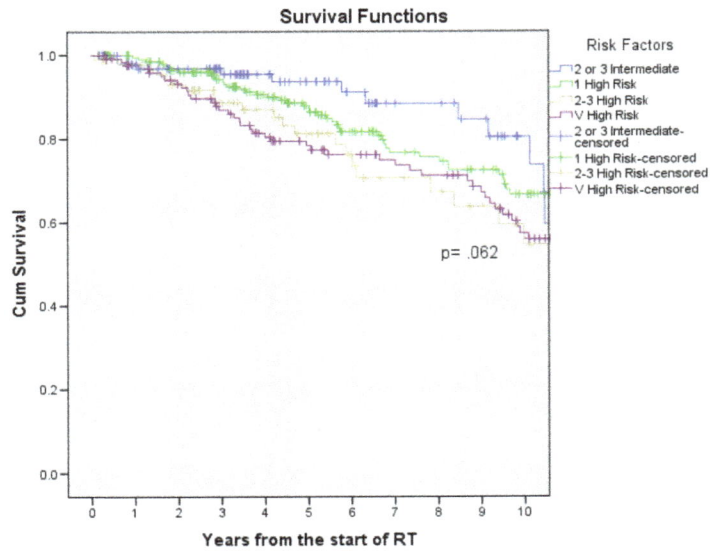

Fig. 1 Kaplan-Meier curves of distant metastases-free survival by high-risk subgroup. Abbreviations: C = censored; O = observed; N = number

The optimal treatment for men with high-risk disease remains debatable, although treatment options include surgery, radiation, and/or ADT [4–8, 17–21]. Currently regardless of the treatment used, there is significant heterogeneity in outcomes from high-risk prostate cancer [18–25]. One potential way to overcome this heterogenity, is by defining high risk by adding several high-risk factors.

This study sought to report on the outcomes of patients with high-risk prostate cancer treated on prospective clinical trials. Numerous randomized trials

have established the combination of EBRT and ADT as one of the standards of care for treating high- risk prostate cancer [4–6, 26, 27]. The optimal duration of hormone therapy remains unknown. However, many trials have shown superior outcomes with a longer duration of ADT [6, 28]. The majority of these earlier clinical trials establishing the value of ADT, used suboptimal radiation doses, typically in the order of 70 Gy [8, 19–21]. Currently, delivery of high-dose EBRT in high-risk prostate cancer is standard of care [4–8].

In our analysis we included patients with multiple intermediate factors as per NCCN criteria, these could be managed as high-risk disease [2]. We felt that they would also act as a good comparative arm for patients with high-risk and very high-risk factors. We sought to incorporate several high-risk factors to help potentially distinguish distinct subgroups within high-risk prostate cancer. We found that a high GS of 8 to 10, higher PSA level and lower radiation dose were significant predictors of shorter DMFS on multivariate analyses. T stage at diagnosis did not predict distant metastasis-free survival. Looking at bRFS high GS of 8 to 10, higher PSA level,

Table 2 5-year rates of DMFS by sub-group

Sub-group	Number of patients	5-year DMFS (%)	95% CI
All patients	421	87.8	84.1–91.5
2–3 Intermediate risk factors	104	93.7	88.2–99.2
1 High risk factor	225	88.0	83.1–92.9
2–3 High risk factors	92	81.2	71.6–90.8
V High Risk	126	78.4	70.8–86.0

Abbreviations: *CI* confidence interval, *DMFS* distant metastases-free survival

Table 3 Patient and treatment characteristics by high-risk cohort

Characteristic	All patients (n = 547)		FHR (n = 225)		UHR (n = 92)		vHigh Risk (n = 126)		FHR vs. UHR p-value
		%		%		%		%	
Age (years)									
Median	67.0		67.4		68.4		67.2		278
Range	46–83		47–83		46–80		48–81		
T Stage (no.)									<.0005
T1b–T2a	132	24	78	35	10	11	0	0	
T2b–T2c	121	22	51	23	10	11	0	0	
T3a	168	31	96	43	72	78	0	0	
T3b-T4	126	23	0	0	0	0	126	100	
PSA (µg/L)									<.0005
Median	14.5		14.1		22.5		14.9		
Mean	20.2		18.3		31.2		21.9		
Range	0.6–263		0.6–69		1.8–263		1.2–127		
PSA Group (no.)									<.0005
< 10 µg/L (no.)		28		33		17	37	29	
10–20 µg/L	151	38	74	34	16	10	44	35	
(no.)	209	34	76	33	9	73	45	36	
≥ 20 µg/L (no.)	187		75		67				
Gleason Score (No.)									<.0005
<7	147	27	80	36	11	12	50	40	
=7	250	46	91	40	24	26	37	29	
>7	150	27	54	24	57	62	39	31	
Radiation dose									
Median (Gy)	74.0		74.0		74.0		70.0		.082
Radiation technique									.123
3D–CRT	432	79	170	76	61	66	112	89	
IMRT	115	21	55	24	31	34	14	11	
Duration of ADT									
Median (months)	8.0		8.0		13.5		8.0		.102
Mean (months)	14.9		16.4		20.8		13.7		
Range (months)	0–72		0–53		4–72		0–68		
Duration of ADT (no)									
None (no.)	11	2	4	2	0	0	1	1	
1–6 months (no.)	181	32	69	31	24	26	44	35	
7–12 months (no.)	195	34	74	33	22	24	50	40	
13–24 months (no.)	10	2	3	1	4	4	2	2	
>24 months (no.)	150	29	75	33	42	46	29	23	

Abbreviations: *FHR* favourable high risk, *UHR* unfavourable high risk, *PSA* prostate-specific antigen, *ADT* androgen deprivation therapy, *3D–CRT* three dimensional conformal radiotherapy, *IMRT* intensity-modulated radiation therapy

lower radiation dose & shorter duration of ADT were significant predictors of shorter bRFS on multivariate analyses.

By doing this, we demonstrated the marked heterogeneity in this disease. Our data suggest that there may be two dichotomous subgroups of high-risk patients. One group with one high-risk factor, whose 5 year DMFS outcomes are similar to the intermediate risk prostate cancer group, may have excellent outcomes with a short duration of ADT and high-dose radiotherapy limited to the prostate and seminal vesicles. On the other hand, patients in the unfavourable high-risk subgroup, patients

Table 4 2-year and 5-year rates of bRFS and DMFS

Sub-group	2-year rate (%)	95% CI	5-year rate (%)	95% CI
bRFS				
FHR	91.6	87.7–95.5	69.2	61.9–76.5
UHR	78.8	70.0–87.6	66.2	54.6–77.8
vHigh Risk	79.4	72.0–86.8	58.2	48.8–67.6
DMFS				
FHR	96.5	94.0–99.0	88.0	83.1–92.9
UHR	93.0	87.5–98.5	81.2	71.6–90.8
vHigh risk	93.2	88.7–97.7	78.4	70.8–86.0

Abbreviations: *bRFS* biochemical relapse-free survival, *CI* confidence interval, *DMFS* distant metastases-free survival

Table 5 Cox proportional hazards regression analysis by high-risk subgroup

End point	Risk-group	Reference category	HR	95% CI	p-value
bRFS	UHR	FHR	1.36	0.89–2.06	0.155
DMFS	UHR	FHR	1.54	0.92–2.57	0.100

Abbreviations: *FHR* favourable high risk, *UHR* unfavourable high risk, *bRFS* biochemical relapse-free survival, *DMFS* distant metastases-free survival, *HR* hazard ratio, *CI* confidence interval

with multiple high-risk features had a poor prognosis despite longer duration of ADT, with risk of metastasis approaching 20% at 5 years. Our results are consistent to outcomes from John Hopkins who reported similar results in a surgical cohort of patients [29] and in patients treated with ADT and high-dose radiotherapy [30]. They identified similar subpopulations of patients with NCCN high-risk men who experienced inferior outcomes following definitive radiation and long-term androgen deprivation therapy (ADT). They noted that the 10-year risk of distant metastasis (DM) of 35%, for

patients with unfavourable high risk disease. This was far worse than NCCN high-risk men whose 10 year risk of distant metastasis (DM) was 13%. Our study adds to this body of evidence with much worse 10-year risk of distant metastasis (DM) in the UHR cohort when compared to the FHR cohort.

Consistent with other reports, a high GS is the strongest driver for bRFS and DMFS (Table 1), particularly when combined with other high-risk factors [3, 21]. Patients with multiple high-risk factors could be ideal candidates for clinical trials investigating more aggressive treatment strategies.

The use of a longer duration of ADT, when given with high-dose radiation, does improve bRFS on multivariate analyses but does not predict DMFS. The median duration of ADT in this study overall was 8 months. Our

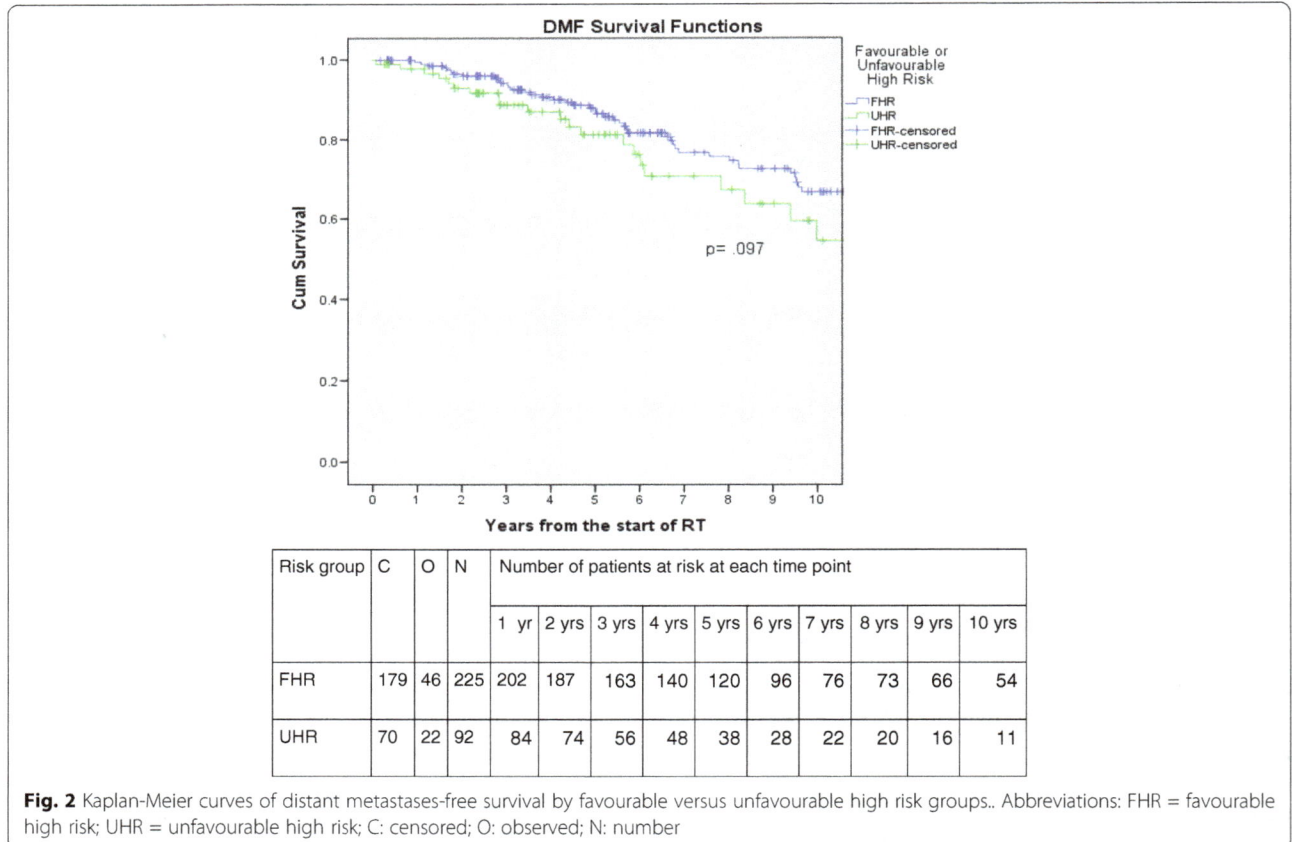

Risk group	C	O	N	Number of patients at risk at each time point									
				1 yr	2 yrs	3 yrs	4 yrs	5 yrs	6 yrs	7 yrs	8 yrs	9 yrs	10 yrs
FHR	179	46	225	202	187	163	140	120	96	76	73	66	54
UHR	70	22	92	84	74	56	48	38	28	22	20	16	11

Fig. 2 Kaplan-Meier curves of distant metastases-free survival by favourable versus unfavourable high risk groups.. Abbreviations: FHR = favourable high risk; UHR = unfavourable high risk; C: censored; O: observed; N: number

findings showing marginal benefit to long term hormones in high risk prostate cancer are consistent with prior publications that have sought to reclassify high-risk prostate cancer [22, 23]. This analysis validates the importance of aggressive local treatment as escalated radiation doses reduce the risk of distant failure consistent with other series [24, 25]. This may have implications for future trial design. Given the lower rate of distant metastasis in the favourable cohort of high-risk prostate cancer, these patients could conceivably be managed in a similar way to unfavourable intermediate risk prostate cancer. Future studies might focus on the unfavourable high-risk prostate cancer group in the design of clinical trials, where a bigger benefit is likely to be seen.

We are aware of the existence of several high-risk definitions. None discriminates accurately between patients who are likely to do well, and patients do worse. We specifically chose to examine the current NCCN high-risk classification because it is widely used and simple in design. We recognize that several clinical factors must be considered when identifying those with an unfavorable prognosis and encourage future studies to incorporate as many predictive markers as possible to better define the high-risk population.

Our study has successfully demonstrated an ability to stratify high-risk prostate cancer into a favorable and unfavourable subgroup. Our favourable subgroup has 5 year DMFS outcomes comparable to unfavourable intermediate risk prostate cancer, and our unfavourable high-risk group have outcomes more in line with very high-risk disease, a cohort which received lower radiation dose and a shorter duration of ADT. Our findings might help to direct future clinical trial design and may help personalize care for individual patients. There are a number of current studies with preliminary results which are specifically looking patients with high risk disease to see if the addition of brachytherapy or enzalutamide may optimize disease control [31, 32].

These results highlight the heterogeneity within high-risk prostate cancer. This is one of the first series from Europe in patients with high-risk prostate cancer treated with radiotherapy that has sought to sub-classify high-risk disease. Other series have been in high-risk prostate cancer patients managed surgically. Three studies have shown that the presence of more high-risk features may predict for worse cancer-specific outcomes among patients with high-risk prostate cancer treated with radical prostatectomy suggesting that there is an additive effect from each individual risk factors [17, 18]. Some North American studies looking at patients with high-risk disease treated with ADT and RT, one of which validated their data against the SEER database, have also managed to sub-classify high-risk disease [22, 23]. However a

significant strength of our study was that we used data from six clinical trials which was prospectively gathered.

There are limitations to our study. First, our results are based on a secondary analysis of the combined data from 6 prostate cancer clinical trials and should be interpreted cautiously. Second, our outcomes in the unfavourable high-risk group are similar to patients in the very high-risk group. However this is in an era before the use of MRI staging, so there may be significant stage migration in a more modern cohort. Finally, picking 5 year DMFS rates as the cut-off may be arbitrary or may mask other salvage treatments.

We await further prospective evaluations for high-risk patients, and encourage future studies to consider the wide heterogeneity in this cohort. Several biomarkers are under investigation as predictive tools but none is clinically available yet, and it remains to be seen how these will translate into the management of patients with prostate cancer [33]. Novel radiographic techniques and molecular markers which help predict relapse following treatment are needed to help us more accurately direct individualised treatment. Until such markers exist, additional clinical information from prostate biopsy, pretreatment PSA velocity, and radiographic findings from endorectal MRI may help to predict better and enable more accurate discrimination between the different risk groups.

Conclusion

In summary, high-risk prostate cancer is a widely heterogeneous disease. In patients treated with high dose radiotherapy and ADT, bGS, PSA level, duration of ADT, and radiation dose were significant predictors for bRFS after adjustment for the effects of the other covariates. With the exception of duration of ADT, these variables were also predictive for DMFS. We identified an unfavorable group of high-risk prostate cancer patients, similar to those with very high-risk disease, with significantly shorter times to distant metastases than the favourable high risk group. We encourage future clinical trials to consider the marked heterogeneity in this disease.

Acknowledgements

D. N. Cagney acknowledges contribution made by Richard Steevens Scholarship 2015 & St. Luke's Institute of Cancer Research Award 2016.

Funding

No Funding for this study. Trials were supervised by ICORG.

Author Contributions

DC, MD, JA – Conceived the study, wrote original manuscript & performed the statistical analysis COS, MF, EN, MS, LMcD, LOS, PT – edited the manuscript, aided in data collection All authors read and approved the final manuscript.

Competing interests

The authors declare that they have no competing interests.

Author details

[1]Department of Radiation Oncology, St. Luke's Radiation Oncology Network, Highfield Road Rathgar, Dublin, Ireland. [2]Clinical Trials Unit, St. Luke's Radiation Oncology Network, Dublin, Ireland.

References

1. D'Amico AV, et al. Biochemical outcome after radical prostatectomy, external beam radiation therapy, or interstitial radiation therapy for clinically localized prostate cancer. JAMA. 1998;280(11):969–74.
2. Prostate, O. and P.A. Washington, National Comprehensive Cancer Network Clinical Practice Guidelines in NCCN, fort. 2015.
3. Tsai HK, et al. Cancer-specific mortality after radiation therapy with short-course hormonal therapy or radical prostatectomy in men with localized, intermediate-risk to high-risk prostate cancer. Cancer. 2006;107(11):2597–603.
4. Bolla M, et al. Long-term results with immediate androgen suppression and external irradiation in patients with locally advanced prostate cancer (an EORTC study): a phase III randomised trial. Lancet (London, England). 2002;360(9327):103–6.
5. Pilepich MV, et al. Androgen suppression adjuvant to definitive radiotherapy in prostate carcinoma–long-term results of phase III RTOG 85-31. Int J Radiat Oncol Biol Phys. 2005;61(5):1285–90.
6. Horwitz EM, et al. Ten-year follow-up of radiation therapy oncology group protocol 92-02: a phase III trial of the duration of elective androgen deprivation in locally advanced prostate cancer. J Cli Oncol Off J Am Soc Clin Oncol. 2008;26(15):2497–504.
7. Kuban DA, et al. Long-term results of the M. D. Anderson randomized dose-escalation trial for prostate cancer. Int J Radiat Oncol Biol Physi. 2008;70(1):67–74.
8. Zelefsky MJ, et al. Long-term results of conformal radiotherapy for prostate cancer: impact of dose escalation on biochemical tumor control and distant metastases-free survival outcomes. Int J Radiat Oncol Biol Phys. 2008;71(4):1028–33.
9. Roach M, et al. Defining biochemical failure following radiotherapy with or without hormonal therapy in men with clinically localized prostate cancer: recommendations of the RTOG-ASTRO phoenix consensus conference. Int J Radiat Oncol Biol Phys. 2006;65(4):965–74.
10. Kaplan EL, Meier P, Am J. Nonparametric estimation from incomplete observations. Stat Assoc. 1958;53:457–81. SRC - GoogleScholar
11. Cox DR, Roy J. Regression models and life tables. Stats Soc. 1972;34: 187–220. SRC - GoogleScholar
12. Thompson I, et al. Guideline for the management of clinically localized prostate cancer: 2007 update. J Urol. 2007;177(6):2106–31.
13. Roach M, et al. Four prognostic groups predict long-term survival from prostate cancer following radiotherapy alone on radiation therapy oncology group clinical trials. Int J Radiat Oncol Biol Phys. 2000;47(3):609–15.
14. Roach M, et al. Defining high risk prostate cancer with risk groups and nomograms: implications for designing clinical trials. J Urol. 2006;176(6 Pt 2):S16–20.
15. Huang J, et al. Percentage of positive biopsy cores: a better risk stratification model for prostate cancer? Int J Radiat Oncol Biol Phys. 2012;83(4):1141–8.
16. Cooperberg MR, et al. The University of California, san Francisco cancer of the prostate risk assessment score: a straightforward and reliable preoperative predictor of disease recurrence after radical prostatectomy. J Urol. 2005;173(6):1938–42.
17. Walz J, et al. Pathological results and rates of treatment failure in high-risk prostate cancer patients after radical prostatectomy. BJU Int. 2011;107(5):765–70.
18. Spahn M, et al. Outcome predictors of radical prostatectomy in patients with prostate-specific antigen greater than 20 ng/ml: a European multi-institutional study of 712 patients. Eur Urol. 2010;58(1):1–7. discussion 10
19. Zietman AL, et al. Comparison of conventional-dose vs high-dose conformal radiation therapy in clinically localized adenocarcinoma of the prostate: a randomized controlled trial. JAMA. 2005;294(10):1233–9.
20. Al-Mamgani A, et al. Update of Dutch multicenter dose-escalation trial of radiotherapy for localized prostate cancer. Int J Radiat Oncol Biol Phys. 2008;72(4):980–8.
21. Nanda A, et al. Gleason pattern 5 prostate cancer: further stratification of patients with high-risk disease and implications for future randomized trials. Int J Radiat Oncol Biol Phys. 2009;74(5):1419–23.
22. Tendulkar RD, et al. Redefining high-risk prostate cancer based on distant metastases and mortality after high-dose radiotherapy with androgen deprivation therapy. Int J Radiat Oncol Biol Phys. 2012;82(4):1397–404.
23. Muralidhar V, et al. Definition and validation of "favorable high-risk prostate cancer": implications for personalizing treatment of radiation-managed patients. Int Oncol Biol Phys 93. 2015;4:828–35. SRC - GoogleScholar
24. Cahlon O, et al. Ultra-high dose (86.4 Gy) IMRT for localized prostate cancer: toxicity and biochemical outcomes. Int J Radiat Oncol Biol Phys. 2008;71(2):330–7.
25. Liauw SL, et al. Dose-escalated radiotherapy for high-risk prostate cancer: outcomes in modern era with short-term androgen deprivation therapy. Int J Radiat Oncol Biol Phys. 2010;77(1):125–30.
26. Amico A V D', Manola J, Loffredo M. 6-month androgen suppression plus radiation therapy vs radiation therapy alone for patients with clinically localized prostate cancer a randomized controlled trial. JAMA. 2004;292: 821–7. SRC-GoogleScholar
27. Bolla M, et al. Duration of androgen suppression in the treatment of prostate cancer. The New England J Med. 2009;360(24):2516–27.
28. Dearnaley DP, et al. Escalated-dose versus standard-dose conformal radiotherapy in prostate cancer: first results from the MRC RT01 randomised controlled trial. Lancet Oncol. 2007;8(6):475–87.
29. Sundi, et al. Very-high-risk localized prostate cancer: definition and outcomes. Prostate Cancer Prostatic Dis. 2014;17(1 SRC-GoogleScholar):57–63.
30. Narang AK, et al. Very high-risk localized prostate cancer: outcomes following definitive radiation. Int J Radiat Oncol Biol Phys. 2016;94(2):254–62.
31. Morris MJ, et al. Radiographic progression-free survival as a response biomarker in metastatic castration-resistant prostate cancer: COU-AA-302 results. J Clin Oncol: Official J Am Soc Clin Oncol. 2015;33(12):1356–63.
32. Williams SG, et al. Randomised phase 3 trial of enzalutamide in androgen deprivation therapy (ADT) with radiation therapy for clinically localised high-risk or node-positive prostate cancer: ENZARAD (ANZUP 1303). 2016;TPS5086-TPS5086.
33. Roach M, Waldman F, Pollack A. Predictive models in external beam radiotherapy for clinically localized prostate cancer. Cancer. 2009;115(13 Suppl):3112–20.

The usefulness of flexible cystoscopy for preventing double-J stent malposition after laparoscopic ureterolithotomy

Jae-Yoon Kim, Seok-Ho Kang, Jun Cheon, Jeong-Gu Lee, Je-Jong Kim and Sung-Gu Kang*

Abstract

Background: The aim of this study was to evaluate the role of flexible cystoscopy in preventing malpositioning of the ureteral stent after laparoscopic ureterolithotomy in male patients.

Methods: From April 2009 to June 2015, 97 male patients with stones >1.8 cm in the upper ureter underwent intracorporeal double-J stenting of the ureter after laparoscopic ureterolithotomy performed by four different surgeons. In the last 50 patients who underwent laparoscopic ureterolithotomy flexible cystoscopy was performed through the urethral route to confirm the position of the double-J stent, while in the first 47 correct positioning of the stent was confirmed through postoperative KUB. The demographic data and perioperative outcomes were reviewed retrospectively. Penalized logistic regression analysis was used to evaluate the effects of flexible cystoscopy.

Results: Upward malpositioning of the ureteral stent was found in 9 of the 47 (19.1%) patients who underwent surgery without flexible cystoscopy. Among the 50 most recent patients who underwent surgery with flexible cystoscopy through the urethral route, upward malpositioning was observed in 10 (20%) patients. The factors preventing upward malpositioning of the double-J catheter in multivariate analysis were surgeon ($p = 0.039$) and use of flexible cystoscopy ($p = 0.008$).

Conclusion: Flexible cystoscopy is a simple, safe, quick, and effective method to identify and correct malpositioning of double-J stents, especially in male patients.

Keywords: Laparoscopy, Stone disease, Ureteral calculus, Ureteral stent

Background

The treatment of large upper ureteral stones is still controversial [1, 2]. The American Urological Association (AUA) and the European Association of Urology (EAU) recommend that laparoscopic stone removal may be considered in rare cases in which shockwave lithotripsy (SWL), ureteroscopic lithotripsy (URS), and percutaneous nephrolithotomy fail or are unlikely to be successful [1–5]. In a recent meta-analysis of treatment of large proximal ureteral stones, Torricelli et al. reported that the outcomes of laparoscopic ureterolithotomy (LUL) for larger upper ureteral stones are favorable compared with

those of URS, and LUL should be considered as a first-line option when flexible ureteroscopy is not available [6]. After such surgery, many surgeons prefer placing a double-J stent, a ureteral catheter that is passed through the ureter from the kidney to the bladder [7, 8]. Although double-J stent placement after LUL remains controversial, many urologists believe that it may help prevent postoperative urinary leakage [9].

Intracorporeal double-J stenting is technically difficult, and malpositioning often occurs after surgery in clinical practice [10]. However, the actual rate of malpositioning of stents has not been reported yet. Although clinicians use different ways to place double-J stents precisely, accurate stent placement before the closure of the ureteral incision might be difficult to confirm.

* Correspondence: kkangsung7@korea.ac.kr
Department of Urology, Korea University College of Medicine, 73 Inchon-Ro, Sungbuk-gu, Seoul 136-705, Republic of Korea

Upward malpositioning of the stent after surgery may necessitate removal of the stent using a ureteroscope. It is difficult to remove stents in the outpatient setting without anesthesia to reduce pain and discomfort, especially in male patients.

In this study, we used flexible cystoscopy through the urethral route before closure of the ureteral incision to confirm that the double-J stent was placed correctly in the bladder of male patients. Upon identification of upward malpositioning of the ureteral stent, position adjustments were performed by intracorporeally manipulating the ureteral stent through the incision site of the ureter. The aim of this study was to determine the malpositioning rate and predicting factors associated with upward malpositioning of intracorporeal double-J stents after LUL and to evaluate the usefulness of flexible cystoscopy in preventing such malpositioning in male patients.

Methods

From April 2009 to June 2015, a total of 97 male patients with large stones (>1.8 cm in size) of the upper ureter underwent LUL. In all patients, intracorporeal double-J stents were placed after surgery. In the first 47 patients, the surgery was finished without verification of double-J stent placement (this was done on postoperative imaging). In the latest 50 consecutive patients, flexible cystoscopy was performed through the urethral route before closure of the ureteral incision to determine whether the double-J stent was correctly placed in the bladder (Fig. 1).

Patient demographic data such as age, height, weight, body mass index, stone level, stone size, degree of hydronephrosis, and previous ureteric procedures were reviewed retrospectively. The levels and sizes of stones were determined using kidney-ureter-bladder (KUB) radiography or computed tomography. The degree of hydronephrosis was determined using a scale from 0 to 4 according to the Society of Fetal Ultrasound grade system [11]. Perioperative data, including surgeon, surgical approach, and use of flexible cystoscopy, were also collected retrospectively. Perioperative outcomes such as operative

time, upward malpositioning rate, and additional time for flexible cystoscopy were reviewed. We defined upward malpositioning as placement of the double-J stent such that its tip is straight instead of being curled on postoperative KUB radiography. Accordingly, we reviewed all postoperative follow-up KUB images.

To identify factors predicting malpositioning, logistic regression analysis was conducted with SPSS, version 22.0. To evaluate the effects of flexible cystoscopy in reducing the malpositioning rate, penalized logistic regression analyses were performed with SAS 9.4, with a $p < 0.05$ considered to represent a statistically significant difference.

Intracorporeal double-J stent insertion after laparoscopic ureterolithotomy

After placing the patient in a semilateral position, a skin and fascial incision was made laterally to the rectus muscle at the level of the umbilicus, and a 10-mm balloon trocar was inserted into the abdominal cavity. Subsequently, with the pneumoperitoneum maintained at 12 mmHg using CO_2, two more trocars (10 and 5 mm) were introduced under laparoscopic view parallel to the first trocar. At the beginning of the procedure, the descending colon was reflected from its retroperitoneal attachment and moved medially to identify the ureter. Each stone was identified as a prominent bulge on a suspicious lesion. To prevent upward movement of the stone, careful dissection was performed while avoiding touching the ureter directly. A needle holder with a broken 15th blade tip was used to incise the ureter overlying the stone, which enabled a sharp, precise ureteral incision at the level of the stone. Subsequently, the stone was removed with a grasper. The ureter was then catheterized using a standard 6F double-J stent with both long and short guidewires inserted through two separate side holes of the stent that were closed at both ends. Then, the prepared stent was inserted in a bidirectional manner through the ureterotomy site, and the two guidewires were extracted.

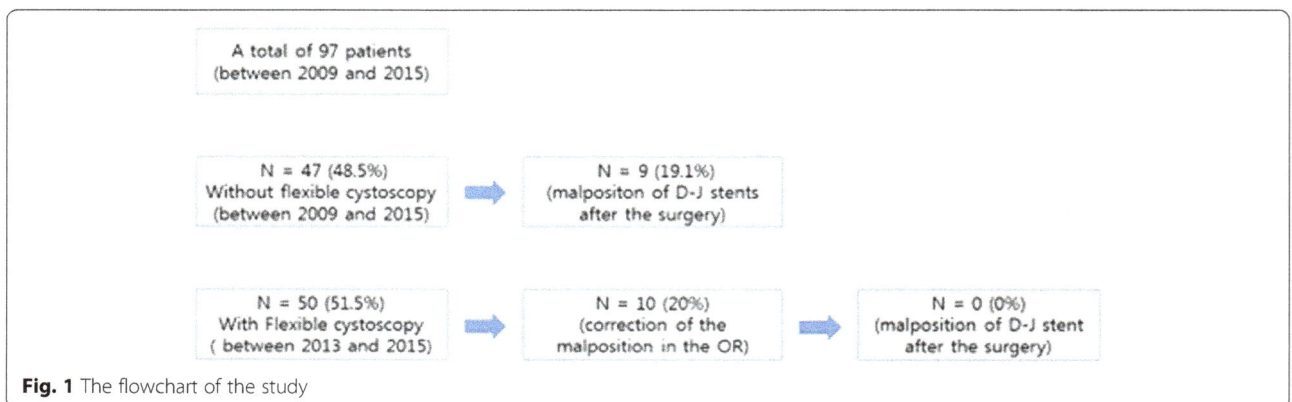

Fig. 1 The flowchart of the study

Laparoscopic adjustment of double-J stent with flexible cystoscopy

From April 2013 to June 2015, the last 50 patients with large upper ureteral stones underwent LUL with flexible cystoscopy to confirm the correct positioning of the double-J stent. After intracorporeal insertion of the double-J catheter, additional endoscopic monitoring with flexible cystoscopy was performed. The surgeon manipulating the double-J catheter used monitor A, while an assistant inserted a flexible cystoscope into the bladder through the urethral route and determined whether the double-J stent was correctly placed in the bladder using monitor B before suturing the site of ureterotomy (Fig. 2). If the stent was well-placed, the flexible cystoscope was withdrawn. If the double-J stent was not visualized in the bladder, the surgeon pushed the stent inferiorly using a laparoscopic instrument and monitor A until the stent came out through the ureteral orifice on monitor B (Additional file 1). After placement of the stent, the ureteral incision was closed with 4–0 Vicryl interrupted sutures.

Results

The preoperative patient demographics are summarized in Table 1. The mean age was 53.46 ± 13.72 years. The mean stone size was 1.87 ± 0.33 cm, and all patients had upper ureteral stones. In 16 (16.5%) cases, the stones were of level L2 or below, whereas in the remaining 81 (83.5%) cases the level exceeded L2. One patient (1%)

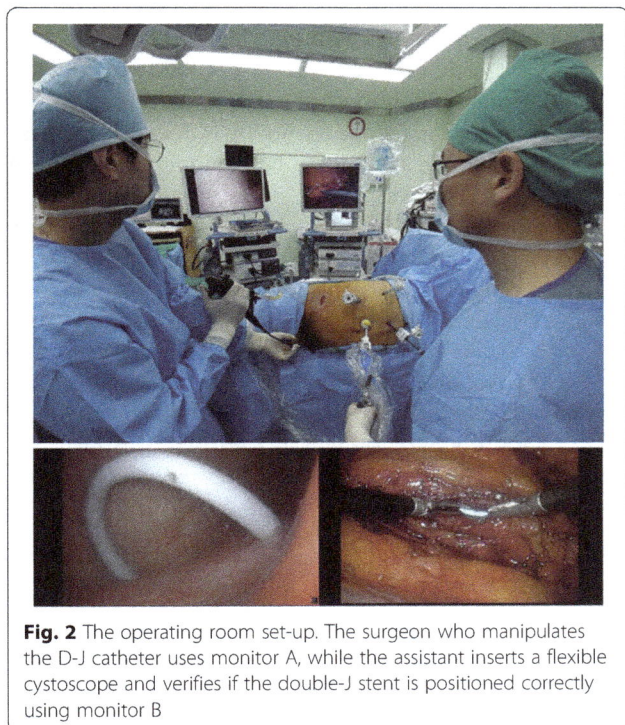

Fig. 2 The operating room set-up. The surgeon who manipulates the D-J catheter uses monitor A, while the assistant inserts a flexible cystoscope and verifies if the double-J stent is positioned correctly using monitor B

Table 1 Patient demographics and clinical characteristics

Variable	Quantity/Value
Age (years)	55 (21–81)
Sex	
Male	97 (100%)
Height (cm)	165.03 ± 10.29 (141–197)
Weight (kg)	68.15 ± 13.17 (38.7–121)
BMI	24.87 ± 3.07 (17.04–32.89)
Stone level	
Upper ureter (groups divided via L2 level)	97 (100%)
L2 level or below	16 (16.5%)
Above L2 level	81 (83.5%)
Stone size (cm)	1.87 ± 0.33 (1.52–2.42)
Degree of hydronephrosis	
Grade 0	1 (1.0%)
Grade 1	26 (26.8%)
Grade 2	39 (40.2%)
Grade 3	17 (17.5%)
Grade 4	14 (14.4%)
Previous history of the ureteral procedure	
None	65 (67.0%)
SWL	23 (23.7%)
URSL	12 (12.4%)

Data are presented as n (%), mean ± SD (range) or median (range)
BMI Body Mass Index, *SWL* Shock Wave Lithotripsy, *URSL* Ureteroscopic Lithotripsy

had hydronephrosis of grade 0, 26 (26.8%) of grade 1, 39 (40.2%) of grade 2, 17 (17.5%) of grade 3, and 14 (14.4%) of grade 4. Medical history review revealed that 23 patients (23.7%) had undergone SWL and 12 patients (12.4%) had undergone URS.

The perioperative data and outcomes are presented in Table 2. The mean operative time was 137.33 ± 52.44 min; 84 patients were treated using the transperitoneal approach and 13 patients using the retroperitoneal approach. The surgeries were performed by four surgeons (40, 26, 20, and 11 cases).

On postoperative KUB radiography, we identified upward malpositioning of ureteral stents in 9 of the 47 (19.1%) patients who underwent surgery without flexible cystoscopy. Among the 50 most recent patients who underwent surgery with flexible cystoscopy through the urethral route, upward malpositioning was identified in 10 (20%). In these 10 patients, the upward malpositioning of the double-J stent was laparoscopically corrected, and there were no patients with upward malpositioning after surgery until the removal of the stents. The mean additional operative time required for flexible cystoscopy was 4 min and 30 s.

In univariate analysis, presence of hydronephrosis ($p = 0.044$) predicted upward malpositioning (Table 3).

Table 2 Perioperative data and outcomes

Variable	Quantity/Value
Operation time (min.)	137 ± 52.44 (45–280)
EBL (ml)	58.6 ± 15.78 (20–90)
Method of surgical approach	
Transperitoneal	84 (86.6%)
Retroperitoneal	13 (13.4%)
Surgeon	
1	40 (41.2%)
2	26 (26.8%)
3	20 (20.6%)
4	11 (11.3%)
Upward malpositioning after surgery without using flexible cystoscopy	9/47 (19.1%)
Flexible cystoscopy use	50/97
Case adjusted by flexible cystoscopy	10/50(20%)
Upward malpositioning after surgery using flexible cystoscope	0/50 (0%)
Mean added time for flexible cystoscopy (min.)	4 min 30s

Data are presented as n (%), mean ± SD (range) or median (range)
EBL Estimated Blood Loss

Table 3 Univariate logistic regression analysis of variables affecting upward malpositioning of ureteral stents (SPSS version 22)

Variable	Odds ratio	95% Confidence Interval	P-value
Age	0.979	0.945–1.015	0.246
Height (cm)	0.991	0.945–1.039	0.706
Weight (kg)	1.010	0.975–1.047	0.584
BMI	1.084	0.923–1.274	0.324
Stone level (groups divided via L2 level)	0.379	0.119–1.205	0.100
Stone size (cm)	1.433	0.533–3.849	0.475
Degree of hydronephrosis			0.044
Previous history of the ureteral procedure	0.567	0.187–1.719	0.316
SWL	0.467	0.124–1.755	0.259
URSL	1.241	0.304–5.064	0.764
Operation time (min.)	1.003	0.994–1.012	0.552
Transperitoneal VS retroperitoneal	2.656	0.766–9.207	0.123
Surgeon type			0.077
2	0.338	0.097–1.176	0.088
3	0.098	0.012–0.809	0.031
4	0.413	0.078–2.180	0.297
Flexible cystoscopy use	0	0	0.997

BMI Body Mass Index, SWL Shock Wave Lithotripsy, URSL Ureteroscopic Lithotripsy

In multivariate penalized logistic regression analysis, surgeon (0.039) and flexible cystoscopy (0.008) were significant factors preventing malpositioning (Table 4).

Discussion

Several modalities are available for the treatment of large upper ureteral stones [12–17]. Although controversial, SWL and URS have been recommended by the AUA and EAU guidelines as the first choice for proximal large ureteral stones, whereas LUL has been used as one of the options in the management of upper urinary tract stones [5, 6]. With regard to the dimension of large proximal ureteral stones, it seems that there is no clear definition. In a recent meta-analysis, Torricelli et al. analyzed six randomized controlled trials for large upper ureteral stones. These six studies used different inclusion criteria in terms of stone size: two studies used 10 mm [13, 16], whereas the other three used 12 mm [17], 15 mm [12], and 20 mm [14]. In our study, we analyzed patients with stones exceeding 15 mm in size. The main advantage of LUL is the high probability of removing impacted stones in one session without additional procedures, whereas SWL and ureteroscopic approaches are characterized by higher risks of remnant stones, stone-free failure (especially in cases of large stones), impacted stones, and hard stones.

Although many surgeons prefer to insert double-J stents after LUL, there is controversy about whether ureteral stenting is necessary. Hammady et al. [18] performed a randomized controlled study and concluded that LUL without stent insertion is safe, cost-effective, and relatively quick. In addition, LUL without stenting does not require auxiliary procedures for removing the stent afterwards. On the other hand, Karami et al. [9] reported that placing a stent during LUL does not increase the operation time and may play an important role in preventing urinary leakage. In our study, there were no patients with flank pain or increased postoperative drainage after LUL with double-J stent placement.

The procedures used to insert the double-J stent intracorporeally after LUL are challenging and time consuming for inexperienced surgeons [10]. Therefore, various methods have been described to accomplish this successfully. In one of the most commonly used techniques, a retrograde double-J stent is placed beneath the stone using cystoscopy before LUL and advanced after stone removal [19–24].

Table 4 Penalized logistic regression analysis of variables affecting upward malpositioning of ureteral stents (SAS version 9.4)

Variable	Odds ratio	95% Confidence Interval	P-value
Surgeon			0.039
Flexible cystoscopy use	0.02	<0.001–0.35	0.008

Chen et al. [10] evaluated the feasibility of ureteroscope-assisted ureteral double-J stenting after LUL and found that it was a simple and safe alternative method of correct stent placement. However, retrograde cystoscopic or ureteroscopic stenting requires additional position changes. Moreover, cystoscopic retrograde stenting is associated with risks due to advancing the suture site without direct visualization. Alongside these retrograde cystoscopic or ureteroscopic stenting techniques, several intracorporeal stenting techniques have previously been described [25–28]. However, these techniques require fluoroscopic confirmation of correct placement after closing the ureter. It is difficult to place the film between the patient's body and the operation table to take an intraoperative KUB image when the patient is draped. Additionally, it takes substantial time to obtain KUB radiography results. Moreover, upon recognition using KUB radiography and correction of a malpositioned double-J stent, another KUB image would be necessary to confirm correct positioning. Therefore, readjustment of the stent using intraoperative KUB radiography for guidance may be technically difficult and increase operative time, potentially leading to stent failure. In this regard, our technique does not require position changes or fluoroscopic confirmation. Furthermore, the additional time required for flexible cystoscopy was <2 min if the stent was correctly placed in the bladder. Even when the stent was not adequately placed in the bladder, the mean additional time for readjustment was only 4 min. Flexible cystoscopy is an especially suitable method for male patients who might experience moderate pain if ureteroscopic removal of the stent is needed after LUL because of its upward malpositioning.

Surgeon and use of flexible cystoscopy were significant predicting factors for upward malpositioning. To our knowledge, no previous studies related to malpositioning of double-J stents have addressed this question. It makes intuitive sense that the rate of malpositioning differs according to the operator. Experience of the surgeon is important in preventing malpositioning. However, all our surgeons had several cases of upward malpositioning. Additionally, the use of flexible cystoscopy resulted in a 100% success rate, and malpositioning was corrected with a p-value of 0.008 in our study.

We recognize several limitations in this study. The first is that the data were collected from four different surgeons with different surgical experience without randomization. The differences in the number of performed LUL among the surgeons may indicate different levels of experience, resulting in variations in operative time, blood loss, and complication rates.

The second limitation is a lack of precise definition of upward malpositioning of the double-J stent. In fact, criteria for deciding whether the double-J stent is accurately positioned have not been defined in any previous study.

Additionally, in this retrospective study, methods for the removal of the double-J stent after LUL were not described in the medical records in many cases. Therefore, we defined upward malpositioning as placement of the double-J stent such that its tip is straight instead of being curled on postoperative KUB radiography. This strict definition may have contributed to the high rate of malpositioning of double-J stents in this study. This rate would be lower if malpositioning was defined to occur if the double-J stent had to be removed with an ureteroscope after LUL. In fact, flexible cystoscopy through the urethral route determined that the double-J stent was malpositioned in 10 of 50 cases (20%), which supports our assertion that the malpositioning rate in many cases is actually higher.

The third limitation of our study is the small sample size. Thus, future studies with a larger number of patients are needed.

Despite these limitations, our results show that flexible cystoscopy may be a useful method for confirming the placement of ureteral stents in the bladder and reducing malpositioning rates in male patients. The use of flexible cystoscopy after intracorporeal double-J stenting following LUL is an effective, quick, simple, and safe method that does not require position changes.

Conclusions

Intracorporeal double-J stenting during laparoscopic ureterolithotomy is technically difficult, and malpositioning of stents often occurs after surgery. Immediate correction of double-J stent malpositioning based on outcomes of flexible cystoscopy is a simple and effective method that can be used after laparoscopic ureterolithotomy.

Abbreviations
AUA: American Urological Association; EAU: European Association of Urology; EBL: Estimated blood loss; KUB: Kidney-ureter-bladder; LUL: Laparoscopic ureterolithotomy; SWL: Shockwave lithotripsy; URS: Ureteroscopic lithotripsy

Acknowledgments
The authors thank all our participants for their gracious participation in this study.

Funding
This study was supported by a research grant (K1507921) from the Korea University Medical College (Seoul, Korea).

Authors' contributions
JK and SK have made substantial contributions to conception and design, or acquisition of data, or analysis and interpretation of data. SK, JC, JL, and JK have been involved in drafting the manuscript or revising it critically for important intellectual content. Each author should have participated sufficiently in the work to take public responsibility for appropriate portions of the content and agreed to be accountable for all aspects of the work in ensuring that questions related to the accuracy or integrity of any part of the work are appropriately investigated and resolved. And all authors have given final approval for the manuscript to be published.

Competing interests
The authors declare that they have no competing interests.

References

1. Preminger GM, Tiselius HG, Assimos DG, Alken P, Buck AC, Gallucci M, et al. 2007 guideline for the management of ureteral calculi. Eur Urol. 2007;52:1610–31.
2. Bader MJ, Eisner B, Porpiglia F, Preminger GM, Tiselius HG. Contemporary management of ureteral stones. Eur Urol. 2012;61:764–72.
3. Tiselius HG, Ackermann D, Alken P, Buck C, Conort P, Gallucci M. Working party on Lithiasis EAoU. Guidelines on urolithiasis. Eur Urol. 2001;40:362–71.
4. Matlaga BR, Jansen JP, Meckley LM, Byrne TW, Lingeman JE. Treatment of ureteral and renal stones: a systematic review and meta-analysis of randomized, controlled trials. J Urol. 2012;188:130–7.
5. Turk C, Petrik A, Sarica K, Seitz C, Skolarikos A, Straub M, et al. EAU guidelines on interventional treatment for urolithiasis. Eur Urol. 2016;69:475–82.
6. Torricelli FCM, Monga M, Marchini GS, Srougi M, Nahas WC, Mazzucchi E. Semi-rigid ureteroscopic lithotripsy versus laparoscopic ureterolithotomy for large upper ureteral stones: a meta - analysis of randomized controlled trials. Int Braz J Urol. 2016;42:645–54.
7. Skrepetis K, Doumas K, Siafakas I, Lykourinas M. Laparoscopic versus open ureterolithotomy. A comparative study. Eur Urol. 2001;40:32–6. discussion 37
8. Kiyota H, Ikemoto I, Asano K, Madarame J, Miki K, Yoshino Y, et al. Retroperitoneoscopic ureterolithotomy for impacted ureteral stone. Int J Urol. 2001;8:391–7.
9. Karami H, Javanmard B, Hasanzadeh-Hadah A, Mazloomfard MM, Lotfi B, Mohamadi R, et al. Is it necessary to place a double J catheter after laparoscopic ureterolithotomy? A four-year experience. J Endourol. 2012;26:1183–6.
10. Chen IH, Tsai JY, Yu CC, Wu T, Huang JK, Lin JT. Ureteroscope-assisted double-J stenting following laparoscopic ureterolithotomy. Kaohsiung J Med Sci. 2014;30:243–7.
11. Fernbach SK, Maizels M, Conway JJ. Ultrasound grading of hydronephrosis: introduction to the system used by the Society for Fetal Urology. Pediatr Radiol. 1993;23:478–80.
12. Basiri A, Simforoosh N, Ziaee A, Shayaninasab H, Moghaddam SMMH, et al. Retrograde, antegrade, and laparoscopic approaches for the management of large, proximal ureteral stones: a randomized clinical trial. J Endourol. 2008;22:2677–80.
13. Fang YQ, Qiu JG, Wang DJ, Zhan HL, Situ J. Comparative study on ureteroscopic lithotripsy and laparoscopic ureterolithotomy for treatment of unilateral upper ureteral stones. Acta Cir Bras. 2012;27:266–70.
14. Kumar A, Vasudeva P, Nanda B, Kumar N, Jha SK, Singh H. A prospective randomized comparison between laparoscopic ureterolithotomy and semirigid ureteroscopy for upper ureteral stones >2 cm: a single-center experience. J Endourol. 2015;29:1248–52.
15. Liu YH, Zhou ZY, Xia A, Dai HT, Guo LJ, Zheng J. Clinical observation of different minimally invasive surgeries for the treatment of impacted upper ureteral calculi. Pak J Med Sci. 2013;29:1358–62.
16. Neto ACL, Korkes F, Silva JL, Amarante RD, Mattos MHE, Tobias-Machado M, et al. Prospective randomized study of treatment of large proximal ureteral stones: extracorporeal shock wave lithotripsy versus ureterolithotripsy versus laparoscopy. J Urol. 2012;187:164–8.
17. Shao YA, Wang DW, Lu GL, Shen ZJ. Retroperitoneal laparoscopic ureterolithotomy in comparison with ureteroscopic lithotripsy in the management of impacted upper ureteral stones larger than 12 mm. World J Urol. 2015;33:1841–5.
18. Hammady A, Gamal WM, Zaki M, Hussein M, Abuzeid A. Evaluation of ureteral stent placement after retroperitoneal laparoscopic ureterolithotomy for upper ureteral stone: randomized controlled study. J Endourol. 2011;25:825–30.
19. Goel A, Hemal AK. Upper and mid-ureteric stones: a prospective unrandomized comparison of retroperitoneoscopic and open ureterolithotomy. BJU Int. 2001;88:679–82.
20. Nouira Y, Kallel Y, Binous MY, Dahmoul H, Horchani A. Laparoscopic retroperitoneal ureterolithotomy: initial experience and review of literature. J Endourol. 2004;18:557–61.
21. Bellman GC, Smith AD. Special considerations in the technique of laparoscopic ureterolithotomy. J Urol. 1994;151:146–9.
22. Micali S, Moore RG, Averch TD, Adams JB, Kavoussi LR. The role of laparoscopy in the treatment of renal and ureteral calculi. J Urol. 1997;157:463–6.
23. Turk I. Laparoscopic ureterolithotomy: the Edinburgh experience. BJU Int. 2000;86:147–8.
24. Feyaerts A, Rietbergen J, Navarra S, Vallancien G, Guillonneau B. Laparoscopic ureterolithotomy for ureteral calculi. Eur Urol. 2001;40:609–13.
25. Gaur DD, Joshi NR, Dubey M, Acharya UP. A simple technique for retroperitoneal laparoscopic JJ stenting of the ureter. BJU Int. 2003;91:725–6.
26. Khan M, Khan F. Innovative technique for ureteral stenting during retroperitoneal laparoscopic ureterolithotomy. J Endourol. 2005;19:994–6.
27. Fan T, Xian P, Yang L, Liu Y, Wei Q, Li H. Experience and learning curve of retroperitoneal laparoscopic ureterolithotomy for upper ureteral calculi. J Endourol. 2009;23:1867–70.
28. Choi KH, Yang SC, Lee JW, Rha KH, Han WK. Laparoendoscopic single-site surgery for ureterolithotomy: focus on intracorporeal stenting and suturing. Urology. 2010;76:1283–7.

Presence of transient hydronephrosis immediately after surgery has a limited influence on renal function 1 year after ileal neobladder construction

Takuma Narita[1], Shingo Hatakeyama[1]* (iD), Takuya Koie[1], Shogo Hosogoe[1], Teppei Matsumoto[1], Osamu Soma[1], Hayato Yamamoto[1], Tohru Yoneyama[2], Yuki Tobisawa[1], Takahiro Yoneyama[1], Yasuhiro Hashimoto[2] and Chikara Ohyama[1,2]

Abstract

Background: Urinary tract obstruction and postoperative hydronephrosis are risk factor for renal function deterioration after orthotopic ileal neobladder construction. However, reports of relationship between transient hydronephrosis and renal function are limited.
We assess the influence of postoperative transient hydronephrosis on renal function in patients with orthotopic ileal neobladder construction.

Methods: Between January 2006 and June 2013, we performed radical cystectomy in 164 patients, and 101 received orthotopic ileal neobladder construction. This study included data available from 64 patients with 128 renal units who were enrolled retrospectively. The hydronephrosis grade of each renal unit scored 0–4. The patients were divided into 4 groups according to the grade of hydronephrosis: control, low, intermediate, and high. The grade of postoperative hydronephrosis was compared with renal function 1 month and 1 year after surgery.

Results: There were no significant differences in renal function before surgery between groups. One month after surgery, the presence of hydronephrosis was significantly associated with decreased renal function. However, 1 year after urinary diversion hydronephrosis grades were improved significantly, and renal function was comparable between groups. Postoperative hydronephrosis at 1 month had no significant influence on renal function 1 year after ileal neobladder construction. Limitations include retrospective design, short follow-up periods, and a sample composition.

Conclusions: The presence of transient hydronephrosis immediately after surgery may have limited influence on renal function 1 year after ileal neobladder construction.

Keywords: eGFR, Hydronephrosis, Ileal neobladder, Radical cystectomy, Renal function

Background

Urinary diversion after radical cystectomy is mandatory for muscle-invasive bladder cancer patients, and it should ensure protection of the upper urinary tract. Orthotopic ileal neobladder construction following cystectomy has evolved in an attempt to restore anatomy and function as close as possible to the preoperative state. Several risk factors have been reported for the postoperative decline in renal function [1–4]. Recent retrospective studies suggested that risk factors associated with renal function decline are urinary tract obstruction [2] and postoperative hydronephrosis [4]. However, the progression of hydronephrosis and renal function after ileal neobladder construction are not well defined, and there are few reports describing the relationship between transient hydronephrosis and renal function following radical cystectomy and orthotopic ileal neobladder construction. Moreover, the association between transient hydronephrosis and

* Correspondence: shingoh@hirosaki-u.ac.jp
[1]Department of Urology, Hirosaki University Graduate School of Medicine, 5 Zaifu-cho, Hirosaki 036-8562, Japan
Full list of author information is available at the end of the article

renal function was not studied. Therefore, the aim of this study was to investigate the effect of postoperative hydronephrosis on renal function in patients with orthotopic ileal neobladder construction. Specifically, we compared the grade of postoperative hydronephrosis with renal function 1 month and 1 year after surgery.

Methods

Ethics statement

This study was performed in accordance with the ethical standards of the Declaration of Helsinki, and approved by an ethics review board of Hirosaki University School of Medicine (The authorization number: 2015–047). The participants in this study provide their verbal informed consent when hospitalized, and it was recorded in medical chart. Pursuant to the provisions of the ethics committee and the ethic guideline in Japan, written consent was not required in exchange for public disclosure of study information in the case of retrospective study. The study information was open for the public consumption at http://www.med.hirosaki-u.ac.jp/~uro/html/IRB/IRBdoc.html.

Patient selection

Between January 2006 and June 2013, we performed radical cystectomy in 164 patients, and 101 received orthotopic ileal neobladder construction. Of these, 34 patients without serum creatinine levels and/or computed tomography (CT) imaging within 1 year after surgery as well as three with unilateral nephroureterectomy were excluded. As a result, 64 patients with 128 of renal-units were enrolled in this retrospective study. Tumor stage and grade were assigned according to the 2009 TNM classification of the Union of International Cancer Control [5].

Evaluation of hydronephrosis grade and classification

The hydronephrosis grade of each renal unit was evaluated by CT imaging, and scored according to the hydronephrosis grading scale: grade 0, no dilatation (G0); grade 1, pelvic dilatation only (G1); grade 2, mild caliceal dilatation (G2); grade 3, severe caliceal dilatation (G3); grade 4, renal parenchymal atrophy (G4) (Fig. 1a), as described previously [6, 7]. It was measured by single urologist who was blinded to the outcomes. The patients were also stratified into 4 groups according to hydronephrosis grade and status (unilateral or bilateral): no hydronephrosis in bilateral kidney (control group), unilateral hydronephrosis (low), bilateral hydronephrosis with G1 or G2 (intermediate), and bilateral hydronephrosis with G3 or G4 on either side (high) (Fig. 1b). The grade of postoperative hydronephrosis was compared with renal function 1 month and 1 year after surgery.

Evaluation of renal function and clinical parameters

Renal function was evaluated using estimated glomerular filtration rate (eGFR) using a modified version of the abbreviated Modification of Diet in Renal Disease Study formula [8]: eGFR mL/min/1.73 m^2 = 194 × sCr$^{-1.094}$ × age$^{-0.287}$ (×0.739, if female). Each patient was evaluated using preoperative and postoperative eGFR after 1 month and 1 year.

We analyzed the variables including age, gender, Eastern Cooperative Oncology Group Performance Status (ECOG-PS), history of cardiovascular disease, hypertension, diabetes mellitus, renal function (eGFR) clinical and pathological stage, blood loss, operative duration, postoperative complications, and tumor recurrence. We defined pyelonephritis as a positive urine culture and tenderness with fever (axillary temperature > 38.5 °C). Repeated postoperative episodes (at least 2 or more) of acute pyelonephritis were recorded as postoperative complications. Hypertension was defined as any antihypertensive medications intake or preoperative systolic and diastolic blood pressure measurements of >140 and >90 mmHg, respectively. Diabetic patients were defined as those who met the relevant diagnostic criteria, required glycemic control, and/or those with a history of type 2 diabetes.

Surgical procedures

All patients underwent radical cystectomy, orthotopic ileal neobladder construction, and lymphadenectomy procedures. The basic procedure was identical regardless of the surgeon [9, 10]. Orthotopic ileal reservoir construction was performed as described previously [11, 12]. Key points of our procedures were that 1) resected a 40-cm of ileal segment approximately 20 cm proximal to the ileocecal valve, 2) ileal segment loop was arranged in a U shape, 3) an anti-reflux procedure was not performed in ureteroileal anastomosis.

Patient follow-up

Ureteral stents were removed 1 week after surgery under radiographic guidance. An 18-F urethral catheter was removed 3 weeks after orthotopic ileal reservoir construction under radiographic guidance. We performed CT 1 month and 1 year after surgery as a routine work, and patients were discharged 4–6 weeks after surgery. Each patient was assessed every 3 months using ultrasonography to monitor for hydronephrosis; serum electrolytes, blood urea nitrogen, serum creatinine, and liver function were also measured. Subsequent formation of uretero-intestinal stricture was suspected and investigated when hydronephrosis was worsening. CT was performed every 6–12 months for the early detection of tumor recurrence. Urethroscopic examination and urine cytology was performed at 3-month intervals for 2 years.

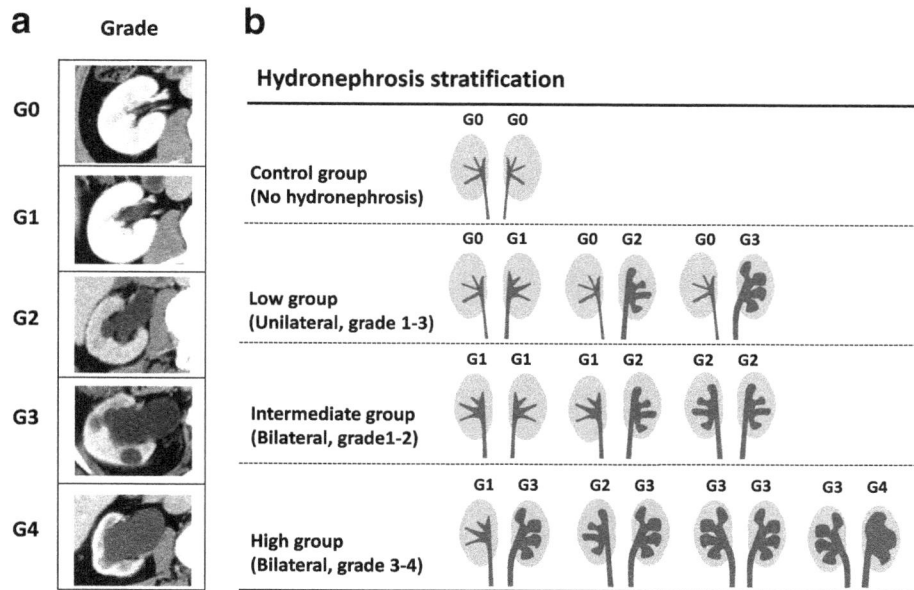

Fig. 1 Hydronephrosis grade and stratification. **a.** The hydronephrosis grade of each renal unit was evaluated by computed tomography (CT) imaging, and scored according to hydronephrosis grading scale: grade 0, no dilatation (G0); grade 1, pelvic dilatation only (G1); grade 2, mild caliceal dilatation (G2); grade 3, severe caliceal dilatation (G3); and grade 4, renal parenchymal atrophy (G4). **b.** Patients were stratified into 4 groups according to hydronephrosis grade and status (unilateral or bilateral): no hydronephrosis in bilateral kidneys (control group), unilateral hydronephrosis (low group), bilateral hydronephrosis with G1 or G2 (intermediate group), and bilateral hydronephrosis with G3 or G4 on either side (high group)

Statistical analysis

Statistical analyses of the clinical data were performed using SPSS ver. 19.0 (SPSS, Inc., Chicago, IL, USA) and GraphPad Prism 5.03 (GraphPad Software, San Diego, CA, USA). Categorical variables were compared using Fisher's exact test or the χ^2 test. Quantitative variables were expressed as mean with standard deviation or median with interquartile ratio (IQR). The differences between groups were compared statistically using Student's t-test for normal distribution. Mann–Whitney U-test was used for the differences between groups with non-normal distribution. The Wilcoxon matched-pairs signed-rank test was used for matched pairs showing non-normal distribution. P values of <0.05 were considered to be statistically significant.

Risk factors for an eGFR <60 mL/min/1.73 m^2 were identified using univariate and multivariate analyses with the logistic regression model, and odds ratios (ORs) with 95% confidence intervals (CI) were calculated after controlling simultaneously for potential confounders. Variables included in the models were age (>65.5 years), gender, history of cardiovascular disease, hypertension, type 2 diabetes, neoadjuvant chemotherapy, pathological T stage (>pT2), pathological lymph nodes involvement, postoperative complications, tumor recurrence, operative duration (>294 min), blood loss (>1380 g), hydronephrosis stratification (>low), and eGFR (<60 mL/min/1.73 m^2).

Results

The clinicopathological characteristics and distributions of the patients are presented in Table 1. A total of 64 patients underwent radical cystectomy and orthotopic ileal neobladder construction. The median age of this cohort was 65.5 years. Sixty-one patients (95%) received 2 cycles of platinum-based neoadjuvant chemotherapy, and cystectomy was done within 1 month after neoadjuvant chemotherapy. There were no patients required clean intermittent catheterization or indwelling catheter after the surgery. One patient required urethral bougie only once because of neobladder-urethral anastomotic stricture.

Postoperative eGFR 1 year after surgery was significantly lower than preoperative eGFR ($P < 0.001$, Wilcoxon matched-pairs signed rank test); the median decrease in 1-year eGFR was 12% in all patient. (control group: 10.8%, low group: 24.2%, intermediate group: 11.0%, high group: 0.0%).

The preoperative and postoperative hydronephrosis grades of 128 renal units are shown in Fig. 2a. The median [first quartile (Q1)–third quartile (Q3)] preoperative, 1-month, and 1-year hydronephrosis grades were 0 (0–0), 2 (0–2), and 0 (0–1), respectively. The overall hydronephrosis grades in 128 renal units were increased significantly at 1 month after surgery, which improved significantly 1 year after surgery (Fig. 2a, $P < 0.001$, Wilcoxon matched-pairs signed rank test).

Table 1 Clinical and pathological patient characteristics

| | All | Hydronephrosis stratification at 1 M | | | | P value |
		Control	Low	Intermediate	High	
n	64	12	11	27	14	
Age[a]	66 (61–71)	63 (55–69)	69 (60–73)	67 (59–71)	69 (63–75)	0.401 [b]
Gender (Male/Female), n=	48 / 16					
ECOG-PS	0.0 (0–0)	0.0 (0–0)	0.0 (0–0)	0.0 (0–0)	0.0 (0–0)	1.000 [b]
Past history, n=						
Cardiovascular disease	6 (9%)	1 ((%)	1 (9%)	3 (11%)	1 (7%)	1.000 [c]
Hypertension	21 (33%)	3 (25%)	3 (27%)	11 (41%)	4 (29%)	0.765 [c]
Diabetes	9 (14%)	1 (8%)	2 (18%)	5 (19%)	1 (7%)	0.729 [c]
Neoadjuvant chemotherapy, n=	61 (95%)	11 (92%)	11 (100%)	26 (96%)	13 (93%)	0.882 [c]
Clinical T stage[a]	2 (2–3)	3 (2–3)	2 (2–3)	2 (2–3)	3 (2–3)	0.580 [b]
Pathological T stage[a]	1 (0–2)	2 (0–2)	1 (0–2)	2 (1–2)	2 (0–2)	0.578 [b]
Pathological N+, n=	2 (3%)	0 (0%)	0 (0%)	1 (4%)	1 (7%)	1.000 [c]
eGFR[a]						
Before surgery	73 (66–87)	77 (75–97)	84 (73–91)	72 (65–88)	69 (62–73)	0.062 [b]
1 month after surgery	60 (53–74)	71 (57–82)	73 (60–88)	58 (52–65)	56 (43–72)	0.029 [b]
1 year after surgery	65 (56–74)	69 (62–76)	63 (53–78)	63 (53–74)	69 (61–75)	0.524 [b]
Hydronephrosis grades[a]						
Before surgery	0 (0–0)	0 (0–1)	0 (0–0)	0 (0–0)	0 (0–0)	0.348 [b]
1 month after surgery	2 (0–2)	0 (0–0)	1 (0–2)	2 (2–2)	3 (3–3)	< 0.001 [b]
1 year after surgery	0 (0–1)	0 (0–0)	0 (0–1)	0 (0–0)	1 (0–1)	0.021 [b]
Complications (any grades), n=	16 (25%)	2 (17%)	3 (27%)	10 (37%)	1 (7%)	0.213 [c]
Complications (Clavien Grade > 3), n=	2 (2%)	0 (0%)	1 (9%)	1 (4%)	0 (0%)	0.261 [b]
Operative duration[a] (min)	294 (266–323)	281 (237–303)	277 (263–300)	322 (273–356)	280 (265–307)	0.015 [b]
Blood loss[a] (g)	1380 (1034–2302)	1345 (576–2211)	1400 (1070–2465)	1470 (926–2350)	1430 (1095–2359)	0.914 [b]
Recurrence (within 1 year), n=	2 (3%)	0 (0%)	2 (18%)	0 (0%)	0 (0%)	0.813 [c]

[a]median (Q1-Q3)

Q1, first quartile; Q3, third quartile; [b] Kruskal–Wallis test; [c] Fisher's exact test

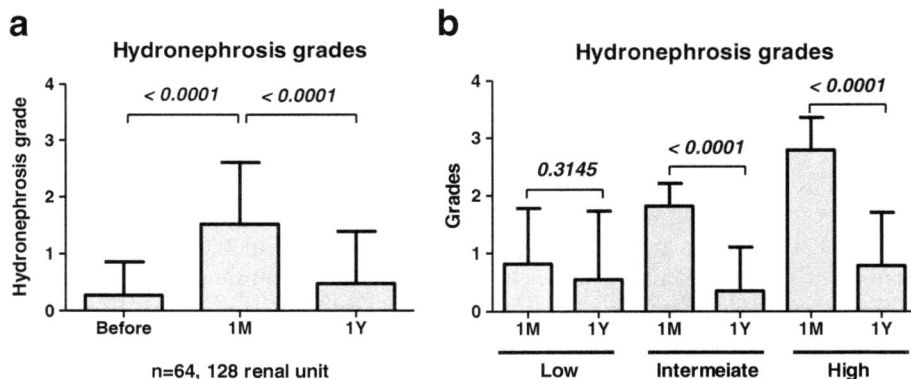

Fig. 2 Preoperative and postoperative hydronephrosis grades. **a**. The overall hydronephrosis grades in 128 renal units were increased significantly 1 month after surgery ($P < 0.001$), but improved significantly 1 year after surgery ($P < 0.001$). **b**. The hydronephrosis grades in the low group did not changed significantly ($P = 0.3145$). The hydronephrosis grades in the intermediate and high groups were significantly increased 1 month after surgery ($P < 0.0001$), but improved significantly 1 year after surgery ($P < 0.001$). Statistical analyses were performed using Wilcoxon matched-pairs signed rank test

The patients were divided into 4 groups according to their hydronephrosis grade 1 month after surgery. The method used for stratification is shown in Fig. 1b. The numbers of patients in the control, low, intermediate, and high group were 12, 11, 27, and 14, respectively. There were no significant differences in patient background before surgery between the groups, except for operative duration (Table 1, P = 0.015, Kruskal–Wallis test). The hydronephrosis grades in the intermediate and high groups were increased significantly 1 month after surgery, which improved significantly 1 year after surgery (Fig. 2b, P < 0.001, Wilcoxon matched-pairs signed rank test).

In the control group, there were no significant changes in renal function before, or 1 month and 1 year after surgery (Fig. 3a). In contrast, the presence of hydronephrosis 1 month after surgery was significantly associated with a decline in renal function in the low and intermediate groups (Fig. 3b, c, Wilcoxon matched-pair signed-rank test). In the high group, renal function, which was decreased significantly 1 month after surgery, was improved significantly 1 year after surgery (Fig. 3d, P = 0.008, Wilcoxon matched-pairs signed rank test). As a result, renal function in the high group became comparable with the other groups 1 year after surgery

(Fig. 4b, P = 0.8774, Mann–Whitney U test), which was significantly lower than that in the control group 1 month after surgery (Fig. 4a, P = 0.0448, Mann–Whitney U test). Using multivariate analysis, age (>65.5 years, OR 1.2, P = 0.03), male (OR 0.7, P = 0.03), postoperative eGFR <60 mL/min/1.72 m^2 at 1 month (OR 9.0, P = 0.01) and operative duration >294 min (OR 6.2, P = 0.02) were selected as risk factors for significantly associated with eGFR <60 mL/min/1.72 m^2 after radical cystectomy and orthotopic ileal neobladder construction, whereas presence of transient bilateral hydronephrosis (intermediate and high groups) was not selected (OR 0.4, P = 0.36, 95% CI 0.7–1.1) (Table 2).

Discussion
In the present study, we compared the grade of postoperative hydronephrosis to renal function at 1 month and 1 year after orthotopic ileal neobladder construction to assess the influence of postoperative transient hydronephrosis on renal function in patients with ileal neobladder construction. Our results suggest that transient postoperative hydronephrosis at 1 month had no significantly effect on renal function 1 year after ileal neobladder construction. Transient hydronephrosis may be caused by transient edema at anastomosis and reduced compliance of the

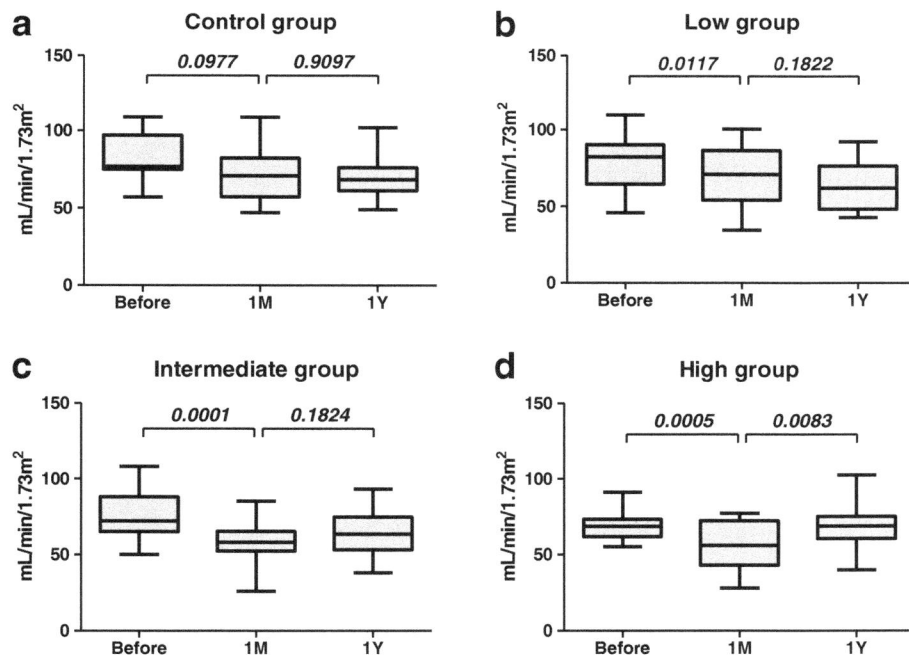

Fig. 3 Preoperative and postoperative eGFR. **a**. No significant changes were observed in renal function before surgery and 1 month after surgery (P = 0.0977) or 1 month and 1 year after surgery (P = 0.9097) in the control group. **b and c**. The presence of mild hydronephrosis 1 month after surgery was significantly associated with renal function decline in the low (P = 0.0117) and intermediate (P = 0.0001) groups. Renal function became stable 1 year after surgery. **d**. The presence of severe hydronephrosis 1 month after surgery was significantly associated with a decline in renal function in the high group (P = 0.0005). However, renal function recovered significantly 1 year after surgery (P = 0.0083). Statistical analyses were performed using Wilcoxon matched-pairs signed-rank test

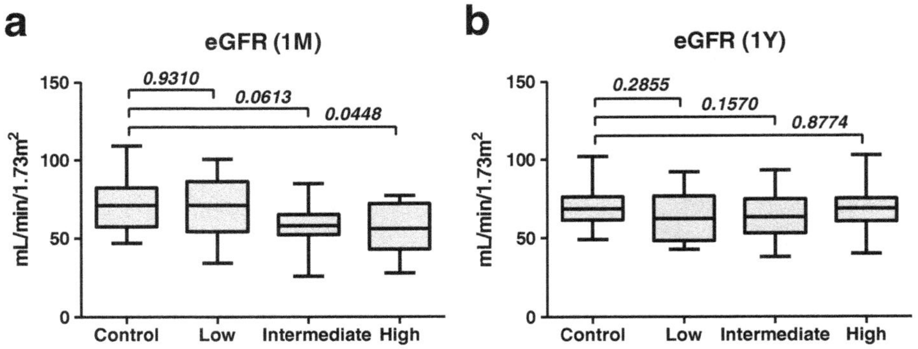

Fig. 4 Intergroup postoperative eGFR differences compared with control. **a**. One month after surgery, postoperative eGFR was significantly lower in the high group. **b**. One year after surgery, postoperative eGFR was not significantly different between the high and control groups. Statistical analyses were performed using Mann–Whitney U test

neobladder. However, the significance and implication of postoperative hydronephrosis is controversial. Several previous studies reported that the postoperative decline in renal function and hydronephrosis were associated [4] and unassociated [2] after orthotopic ileal neobladder construction. Because most clinical reports describing renal function and postoperative hydronephrosis after orthotopic ileal neobladder construction are retrospective and cross-sectional, detailed information describing postoperative hydronephrosis are limited, and conclusions are impeded by differences in patient backgrounds, selection bias, and the surgical techniques used. Therefore, it is difficult to prove our hypothesis in the present study. Further prospective study is necessary to verify our findings.

In the present study, we developed original hydrone-phrosis grading system influencing on total renal function. We stratified patients into five categories (Grade 0 to 4) depending on hydronephrosis status on both sides (Fig. 1). Because the impact of unilateral grade 3 or 4 hydronephrosis on renal function remain unclear, we tried to make optimal stratification for unilateral grade 3 or 4 hydronephrosis. As a result, we found that unilateral grade 3 or 4 was suitable for the low group because these patients did not reduce renal function after urinary diversion. This might be due to the compensate recovery of contralateral kidney. However, it is unknown whether this hydronephrosis grading system is effective for other studies. Further studies with larger sample sizes are needed on this issue.

Radical cystectomy and urinary diversion remain the standard treatment modality for muscle-invasive bladder cancer patients. However, these are associated with the significant risks of perioperative and long-term morbidity and mortality [13, 14], including a subsequent decline in renal function [15–17]. The goals of urinary diversion after radical cystectomy have evolved from protecting the proximal portions of the tract to functional anatomical restoration because patients with urinary diversion

are at a notably higher risk of decline in renal function [18–20]. In general, renal function is favorably preserved after continent urinary diversion compared with after conduit urinary diversion [21]; the incidence of a decline in renal function after continent urinary diversion has been reported range from 3 to 25% over 10 years [2, 4]

Table 2 Univariate and multivariate logistic regression analyses of the risk factors for eGFR <60 mL/min/1.73 m^2 at 1 year after surgery

Univariate	Risk factors	P value	Odds ratio	95% CI
Age	> 65.5 years	0.11	2.4	0.8–7.3
Gender	Male	1.00	1.0	0.3–3.4
Past history of				
Cardiovascular disease	Positive	0.43	0.4	0.0–3.8
Hypertension	Positive	0.75	0.8	0.3–2.6
Diabetes	Positive	0.36	1.9	0.5–8.2
Pathological T stage	pT3, 4	0.68	0.7	0.1–3.8
Pathological N status	pN+	0.57	2.3	0.1–38.1
Hydronephrosis at 1 M	> low	0.22	2.1	0.6–6.7
Neoadjuvant chemotherapy	received	0.94	0.9	0.1–10.6
Preoperative eGFR	< 60	0.03	7.0	1.2–40
Postoperative eGFR at 1 M	< 60	0.00	7.7	2.2–27
Complications (any grade)	Positive	0.53	1.5	0.4–4.8
Operative duration	> 294	0.04	3.4	1.1–10
Blood loss (g)	> 1380	0.11	2.4	0.8–7.3
Recurrence	Positive	0.57	2.3	0.1–38.1
Multivariate	Risk factors	P value	Odds ratio	95% CI
Age	> 65.5 years	0.03	1.2	1.1–1.5
Gender	Male	0.03	0.7	0.5–0.9
Hydronephrosis at 1 M	> low	0.36	0.4	0.7–1.1
Preoperative eGFR	< 60	0.25	3.7	0.4–34.0
Postoperative eGFR at 1 M	< 60	0.01	9.0	1.9–42.4
Operative duration	> 294	0.02	6.2	1.3–29.3

In several reports, decline in renal function was observed immediately after radical cystectomy and urinary diversion, but stabilized afterward within 1–2 months [4, 17]. However, limited evidence is available describing the effects of orthotopic ileal neobladder construction on renal function after radical cystectomy. Several risk factors have been reported for the postoperative decline in renal function, including urinary tract obstruction, pyelonephritis, diabetes, and hypertension [1–4]. It is reasonable to suggest that urinary tract obstruction has a significant impact on the postoperative decline in renal function; however, the evidence is limited regarding the degree and critical duration of postoperative hydronephrosis for causing unrecoverable damage to renal function after orthotopic ileal neobladder construction.

An additional important factor for protecting the upper urinary tract is ureterointestinal anastomosis. A large number of techniques for ureterointestinal anastomosis have been described [21–23]. The most commonly used techniques for implantation into an ileal segment involve antirefluxing anastomoses (e.g., the afferent loop in the Studer pouch) [24], the Le Duc technique or use of a chimney [20], the split-cuff ureteric nipple [22], and the serous-lined extramural tunnel [23]. However, comparisons between studies are challenging because of differences in patient age, underlying disorders, the use of radiotherapy, and preoperative/postoperative routines. To date, no single method has proved superior to others. Therefore, further studies are needed to address this issue.

This study has several limitations, including the small sample size, short follow-up periods, anastomosis techniques, its retrospective nature, and a sample composition that excluded many patients in whom CT imaging was not performed within 1 month. In addition, we were unable to control all variables, including selection bias, operative duration, influence of neoadjuvant chemotherapy, split renal function, continence status, uro-dynamic testing data, and other unmeasurable confounding factors. Statistical power was also insufficient due to the small sample size. Furthermore, long-term follow-up is necessary to address the long-term influences of transient hydronephrosis after orthotopic ileal neobladder construction, particularly in patients with severe bilateral hydronephrosis. Despite these limitations, this study was the first report to assess the influence of postoperative hydronephrosis on renal function at 1 month and 1 year after surgery. The data revealed no differences in postoperative renal function, regardless of the degree of postoperative transient hydronephrosis after radical cystectomy and orthotopic ileal neobladder construction.

Conclusion

In conclusion, the presence of transient hydronephrosis immediately after surgery may have limited influence on renal function at 1 year after orthotopic ileal neobladder construction. Further investigation by well-designed randomized prospective studies is necessary to assess the influence between postoperative hydronephrosis and renal function in patients with orthotopic ileal neobladder construction.

Abbreviations
CI: Confidence intervals; CT: Computed tomography; ECOG-PS: Eastern cooperative oncology group performance status; eGFR: Estimated glomerular filtration rate; ORs: Odds ratios; Q1: First quartile; Q3: Third quartile

Acknowledgements
This research was supported by Hirosaki University Hospital and the urological ward nursing staff. We are thankful to our clinical clerk Yuki Fujita who provided expertise that greatly assisted the research.

Financial disclosure
This work was supported by the Japan Society for the Promotion of Science (No. 23791737, 15H02563, 15 K15579, 17 K11118, 17 K11119, 17 K16768, 17 K16770, and 17 K16771).

Authors' contributions
All authors read and approved the final manuscript. TN: acquisition, analysis, interpretation of data, and drafting the manuscript. SH: responsible for the concept and design of the study, analysis and interpretation of data, drafting the manuscript. TK: acquisition, analysis and interpretation of data, revising it critically for important intellectual content, supervision of the research. SH: acquisition, analysis and interpretation of data. TM: acquisition, analysis and interpretation of data. OS: acquisition, analysis and interpretation of data. HY: acquisition, analysis and interpretation of data, revising it critically for important intellectual content. TY: acquisition, analysis and interpretation of data, revising it critically for important intellectual content. YT: acquisition, analysis and interpretation of data, revising it critically for important intellectual content. TY: acquisition, analysis and interpretation of data, revising it critically for important intellectual content. YH: acquisition, analysis and interpretation of data, revising it critically for important intellectual content. CH: acquisition of funding, conception and design, revising it critically for important intellectual content, supervision of the research.

Authors' information
TN: postgraduate student, SH: assistant professor, TK: associate professor, SH: postgraduate student, TM: postgraduate student, OS: postgraduate student, YH: associate professor, TY: associate professor, YT: associate professor, TY: associate professor, YH: associate professor, CO: professor and chairman, Department of Urology, Hirosaki Graduate School of Medicine.

Competing interests
The authors declare that they have no competing interests.

Author details
¹Department of Urology, Hirosaki University Graduate School of Medicine, 5 Zaifu-cho, Hirosaki 036-8562, Japan. ²Department of Advanced Transplant and Regenerative Medicine, Hirosaki University Graduate School of Medicine, Hirosaki, Japan.

References

1. Samuel JD, Bhatt RI, Montague RJ, Clarke NW, Ramani VA. The natural history of postoperative renal function in patients undergoing ileal conduit diversion for cancer measured using serial isotopic glomerular filtration rate and 99m technetium-mercaptoacetyltriglycine renography. J Urol. 2006; 176(6 Pt 1):2518–22. discussion 2522

2. Jin XD, Roethlisberger S, Burkhard FC, Birkhaeuser F, Thoeny HC, Studer UE. Long-term renal function after urinary diversion by ileal conduit or orthotopic ileal bladder substitution. Eur Urol. 2012;61(3):491–7.

3. Osawa T, Shinohara N, Maruyama S, Oba K, Abe T, Maru S, Takada N, Sazawa A, Nonomura K. Long-term renal function outcomes in bladder cancer after radical cystectomy. Urol J. 2013;10(1):784–9.

4. Eisenberg MS, Thompson RH, Frank I, Kim SP, Cotter KJ, Tollefson MK, Kaushik D, Thapa P, Tarrell R, Boorjian SA. Long-term renal function outcomes after radical cystectomy. J Urol. 2014;191(3):619–25.

5. Sobin LH, Gospodarowicz MK, Wittekind C. International union against cancer., ebrary inc.: TNM classification of malignant tumours, 7th edn. Chichester, west Sussex, UK. Hoboken: Wiley-Blackwell; 2009.

6. Cho KS, Hong SJ, Cho NH, Choi YD. Grade of hydronephrosis and tumor diameter as preoperative prognostic factors in ureteral transitional cell carcinoma. Urology. 2007;70(4):662–6.

7. Ito Y, Kikuchi E, Tanaka N, Miyajima A, Mikami S, Jinzaki M, Oya M. Preoperative hydronephrosis grade independently predicts worse pathological outcomes in patients undergoing nephroureterectomy for upper tract urothelial carcinoma. J Urol. 2011;185(5):1621–6.

8. Matsuo S, Imai E, Horio M, Yasuda Y, Tomita K, Nitta K, Yamagata K, Tomino Y, Yokoyama H, Hishida A. Revised equations for estimated GFR from serum creatinine in Japan. Am J Kidney Dis. 2009;53(6):982–92.

9. Koie T, Ohyama C, Yamamoto H, Hatakeyama S, Kudoh S, Yoneyama T, Hashimoto Y, Kamimura N. Minimum incision endoscopic radical cystectomy in patients with malignant tumors of the urinary bladder: clinical and oncological outcomes at a single institution. Eur J Surg Oncol. 2012;38(11):1101–5.

10. Kubota Y, Nakaigawa N. Essential content of evidence-based clinical practice guidelines for bladder cancer: the Japanese Urological Association 2015 update. Int J Urol. 2016;23(8):640–5.

11. Koie T, Hatakeyama S, Yoneyama T, Ishimura H, Yamato T, Ohyama C. Experience and functional outcome of modified ileal neobladder in 95 patients. Int J Urol. 2006;13(9):1175–9.

12. Koie T, Hatakeyama S, Yoneyama T, Hashimoto Y, Kamimura N, Ohyama C. Uterus-, fallopian tube-, ovary-, and vagina-sparing cystectomy followed by U-shaped ileal neobladder construction for female bladder cancer patients: oncological and functional outcomes. Urology. 2010;75(6):1499–503.

13. Shabsigh A, Korets R, Vora KC, Brooks CM, Cronin AM, Savage C, Raj G, Bochner BH, Dalbagni G, Herr HW, et al. Defining early morbidity of radical cystectomy for patients with bladder cancer using a standardized reporting methodology. Eur Urol. 2009;55(1):164–74.

14. Shimko MS, Tollefson MK, Umbreit EC, Farmer SA, Blute ML, Frank I. Long-term complications of conduit urinary diversion. J Urol. 2011;185(2):562–7.

15. Lawrentschuk N, Colombo R, Hakenberg OW, Lerner SP, Mansson W, Sagalowsky A, Wirth MP. Prevention and management of complications following radical cystectomy for bladder cancer. Eur Urol. 2010;57(6):983–1001.

16. Hautmann RE, de Petriconi RC, Volkmer BG. 25 years of experience with 1,000 neobladders: long-term complications. J Urol. 2011;185(6):2207–12.

17. Hatakeyama S, Koie T, Narita T, Hosogoe S, Yamamoto H, Tobisawa Y, Yoneyama T, Yoneyama T, Hashimoto Y, Ohyama C. Renal function outcomes and risk factors for stage 3B chronic kidney disease after urinary diversion in patients with muscle invasive bladder cancer. PLoS One. 2016; 11(2):e0149544.

18. Canter D, Viterbo R, Kutikov A, Wong YN, Plimack E, Zhu F, Oblaczynski M, Berberian R, Chen DY, Greenberg RE, et al. Baseline renal function status limits patient eligibility to receive perioperative chemotherapy for invasive bladder cancer and is minimally affected by radical cystectomy. Urology. 2011;77(1):160–5.

19. Hautmann RE. Urinary diversion: ileal conduit to neobladder. J Urol. 2003; 169(3):834–42.

20. Hautmann RE, de Petriconi R, Gottfried HW, Kleinschmidt K, Mattes R, Paiss T. The ileal neobladder: complications and functional results in 363 patients after 11 years of followup. J Urol. 1999;161(2):422–7. discussion 427-428

21. Kristjansson A, Bajc M, Wallin L, Willner J, Mansson W. Renal function up to 16 years after conduit (refluxing or anti-reflux anastomosis) or continent urinary diversion. 2. Renal scarring and location of bacteriuria. Br J Urol. 1995;76(5):546–50.

22. Studer UE, Danuser H, Thalmann GN, Springer JP, Turner WH. Antireflux nipples or afferent tubular segments in 70 patients with ileal low pressure bladder substitutes: long-term results of a prospective randomized trial. J Urol. 1996;156(6):1913–7.

23. Osman Y, Abol-Enein H, Nabeeh A, Gaballah M, Bazeed M. Long-term results of a prospective randomized study comparing two different antireflux techniques in orthotopic bladder substitution. Eur Urol. 2004;45(1):82–6.

24. Studer UE, Ackermann D, Casanova GA, Zingg EJ. Three years' experience with an ileal low pressure bladder substitute. Br J Urol. 1989;63(1):43–52.

16

Toileting behaviors and overactive bladder in patients with type 2 diabetes

Dongjuan Xu[1,2†], Ran Cheng[1†], Aixia Ma[3], Meng Zhao[1] and Kefang Wang[1*] (ID)

Abstract

Background: Overactive bladder is more prevalent in patients with type 2 diabetes than in those without diabetes. Unhealthy toileting behaviors may be associated with the development and worsening of overactive bladder symptoms. However, little is known about the relationships between toileting behaviors and overactive bladder in patients with diabetes. This study aimed to identify unhealthy toileting behaviors that patients with type 2 diabetes adopted to empty their bladders and investigate the relationships between toileting behaviors and overactive bladder.

Methods: Patients with type 2 diabetes from the endocrinology outpatient department of a hospital in China were recruited. The Toileting Behaviors-Women's Elimination Behavior and Overactive Bladder Symptom Score questionnaires were used to assess the patients' toileting behaviors and overactive bladder symptoms. A multivariate logistic regression model was used to explore the relationships between toileting behaviors and overactive bladder.

Results: Almost 14% of patients with diabetes had overactive bladder. The unhealthiest toileting behavior was premature voiding. In the multivariate logistic regression analysis, premature voiding (OR = 1.286, $p = 0.016$) and straining to void (OR = 1.243, $p = 0.026$) were associated with overactive bladder. There was a greater likelihood of having overactive bladder when patients engaged in unhealthy toileting behaviors (premature voiding and straining to void).

Conclusions: Overactive bladder in patients with type 2 diabetes was more than twofold higher than that in the general population. Thus, overactive bladder is not just an inconsequential condition for patients with diabetes. Unhealthy toileting behaviors, e.g., premature voiding and straining to void, may contribute to the onset or worsening of overactive bladder in patients with diabetes. Identification and awareness of these modifiable behavioral factors during diabetes care is an essential component of primary prevention, alleviation, and management of overactive bladder symptoms.

Keywords: Overactive bladder, Diabetes mellitus, Toileting behaviors

Background

Overactive bladder, defined as "urinary urgency, usually accompanied by frequency and nocturia, with or without urgency urinary incontinence" [1], affects a large proportion of the general adult population. Approximately 455 million people worldwide (almost 11%) experience overactive bladder, and the regional burden of overactive bladder is estimated to be greatest in Asia [2]. A recent large population-based survey conducted in China found that the prevalence of overactive bladder was 6% [3]. Overactive bladder can have a substantial negative effect on patients' quality of life specifically in terms of physical and psychological well-being, social interactions, work productivity, and sexual health [4, 5]. In addition, the direct and indirect costs of overactive bladder could seriously aggravate the economic burden on individuals and healthcare systems [6].

Unhealthy toileting behaviors may be associated with the development and worsening of overactive bladder

* Correspondence: wangkf@sdu.edu.cn
Dongjuan Xu and Ran Cheng are joint first authors of this article.
†Equal contributors
[1]School of Nursing, Shandong University, No.44, Wenhua Xi Road, Jinan, Shandong 250012, China
Full list of author information is available at the end of the article

symptoms. Individuals may empty bladder more frequently than necessary, based on the misconception that frequent voiding avoids bladder incontinence episodes [7]. However, too frequent voiding only signal an urge to empty the bladder despite a smaller volume of urine [8], which can precipitate or exacerbate bladder dysfunction [9]. Straining to empty the bladder, which involves an abdominal muscle contraction, could increase the peak flow and mean flow rates, as well as decrease the total voiding time [10]. Individuals who use straining to start voiding before the initiation of the micturition reflex may be more likely to develop incontinence and voiding dysfunction [11]. Toileting behavior is a comprehensive concept that includes voiding place, time, position, and style [12]; however, most recent studies on toileting behavior and overactive bladder focused only on one or some aspects of toileting behavior [13, 14]. Previously, Wan et al. examined the relationship between toileting behaviors and lower urinary tract symptoms among female nurses and found that three unhealthy toileting behaviors (i.e., premature voiding, delayed voiding, and straining to void) were significantly associated with lower urinary tract symptoms, while no significant association with voiding place or position preference was observed [15]. However, little is known about the relationships between toileting behaviors and overactive bladder in other populations.

Diabetes mellitus has been related to an earlier onset and increased bladder dysfunction severity [16]. Overactive bladder is more prevalent in patients with type 2 diabetes than in the general population [17, 18]. Moreover, higher glycosylated hemoglobin levels increased the risk of overactive bladder in patients with diabetes [19]. Besides diabetes-related factors, a variety of factors were associated with overactive bladder, including age [3, 19], gender [20], marital status [3], fluid intake [21], smoking [22], alcohol drinking [3], physical exercise [23], history of urinary tract infection [24], constipation [25], hypertension/heart failure [26], and obesity [20].

Because of its high prevalence, overactive bladder is an important therapeutic target in patients with type 2 diabetes. Available evidence suggests that behavioral interventions, such as bladder training [27], pelvic floor muscle training and exercise, and urge suppression techniques [28], are effective in extending voiding interval and alleviating urgency and incontinence. Behavioral interventions may also increase the efficacy of pharmacologic treatment for overactive bladder [9]. If unhealthy toileting behaviors can contribute to overactive bladder symptoms, identifying and modifying these unhealthy behaviors, accompanied by other behavioral and pharmacologic treatments, help prevent, eliminate, alleviate, and manage overactive bladder symptoms in patients with type 2 diabetes. Therefore, the purposes of

this study were (1) to investigate the unhealthy toileting behaviors that patients with diabetes adopted to empty their bladders and (2) to identify the relationships between toileting behaviors and overactive bladder in patients with type 2 diabetes.

Methods
Study design and data collection
This is a cross-sectional study with convenience sampling. From May to August 2014, we recruited participants from the endocrinology outpatient department in one of the largest hospitals in Jinan, the capital city of Shandong Province, China. The inclusion criteria were as follows: (1) ≥18 years old, (2) diagnosed as having type 2 diabetes, and (3) willing to participate in the study and capable of understanding study procedure and questions. The exclusion criteria were the following: (1) new-onset neurological disorders (such as stroke, spinal cord damage, Parkinson's disease, and multiple sclerosis), (2) urinary tract infections within the last month of the survey, (3) pelvic organ prolapse, and (4) history of bladder surgery.

The Institutional Review Board of Shandong University approved this study. A self-administered pencil-and-paper survey was used to collect data. Before the survey, trained graduate students obtained written informed consent from each patient with diabetes. The survey was completed anonymously and the patients were assured that their responses would be kept confidential.

Assessment
We obtained the patients' sociodemographic characteristics data, including age, sex, race/ethnicity, education, marital status, living area, and income, and assessed lifestyle-related characteristics, including smoking, alcohol use, tea drinking, fluid intake, and physical exercise. We also collected health-related data consisting of waist circumference, hip circumference, urinary tract infection history, comorbidity, diabetes mellitus duration, and microvascular complications of diabetes (peripheral neuropathy and retinopathy). Moreover, the Charlson comorbidity index (CCI) was used to measure a range of comorbid conditions, such as hypertension, congestive heart failure, or cancer (a total of 20 conditions) [29]. Since all patients in this study had diabetes, diabetes was excluded from the calculation of CCI. Each condition was assigned a weight of 1, 2, 3, or 6, depending on the risk of mortality [29]. The total score, which is the sum of all weighted conditions, was used to predict mortality.

We used the validated Toileting Behaviors-Women's Elimination Behavior (TB-WEB) scale (Chinese version) to evaluate the participants' toileting behaviors [30]. This 17-item scale contains five domains: place preference for voiding, premature voiding, delayed voiding, straining to void, and position preference for voiding. Since position preference for voiding (e.g., "crouching or hovering to empty bladder when not at home") is specific for the female population, we did not include this domain in the study. Detailed descriptions of each item are provided in Table 3. The TB-WEB used a five-point Likert-type scale (from 1 = never to 5 = always) to assess how often patients with diabetes adopted a behavior. An average score was calculated for each domain, and a higher score corresponding to unhealthier toileting behavior. The 4-domain TB-WEB has been validated in male patients [31], and the Cronbach's alpha coefficient of the TB-WEB scale was 0.71 in this study.

We used the Chinese version of Overactive Bladder Symptom Score (OABSS) questionnaire to evaluate overactive bladder symptoms in the past week. OABSS is a reliable and valid questionnaire designed to quantify the four symptoms of overactive bladder: daytime frequency (0–2), nighttime frequency (0–3), urgency (0–5), and urgency incontinence (0–5) [32]. The total score ranges from 0 to 15, and a higher score represents more severe overactive bladder symptoms. The Chinese version of the OABSS scale has been developed and validated in the Chinese population with good reliability and validity [33]. Here, overactive bladder means an urgency symptom score ≥ 2 and a total score ≥ 3.

Statistical analysis

We used descriptive statistics (frequency and percentage for categorical variables, mean and standard deviation for continuous variables) to describe the characteristics of patients with type 2 diabetes. We performed Student's t-tests to compare the differences of each toileting behavior between patients without overactive bladder and those with overactive bladder. We also used a multivariate logistic regression model to explore the relationships between toileting behaviors and overactive bladder, after adjusting for age, sex, race/ethnicity, education, marital status, living area, income, smoking, alcohol use, tea drinking, fluid intake per day, physical exercise, waist-to-hip ratio, urinary tract infection history, CCI, diabetes mellitus duration, and microvascular complications of diabetes (peripheral neuropathy and retinopathy). We performed all statistical analyses using Stata (Version 14.1; StataCorp, College Station, TX). Statistical significance was accepted at $p < 0.05$.

Results

Among the 1025 eligible patients with type 2 diabetes, seven patients were excluded from the analysis because they omitted four or more survey items. The mean age was approximately 59 years (range 20–86 years), and half of the participants were female. The patients had diabetes for about 9 years on average, and more than

half (52%) had diabetic peripheral neuropathy or retinopathy. Nearly 14% of the patients had overactive bladder. Among the overactive bladder patients, approximately 57% had wet overactive bladder and 43% had dry overactive bladder. The patient characteristics are presented in Table 1.

The unhealthiest toileting behavior among patients with diabetes was premature voiding, followed by place preference for voiding, delayed voiding, and straining to void (Table 2). Premature voiding and straining to void were significantly unhealthier in patients with overactive bladder than in those without overactive bladder, as indicated by Student's t-tests. As shown in Table 3, about half of the patients often or always emptied their bladders with little or no need to urinate before sleep (57%) or before leaving home (47%). Approximately 36% of the patients often or always avoided using toilets at someone else's house. With regard to public toilets, 26% of the patients were often or always worried about the cleanness and 24% of the patients avoided using them. More than 15% of patients often or always waited more than 4 h to urinate at work, and 13% of the patients often or always pushed down or strained to finish emptying their bladder.

After adjusting for control variables, positive associations between unhealthy toileting behaviors (premature voiding and staining to void) and overactive bladder were found among patients with diabetes (Table 4). The more the patients empty their bladder with little or no need to void and pushed down or strained to void, the greater the likelihood of having overactive bladder. There were no significant associations between toileting behaviors (place preference for voiding and delayed voiding) and overactive bladder. In addition, age, waist-to-hip ratio, CCI, and diabetic peripheral neuropathy or retinopathy were positively associated with overactive bladder, while female and married patients with diabetes were less likely to have overactive bladder.

Discussion

A large sample survey of patients with type 2 diabetes was conducted to identify unhealthy toileting behaviors and further investigate their relationships with overactive bladder. The present study adds to the small body of work that extends research focused on only one or some aspects of toileting behavior to comprehensively examine it using a valid instrument. We found that the prevalence of overactive bladder in patients with diabetes was nearly 14%, which is more than twofold higher than that in the general population in China [3]. Moreover, the more the patients with diabetes engage in unhealthy toileting behaviors (e.g., premature voiding and straining to void), the greater the likelihood of having overactive bladder. Thus, our findings provide significant

Table 1 Characteristics of patients with type 2 diabetes mellitus (*n* = 1018)

Variables	Mean ± SD or *n* (%)
Age (years)	59.1 ± 11.7
Sex	
Female	509 (50.0)
Male	509 (50.0)
Race/ethnicity	
Han	981 (96.4)
Other	37 (3.6)
Education	
Elementary school or lower	228 (22.4)
Middle school	232 (22.8)
High school	306 (30.1)
College or higher	252 (24.7)
Marital status	
Married	920 (90.4)
Single/divorced/widowed	98 (9.6)
Living area	
Urban	770 (75.6)
Rural	248 (24.4)
Income (RMB (USD)/month)	
≤3000 (451)	620 (60.9)
>3000 (451)	398 (39.1)
Smoker	
Yes	345 (33.9)
No	673 (66.1)
Alcohol drinker	
Yes	308 (30.3)
No	710 (69.7)
Tea drinker	
Yes	732 (71.9)
No	286 (28.1)
Fluid intake (ml/day)	
≤2500	546 (53.6)
>2500	472 (46.4)
Exercise	
Yes	397 (39.0)
No	621 (61.0)
Waist-to-hip ratio (WHR)	0.9 ± 0.1
Urinary tract infection history [a]	
Yes	93 (9.1)
No	925 (90.9)
Charlson comorbidity index (CCI)	1.7 ± 1.0
Diabetes mellitus duration (years)	9.0 ± 7.4

Table 1 Characteristics of patients with type 2 diabetes mellitus (*n* = 1018) (Continued)

Diabetic peripheral neuropathy or retinopathy	
Yes	533 (52.4)
No	485 (47.6)
overactive bladder	
No overactive bladder	878 (86.3)
Dry overactive bladder	60 (5.9)
Wet overactive bladder	80 (7.9)

SD standard deviation, *RMB* Chinese Yuan, *USD* United States dollar
[a]Patients with type 2 diabetes who had a urinary tract infection at least one month before the survey

implications in the prevention, alleviation, and management of overactive bladder symptoms during diabetes care.

The findings indicated that the most common unhealthy toileting behavior among patients with diabetes was premature voiding. Approximately half of them often or always emptied their bladder with little or no need to void before sleep or before leaving home. Moreover, premature voiding was significantly associated with overactive bladder in patients with diabetes, which is in line with the finding by Wan et al., who found a positive association between premature voiding and lower urinary tract symptoms in female nurses [15]. In addition, too frequent voiding with little or no need to urinate may have no harmful effects in the short term; however, engaging in this behavior leads to increased bladder sensitivity to lower volumes of urine, reduced bladder capacity, and eventually detrusor instability in the long term [8, 9].

We also found that straining to void, although the least common unhealthy toileting behavior, had a positive association with overactive bladder in patients with type 2 diabetes. This finding confirms that from a study of female nurses with regard to straining to void and lower urinary tract symptoms [15]. Pushing down or straining was often or always employed by patients with diabetes to begin urinating (7.0%), keep urine flowing (6.4%), empty bladder more quickly (5.7%), and finish emptying bladder (13.4%). Abdominal straining to void is considered unhealthy by researchers because of its association with poor outcomes, such as fecal and/or urinary incontinence [34], dysfunctional voiding [13], and prolonged postoperative catheterization [35]. Pauwels et al. indicated that if straining was used to begin voiding before the initiation of the micturition reflex and as the only way to empty bladder, voiding problems and incontinence are more likely to occur [11].

In this study, delayed voiding and place preference for voiding were not significantly associated with overactive bladder in patients with diabetes; the patients with

Table 2 Comparison of toileting behaviors between patients with diabetes with and without overactive bladder

Toileting behavior	Overall sample (n = 1018)	No OAB (n = 878)	OAB (n = 140)	p value
Premature voiding	2.41 ± 1.00	2.37 ± 0.98	2.68 ± 1.04	0.001
Place preference for voiding	2.18 ± 1.14	2.18 ± 1.14	2.14 ± 1.13	0.710
Delayed voiding	2.06 ± 0.74	2.05 ± 0.73	2.15 ± 0.77	0.142
Straining to void	1.49 ± 0.88	1.45 ± 0.84	1.74 ± 1.04	0.002

The numbers are expressed as mean ± standard deviation
OAB overactive bladder

overactive bladder had almost the same scores for the two unhealthy toileting behaviors as those of patients without overactive bladder. Nevertheless, delayed voiding and place preference for voiding were common in patients with diabetes. Moreover, suppressing the urge to void may have no detrimental effect in the short term; however, long-term suppression may threaten bladder's health [14]. Avoiding using public toilets or toilets at someone else's house may lead to premature or delayed voiding [36]. Thus, educating patients to adopt healthy toileting behaviors to improve and maintain their optimal bladder health is essential.

Besides unhealthy toileting behaviors, we found another significant modifiable factor associated with overactive bladder in patients with diabetes, i.e., waist-to-hip ratio. Waist-to-hip ratio, as a measure of obesity or health, has been shown to be a better predictor of

cardiovascular disease [37], diabetes [38], and hypercholesterolemia [39] compared with body mass index and waist circumstance. Our finding is similar to studies that showed obesity to be a risk factor of overactive bladder and weight loss to be related to improvements in incontinence status [20, 40]. Weight loss has a beneficial effect on general health and quality of life; thus, it should be encouraged universally. In addition, diabetic peripheral neuropathy or retinopathy, which is the consequence of poor blood glucose control, was found to be associated with overactive bladder. Similarly, Chiu et al. showed that the increased risk of overactive bladder in patients with diabetes could be attributed to higher glycosylated hemoglobin levels [19]. Furthermore, overactive bladder may also result from a number of conditions or comorbidities, such as hypertension, heart failure, cerebrovascular disease, dementia, and renal diseases [26], which

Table 3 Toileting behaviors among patients with type 2 diabetes mellitus (n = 1018)

Behavior	Never/Rarely n (%)	Sometimes n (%)	Often/Always n (%)
Premature voiding			
Empty bladder with little or no need to urinate before sleep	348 (34.2)	89 (8.7)	581 (57.1)
Empty bladder with little or no need to urinate before leaving home	412 (40.5)	131 (12.9)	475 (46.7)
Empty bladder with little or no need to urinate "just in case"	701 (68.9)	132 (13.0)	185 (18.2)
Empty bladder with little or no need to urinate at home	938 (92.1)	54 (5.3)	26 (2.6)
Place preference for voiding			
Avoid using toilets at someone else's house	588 (57.8)	63 (6.2)	367 (36.1)
Worry about cleanness of public toilets	650 (63.9)	104 (10.2)	264 (25.9)
Avoid using public toilets	690 (67.8)	82 (8.1)	246 (24.2)
Hold urine until getting home	705 (69.3)	164 (16.1)	149 (14.6)
Delay voiding			
Wait too long (>4 h) to urinate at work	690 (67.8)	172 (16.9)	156 (15.3)
Delay emptying bladder when busy	572 (56.2)	326 (32.0)	120 (11.8)
Wait to empty bladder until unable to hold	788 (77.4)	152 (14.9)	78 (7.7)
Straining to void			
Push down or strain to finish emptying bladder	774 (76.0)	108 (10.6)	136 (13.4)
Push down or strain to begin urinating	883 (86.7)	64 (6.3)	71 (7.0)
Push down or strain to keep urine flowing	885 (86.9)	68 (6.7)	65 (6.4)
Push down or strain to empty bladder more quickly	880 (86.4)	80 (7.9)	58 (5.7)

Table 4 The relationships between toileting behaviors and overactive bladder among patients with type 2 diabetes mellitus (n = 1018)

Variables	OR (95% CI)	SE	p value
Toileting behavior			
Premature voiding	1.286 (1.048–1.579)	0.135	0.016
Straining to void	1.243 (1.026–1.506)	0.122	0.026
Delayed voiding	1.259 (0.969–1.636)	0.168	0.084
Place preference for voiding	0.883 (0.735–1.062)	0.083	0.188
Age	1.027 (1.006–1.049)	0.011	0.013
Sex (female vs. male)	0.484 (0.274–0.854)	0.140	0.012
Race/Ethnicity (Han vs. other)	4.624 (0.979–21.832)	3.662	0.053
Education (ref. = elementary school or lower)			
Middle school	0.831 (0.471–1.466)	0.241	0.522
High school	0.638 (0.360–1.130)	0.186	0.124
College or higher	0.584 (0.308–1.108)	0.191	0.100
Marital status (married vs. unmarried)	0.513 (0.285–0.922)	0.154	0.026
Living area (urban vs. rural)	1.219 (0.706–2.107)	0.340	0.477
Income (>3000 vs. ≤3000)	0.807 (0.523–1.245)	0.178	0.331
Smoker	1.105 (0.659–1.855)	0.292	0.705
Alcohol drinker	0.638 (0.379–1.073)	0.169	0.090
Tea drinker	1.215 (0.781–1.890)	0.274	0.388
Fluid intake (>2500 vs. ≤2500)	1.070 (0.726–1.575)	0.211	0.734
Exercise	0.823 (0.549–1.233)	0.170	0.345
Waist-to-hip ratio (WHR) [a]	1.266 (1.033–1.552)	0.131	0.023
Urinary tract infection history [b]	0.966 (0.496–1.880)	0.328	0.919
Charlson comorbidity index (CCI)	1.183 (1.001–1.397)	0.101	0.049
Diabetes mellitus duration	0.984 (0.955–1.013)	0.015	0.270
Diabetic peripheral neuropathy or retinopathy	1.506 (1.002–2.264)	0.313	0.049

OR odds ratio, CI confidence interval, SE standard error
[a] Standardized waist-to-hip ratio (WHR) was used in the analysis
[b] Patients with type 2 diabetes who had a urinary tract infection at least one month before the survey

supports our result that higher CCI was associated with increased risk of overactive bladder. Our results are consistent with a previous report that overactive bladder increased with age and was more prevalent in men than in women [20].

This study has several limitations. First, we recruited patients in one hospital using a convenience sampling method. Thus, the generalizability of our findings may be limited. To address this, we surveyed a large sample of 1025 patients with diabetes with <1% missing data. Second, because of the cross-sectional design of the survey, a causal relationship between unhealthy toileting behaviors and overactive bladder could not be established. Moreover, in cross-sectional studies, associations could be reversed. For example, patients might adopt certain toileting behaviors to cope with overactive bladder symptoms. However, this may not be the case in our study because we surveyed unhealthy toileting behaviors and later overactive bladder symptoms. Exploring toileting behavior changes after having overactive bladder symptoms and determining whether these changes further worsen or relieve overactive bladder symptoms would be interesting. Third, our findings may be influenced by uncontrolled confounders, such as constipation, benign prostatic hyperplasia, and vaginal or cesarean delivery. Future studies should include these variables in the survey and explore whether the associations between toileting behaviors and overactive bladder vary by gender.

Conclusions

Overactive bladder in patients with type 2 diabetes was more than twofold higher than that in the general population. Thus, overactive bladder is not just an inconsequential condition for patients with diabetes. Furthermore, in patients with diabetes, preserving bladder health is particularly necessary and unhealthy toileting behaviors, especially premature voiding and straining to void, may contribute to the onset or worsening of overactive bladder. Identification and awareness of modifiable behavioral factors during diabetes care is an essential component of primary prevention, alleviation, and management of overactive bladder symptoms.

Abbreviations
CCI: Charlson comorbidity index; OAB: Overactive bladder; OABSS: Overactive Bladder Symptom Score; TB-WEB: Toileting Behaviors-Women's Elimination Behavior

Acknowledgements
The authors thank all of the patients for their participation.

Funding
This work was supported by a grant from the Natural Science Foundation of Shandong Province (ZR2015HM033). The funders had no role in study design, data collection, data analysis, manuscript preparation, and publication decisions.

Authors' contributions
KFW designed the study. RC, AXM and MZ collected the data. DJX analyzed the data. DJX and RC drafted the manuscript. KFW supervised the study and made critical revisions to the paper for important intellectual content. All authors read and approved the final manuscript.

Competing interests
The authors declare that they have no competing interests.

Author details
[1]School of Nursing, Shandong University, No.44, Wenhua Xi Road, Jinan, Shandong 250012, China. [2]School of Nursing, Purdue University, West Lafayette, Indiana 47907, USA. [3]Department of endocrinology, Qilu Hospital of Shandong University, Jinan, Shandong 250012, China.

References
1. Haylen BT, de Ridder D, Freeman RM, et al. An international Urogynecological association (IUGA)/international Continence society (ICS) joint report on the terminology for female pelvic floor dysfunction. Neurourol Urodyn. 2010;29:4–20.
2. Irwin DE, Kopp ZS, Agatep B, et al. Worldwide prevalence estimates of lower urinary tract symptoms, overactive bladder, urinary incontinence and bladder outlet obstruction. BJU Int. 2011;108:1132–8.
3. Wang Y, Xu K, Hu H, et al. Prevalence, risk factors, and impact on health related quality of life of overactive bladder in China. Neurourol Urodyn. 2011;30:1448–55.
4. Irwin DE, Milsom I, Kopp Z, et al. Impact of overactive bladder symptoms on employment, social interactions and emotional well-being in six European countries. BJU Int. 2006;97:96–100.
5. Coyne KS, Sexton CC, Thompson C, et al. The impact of OAB on sexual health in men and women: results from EpiLUTS. J Sex Med. 2011;8:1603–15.
6. Ganz ML, Smalarz AM, Krupski TL, et al. Economic costs of overactive bladder in the United States. Urology. 2010;75:526–32.
7. Naoemova I, De Wachter S, Wyndaele JJ. Comparison of sensation-related voiding patterns between continent and incontinent women: a study with a 3-day sensation-related bladder diary (SR-BD). Neurourol Urodyn. 2008;27:511–4.
8. Sampselle CM. Teaching women to use a voiding diary. Am J Nurs. 2003;103:62–4.
9. Burgio KL. Influence of behavior modification on overactive bladder. Urology. 2002;60:72–6.
10. Devreese AM, Nuyens G, Staes F, et al. Do posture and straining influence urinary-flow parameters in normal women? Neurourol Urodyn. 2000;19:3–8.
11. Pauwels E, De Laet K, De Wachter S, et al. Healthy, middle-aged, history-free, continent women–do they strain to void? J Urol. 2006;175:1403–7.
12. Wang K, Palmer MH. Development and validation of an instrument to assess women's toileting behavior related to urinary elimination: preliminary results. Nurs Res. 2011;60:158–64.
13. Carlson KV, Rome S, Nitti VW. Dysfunctional voiding in women. J Urol. 2001;165:143–7.
14. Zhang C, Hai T, Yu L, et al. Association between occupational stress and risk of overactive bladder and other lower urinary tract symptoms: a cross-sectional study of female nurses in China. Neurourol Urodyn. 2013;32:254–60.
15. Wan X, Wu C, Xu D, et al. Toileting behaviours and lower urinary tract symptoms among female nurses: a cross-sectional questionnaire survey. Int J Nurs Stud. 2017;65:1–7.
16. Karoli R, Bhat S, Fatima J, et al. A study of bladder dysfunction in women with type 2 diabetes mellitus. Indian J Endocrinol Metab. 2014;18:552–7.
17. Ikeda M, Nozawa K. Prevalence of overactive bladder and its related factors in Japanese patients with diabetes mellitus. Endocr J. 2015;62:847–54.
18. Lawrence JM, Lukacz ES, Liu IL, et al. Pelvic floor disorders, diabetes, and obesity in women: findings from the Kaiser Permanente Continence associated risk epidemiology study. Diabetes Care. 2007;30:2536–41.
19. Chiu AF, Huang MH, Wang CC, et al. Higher glycosylated hemoglobin levels increase the risk of overactive bladder syndrome in patients with type 2 diabetes mellitus. Int J Urol. 2012;19:995–1001.
20. Wen JG, Li JS, Wang ZM, et al. The prevalence and risk factors of OAB in middle-aged and old people in China. Neurourol Urodyn. 2014;33:387–91.
21. Callan L, Thompson DL, Netsch D. Does increasing or decreasing the daily intake of water/fluid by adults affect overactive bladder symptoms? J Wound Ostomy Continence Nurs. 2015;42:614–20.
22. de Boer TA, Slieker-ten Hove MC, Burger CW, et al. The prevalence and risk factors of overactive bladder symptoms and its relation to pelvic organ prolapse symptoms in a general female population. Int Urogynecol J. 2011;22:569–75.
23. Ko IG, Lim MH, Choi PB, et al. Effect of long-term exercise on voiding functions in obese elderly women. Int Neurourol J. 2013;17:130–8.
24. Chung JM, Lee SD, Kang DI, et al. Prevalence and associated factors of overactive bladder in Korean children 5-13 years old: a nationwide multicenter study. Urology. 2009;73:63–7.
25. Wu JW, Xing YR, Wen YB, et al. Prevalence of Spina bifida Occulta and its relationship with overactive bladder in middle-aged and elderly Chinese people. Int Neurourol J. 2016;20:151–8.
26. Asche CV, Kim J, Kulkarni AS, et al. Presence of central nervous system, cardiovascular and overall co-morbidity burden in patients with overactive bladder disorder in a real-world setting. BJU Int. 2012;109:572–80.
27. Christofi N, Hextall A. An evidence-based approach to lifestyle interventions in urogynaecology. Menopause Int. 2007;13:154–8.
28. Burgio KL, Goode PS, Johnson TM, et al. Behavioral versus drug treatment for overactive bladder in men: the male overactive bladder treatment in veterans (MOTIVE) trial. J Am Geriatr Soc. 2011;59:2209–16.
29. Charlson ME, Pompei P, Ales KL, et al. A new method of classifying prognostic comorbidity in longitudinal studies: development and validation. J Chronic Dis. 1987;40:373–83.
30. Wan X, Zhang Y, Liu Y, et al. Reliability and validity of the Chinese version of Women's toileting behavior scale among female nurses. Chin J Nurs. 2014;49:782–5.
31. Cheng R, Gao J, Chen LQ, et al. Reliability and validity of the toileting behavior scale in men with diabetes mellitus. J Nurs. 2016;23:8–11.
32. Homma Y, Yoshida M, Seki N, et al. Symptom assessment tool for overactive bladder syndrome– overactive bladder symptom score. Urology. 2006;68:318–23.
33. Hung MJ, Chou CL, Yen TW, et al. Development and validation of the Chinese overactive bladder symptom score for assessing overactive bladder syndrome in a RESORT study. J Formos Med Assoc. 2013;112:276–82.
34. Lacima G, Espuna M, Pera M, et al. Clinical, urodynamic, and manometric findings in women with combined fecal and urinary incontinence. Neurourol Urodyn. 2002;21:464–9.
35. Bhatia NN, Bergman A. Urodynamic predictability of voiding following incontinence surgery. Obstet Gynecol. 1984;63:85–91.
36. Xu D, Chen L, Wan X, et al. Toileting behaviour and related health beliefs among Chinese female nurses. Int J Clin Pract. 2016;70:416–23.
37. de Koning L, Merchant AT, Pogue J, et al. Waist circumference and waist-to-hip ratio as predictors of cardiovascular events: meta-regression analysis of prospective studies. Eur Heart J. 2007;28:850–6.
38. Motamed N, Rabiee B, Keyvani H, et al. The best obesity indices to discriminate type 2 diabetes mellitus. Metab Syndr Relat Disord. 2016;14:249–53.
39. Haregu TN, Oti S, Egondi T, et al. Measurement of overweight and obesity an urban slum setting in sub-Saharan Africa: a comparison of four anthropometric indices. BMC Obes. 2016;3:46.
40. Subak LL, King WC, Belle SH, et al. Urinary incontinence before and after bariatric surgery. JAMA Intern Med. 2015;175:1378–87.

Suprapubic tube versus urethral catheter drainage after robot-assisted radical prostatectomy

17

Suprapubic tube versus urethral catheter drainage after robot-assisted radical prostatectomy

Zhongyu Jian[†], Shijian Feng[†], Yuntian Chen, Xin Wei, Deyi Luo, Hong Li and Kunjie Wang[*]

Abstract

Background: Prostate cancer is one of the most common cancers in the elderly population. The standard treatment is radical prostatectomy (RARP). However, urologists do not have consents on the postoperative urine drainage management (suprapubic tube (ST)/ urethral catheter (UC)). Thus, we try to compare ST drainage to UC drainage after robot-assisted radical prostatectomy regarding to comfort, recovery rate and continence using the method of meta-analysis.

Methods: A systematic search was performed in Dec. 2017 on PubMed, Medline, Embase and Cochrane Library databases. The authors independently reviewed the records to identify studies comparing ST with UC of patients underwent RARP. Meta-analysis was performed using the extracted data from the selected studies.

Results: Seven studies, including 3 RCTs, with a total of 946 patients met the inclusion criteria and were included in our meta-analysis. Though there was no significant difference between the ST group and the UC group on postoperative pain (RR1.73, P 0.20), our study showed a significant improvement on bother or discomfort, defined as trouble in hygiene and sleep, caused by catheter when compared two groups at postoperative day (POD) 7 in ST group (RR2.05, P 0.006). There was no significant difference between the ST group and UC group on urinary continence (RR0.98, P 0.74) and emergency department visit (RR0.61, P 0.11). The rates of bladder neck contracture and other complications were very low in both groups.

Conclusion: Compared to UC, ST showed a weak advantage. So it might be a good choice to choose ST over RARP.

Keywords: Prostate cancer, Prostatectomy, Robotics, Suprapubic catheter, Urethral catheterization

Background

Prostate cancer is one of the most common cancers in the elderly population. In fact, prostate cancer is the most common cancer in male. It was estimated that in 2014, 233,000 men were diagnosed with prostate cancer and 29,480 men died of this disease [1]. Radical prostatectomy (RP) is an effectively therapy for those who are clinically diagnosed with localized prostate cancer [2]. Urethral catheter (UC) is traditionally used in RP, not only for drainage of the bladder but also protecting the anastomosis and promoting the healing process.

Compared to the retropubic approach, robot-assisted radical prostatectomy (RARP) had a lower incidence rate of anastomotic stricture [3]. Some studies reported uneventful early catheter removal after RARP [4, 5]. Therefore, the use of UC might not be as crucial as previously envisaged. On the other hand, complaints about the discomfort associated with UC were commonly seen in the clinic. In order to improve the life quality of patients, some researchers are exploring whether replacing UC with percutaneous suprapubic tube (ST) after RARP is a better choice [6–12].

* Correspondence: wangkj@scu.edu.cn
[†]Equal contributors
Department of Urology, Institute of Urology (Laboratory of Reconstructive Urology), West China Hospital, Sichuan University, No. 37 Guo Xue Xiang, Chengdu, Sichuan 610041, People's Republic of China

The first report of catheter-less technique after RARP was published in 2008, which showed favorable results in terms of postoperative pain and early recovery of continence [6]. Later researches reported conflicting results in postoperative pain after surgery [7, 8]. Until now, there was no consents or systematic review focusing on ST and UC after RARP. We searched and analyzed the data from the literatures to compare postoperative pain, urinary continence and other related outcomes between ST and UC after RARP surgery.

Methods
Search strategy
A systematic search was performed in Dec. 2017 on PubMed, Medline, Embase and Cochrane Library databases. The following MeSH terms and their combinations were searched in [Title/Abstract]: suprapubic, catheter, catheterization, tube, robotic, radical, prostatectomy, prostate cancer.

Inclusion and exclusion criteria
The inclusion criteria were studies comparing UC and ST for RARP, including randomized controlled trials (RCT), case-control and cohort studies. Our study was limited to human subjects, gender (male), and languages (English and Chinese). Conference abstracts, case reports, letters or reviews were excluded from further analysis.

Data extraction
Two authors reviewed the titles, abstracts and full texts of included studies independently. If disagreement appeared, a senior author was asked to make the final decision. Data was extracted from the included eligible studies. If data was presented as pictures rather than numbers, GetData Graph Digitizer (version 2.26) was used to extract relevant data. The information extracted from the study are listed below: postoperative pain, bother or discomfort by catheter, urinary continence, bladder neck contracture (BNC), emergency department visit and complications.

Quality assessment and statistical analysis
The quality of RCTs was assessed using the Cochrane risk of bias tool. The quality of case-control studies was assessed using the modified Newcastle-Ottawa scale (The total score is nine, studies score six or above were considered as high quality). Data analysis was performed with Review Manager (RevMan 5.3, Cochrane Collaboration, Oxford, UK).

The risk ratio (RR) and weighted mean difference (WMD) were used to compare dichotomous and continuous variables, respectively. And the 95% confidence intervals of the statistics were presented. Heterogeneity was tested using the chi-square test. A random effects model was utilized if $I^2 > 50\%$, otherwise the fixed-effects model was used. $P < 0.05$ was defined as statistically significant different.

Results
Description of included studies and quality assessment
A total of 502 articles were acquired through literature search and screened for eligibility. 212 articles were identified after removal of duplicates in the four database mentioned above. 199 articles were excluded because they were not focused on the comparison between UC and ST of RP after screening the titles and abstracts. Three studies were excluded because they were comments. One descriptive study only focused on ST, and another study about retropubic radical prostatectomy (RRP) were also excluded. We also excluded one study for it did not contain required data in numeric format, but present using figure, which did not show the standard deviation. Finally, seven studies with 946 patients were included in this systematic review (Fig. 1).

The characteristics of the included studies were shown in Table 1. Among these studies, three were RCTs reaching the level of evidence 1b [8, 11, 12]. One cohort, non-randomized study reached the level of evidence 2b [6]. Two case-control studies compared contemporary series of patients reached the level of evidence 3b [9, 10]; and one case-control study using historical series as controls reached the level of evidence 4 [7].

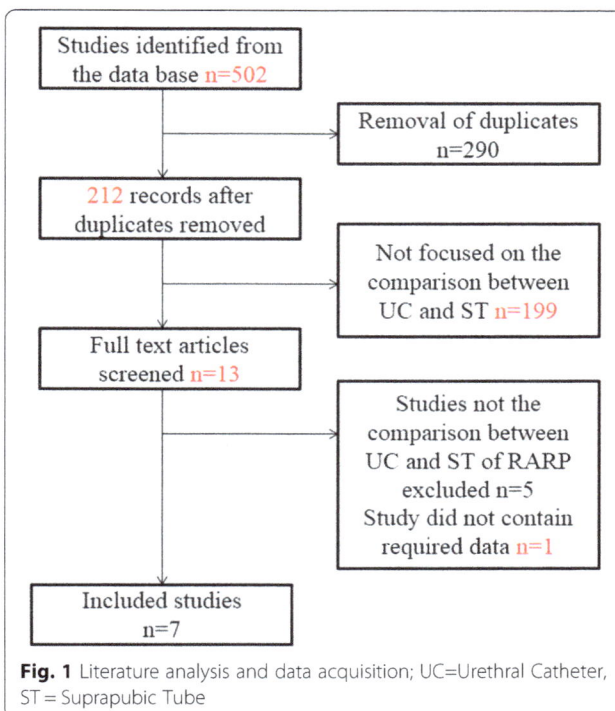

Fig. 1 Literature analysis and data acquisition; UC=Urethral Catheter, ST = Suprapubic Tube

Table 1 Characteristics of included studies

Study	LOE	Design	N		follow up	Time for removal of UC and ST		Pain	Continence definition	Quality
			UC	ST		UC	ST			
Tewari A 2008 [6]	2b	pro	20	10	6 months	POD 7	POD 7	questionnaire	0–1pad/day	8
Krane LS 2009 [7]	4	Retro	50	202	6–12 months	POD 7	POD 7	FPS-R scale (0–10)	0–1pad/day	6
Prasad SM 2014 [8]	1b	pro-random	29	29	N	POD 7	POD 7 (UC removed POD1)	VAS scale (0–10)	N	RCT
Afzal MZ 2015 [9]	3b	Retro	174	51	N	POD 8	POD 6–9 (UC removed POD1)	N	0–1pad/day	7
Morgan MS 2016 [10]	3b	Retro	65	94	>3 months	POD 7–10	POD 9–10 (UC removed POD1)	questionnaire	N	7
Martinschek A 2016 [11]	1b	pro-random	35	27	1 year	N	N	VAS scale (0–10)	N	RCT
Harke N [12]	1b	pro-random	80	80	2 years	POD 5	N (UC removed POD1)	NRS (0–10)	0–1pad/day	RCT

ST Suprapubic tube, *UC* urethral catheter; *Pro* prospective, *Random* randomised, *Retro* retrospective, *LoE* level of evidence, *POD* postorerative day, *N* not gived, *VAS* visual analog scale, *NRS* numeric rating scale, *FPS-R scale* Faces Pain Score-Revised, *RCT* randomized controlled trail

Postoperative pain

A total of six studies reported postoperative pain at postoperative Day (POD) 6 [7, 11, 12] or POD 7 [6, 8, 10]. We divided the patients into two groups (with pain and without pain). Three articles eligible for the meta-analysis (441 patients) were shown in the Fig. 2a [6, 7, 10]. There was no significant difference between UC and ST group (RR1.73; 95% CI 0.75, 3.95; P 0.20) (Fig. 2a).

Four studies reported postoperative pain at POD 1 [8, 11, 12] or POD 2. [7] Meta-analysis of the first three RCTs (280 patients) showed that ST group had not significantly decreased pain at POD 1 compared to the

UC group (WMD 0.06; 95% CI -0.47, 0.59; P 0.79) (Fig. 2b). The fourth study [7] reported that patients in the ST group had significantly decreased pain at POD 2 compared to the UC group ($P < 0.001$).

Bother or discomfort by catheter

Bother or discomfort was defined as the trouble from the hygiene and sleep. The meta-analysis of three studies (247 patients) [6, 9, 10] showed a statistically significant advantage on the rate of bother or discomfort in favour of the ST compared to UC at POD 7 (RR2.05; 95% CI 1.23,3.44; P 0.006) (Fig. 3).

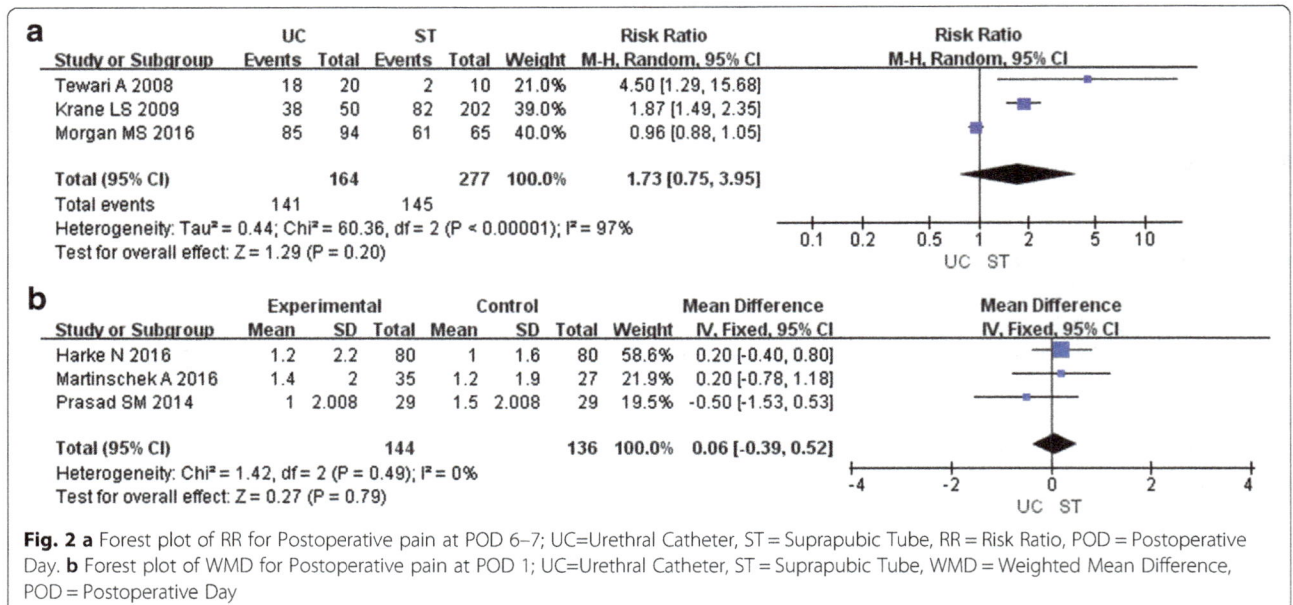

Fig. 2 a Forest plot of RR for Postoperative pain at POD 6–7; UC=Urethral Catheter, ST = Suprapubic Tube, RR = Risk Ratio, POD = Postoperative Day. **b** Forest plot of WMD for Postoperative pain at POD 1; UC=Urethral Catheter, ST = Suprapubic Tube, WMD = Weighted Mean Difference, POD = Postoperative Day

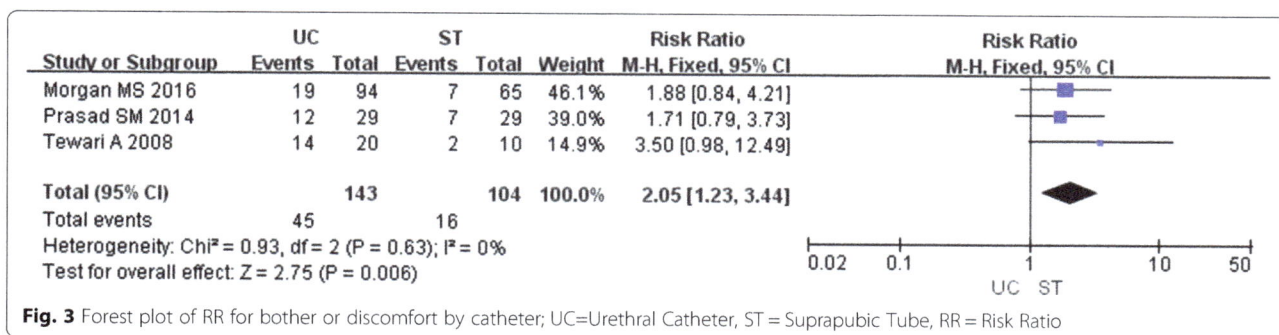

Fig. 3 Forest plot of RR for bother or discomfort by catheter; UC=Urethral Catheter, ST = Suprapubic Tube, RR = Risk Ratio

Urinary incontinence

A total of 507 patients in three studies were included in the meta-analysis for urinary continence [6, 7, 9] (Fig. 4). Results of urinary continence showed no difference between UC group and ST group at 6 weeks after the surgery (RR0.93; 95% CI 0.84, 1.02; P 0.13).

Emergency department visit and complications

Three studies containing 442 patients in assessed the emergency department visit and complications in their studies. The result showed that there was no significant difference between the UC and ST group on the rate of emergency department visit (Fig. 5) (RR0.61; 95% CI 0.33,1.11; P 0.11) [8–10]. Two studies showed no significant difference on bladder spasms between the UC and ST group, 3/10 vs 8/20 ($P > 0.05$) [6] and 56/94 vs 40/65 (P 0.90) [10] respectively.

Publication bias and sensitivity analysis

Figure 6 shows a funnel plot of the studies included in this meta-analysis that reported urinary continence. All studies were evenly distributed inside the 95% CIs, which indicated no obvious publication bias. The funnel plots of the studies reported pain, bother and emergency department visit showed the same results as the urinary continence.

Three RCT studies used visual analog scale (VAS) to evaluate the postoperative pain [8, 11, 12]. Meta-analysis of these three studies revealed no significant difference

between the UC and ST group (WMD 0.06; 95% CI -0.39, 0.52; P 0.79) regarding the postoperative pain.

Discussion

A recent systematic review including 42 trials indicated an advantage on suprapubic catheterization in terms of asymptomatic bacteriuria and pain compared to the urethral catheterization [13]. To our knowledge, UC was traditionally used in RP not only for the drainage of bladder but also for protecting the anastomosis and promoting healing. Lately, several studies have tried to use ST instead of UC after robot-assisted RARP to improve patient life quality. Outcomes of these studies were conflicting, and we systematically searched and collected the studies that compared UC and ST after RARP, and presented the first systematic review and meta-analysis on this topic.

The postoperative pain was a controversial topic [7, 8]. Our study demonstrated that there was no significant difference between the UC and ST group on postoperative pain at POD 7. The other three RCT studies showed similar result too [8, 11, 12]. Prasad et al. stated that the most severe discomfort of catheter was experienced in the evening on surgery day due to bladder spasms induced by the presence of foreign body. The next morning, discomfort from the catheter was eased considerably [14]. Postoperative pain at POD 1 also showed no significant difference between the two groups [8]. But when considering the penile pain, the UC group seemed to be more severe than the ST group according to Morgan

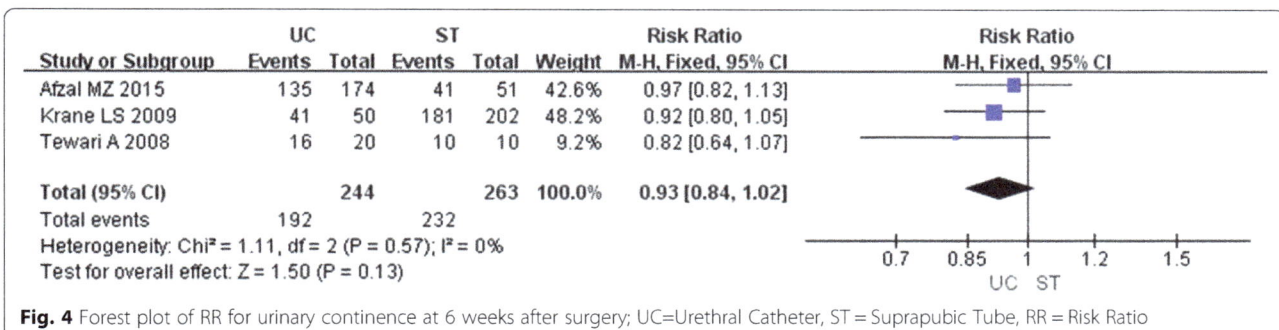

Fig. 4 Forest plot of RR for urinary continence at 6 weeks after surgery; UC=Urethral Catheter, ST = Suprapubic Tube, RR = Risk Ratio

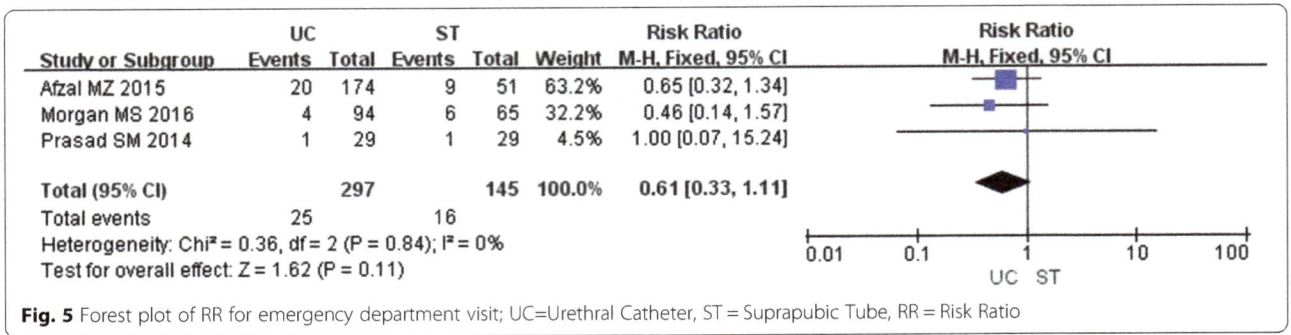

Fig. 5 Forest plot of RR for emergency department visit; UC=Urethral Catheter, ST = Suprapubic Tube, RR = Risk Ratio

et al. [10]. Another recently published study also demonstrated the postoperative pain is superior in ST group than in UC in POD 1 to 5. However, in POD 6, the difference were not statistically different in two groups anymore, which is consistent with our results [12]. So the postoperative pain maybe not associated with the kind of catheterization in the long term, but ST might have advantage in the short term.

Not surprisingly, our results showed a statistically significant advantage on the rate of bother or discomfort in favor of the ST group over the UC group at POD 7. As we all known, the catheterization will influence patients' quality of life including sleep, generally hygiene and genital hygiene, in a bad way. Only one study evaluated the bother at POD 1 to 6, and the results were similar between two groups. Therefore, patients with UC were more bothersome than ST [11].

Regard to incontinence, Krane et al. assessed the urinary incontinence at 2 days, 7 days and 90 days [7]. 23 (46%) patients with UC and 101 (50%) patients with ST were continent at 2 days postoperatively. At 90 days, 41 (92%) of patients with UC and 181 (90%) of patients of ST were recovered from incontinence. But all of the

above incontinence results showed no significant difference ($P > 0.2$ for all time points). Tewari also evaluated the percentage of patient urinary continence of UC and ST at 1 and 12 weeks, and the differences were not statistically significant, 20% vs 20% and 100% vs 98% respectively [6]. Another study showed a trend in favor of ST at five days after surgery (UC 3.1 ± 2.4 vs ST 1.6 2.6; P 0.0752) using urinary pads [11]. A longer follow-up study also found no difference between the two groups at twelve and twenty-four months [12]. These result cannot be combined using meta-analysis due to obvious heterogeneity. According to other previous researches, Sammon et al. found that patients using ST after RARP achieved earlier recovery of incontinence [15]. Moreover, a long-term follow-up study showed the recovery from urinary incontinence was prompted with. 68.7% of continence rate at 4 weeks and 82.6% at 8 weeks after surgery [16]. The rates of recovery from incontinence in the three studies included in our meta-analysis were all very high, 100%, 81% and 82% respectively [6, 7, 9]. But when compared to UC, ST showed no significant advantage in terms of recovery from incontinence at 6 weeks, which is similar to our

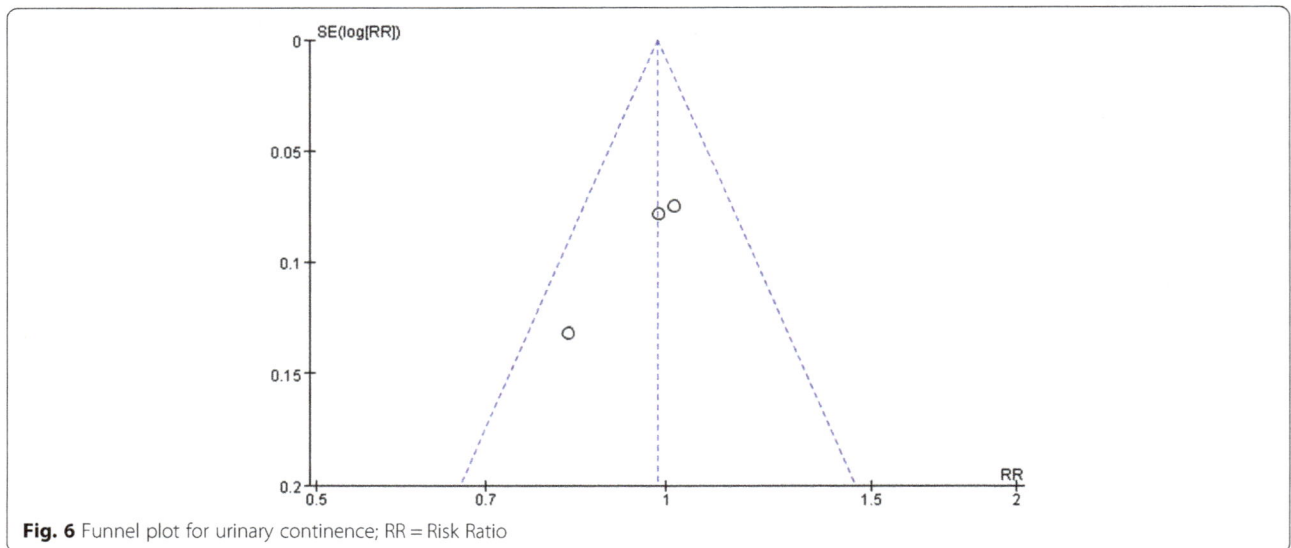

Fig. 6 Funnel plot for urinary continence; RR = Risk Ratio

meta-analysis results. It is still unclear about the mechanism of ST helps early continence, and this proposition need to be further examined with high quality evidence in the future.

In our included studies, six of them with 745 patients measured the incidence of bladder neck contracture at 6 months to 2 years after surgery [6–8, 11, 12]. BNC appeared in two patients (2/35) in the UC group, but none of the patient in the ST group (0/27) from the study of Martinschek et al. [11]. In the study of Harke et al., [12] urethral stricture appeared in one patient in each group. The patients in the rest of the studies and groups had no BNC. Among all included studies, only two patients (2/35) in the UC group had BNC, while no patient in ST group (0/37) had BNC [11]. Open and laparoscopic/ robotic surgeries suggested that early removal of urethral catheter (2 to 4 days following surgery) did not increase the rate of bladder neck contracture [16, 17]. Meanwhile, urethral stricture appeared in one patient in each group [12]. The patients in the rest of the studies and groups showed no BNC through with a follow-up ranged from 6 months to 1 year. Therefore, the safety of ST regarding to BNC was trustworthy.

In general, complication is important in the evaluation of the safety of a technique. Thus, emergency department visit and complications of both technique is relatively important. There was no significant difference between the UC and the ST group on the rate of emergency department visit in our study. Tewari et al. reported that none of the patients in both groups had retention requiring irrigation [6]. The study of Krane et al. showed that 10(5%) patients required urethral catheterization because of ST dislodgement ($n = 5$, 2.5%) or urinary retention ($n = 5$, 2.5%), and additionally three (6%) patients need recatheterization after removing urethral catheter due to urinary retention [7]. Afzal et al. found that eight patients with UC (5%) and 6 patients with suprapubic catheter (11%) had catheter-related problems after RARP (P 0.18), which are urinary retention after catheter removal, ST malfunction and clot retention [9]. In another study, complication rate was not significantly different between UC (4.3%) and ST (4.6%) group (P 0.9) [10]. Similarly, Urinary retention requiring catheterization after catheter removal happened once in each of the two groups and catheter blockage with resulting urinary retention occurred twice in each group [11]. Only one article mentioned the bacteriuria (defined as $>10^5$ bacteria/ml of urine) which was found in 10.3% (UC) and 5.1% (ST) of the patients (P 0.35). Among them, two patient required antibiotic treatment [12]. Two studies' results showed no significant difference on bladder spasms between the UC and the ST group [6, 10]. The rate of urinary retention was very low (<5%) in these studies [6, 7, 11]. These evidence suggested that ST and UC were both safe after RARP.

There were also some limitations in our study. First, the included RCTs had small sample sizes, and the level of evidence of other included studies was relatively low. Second, the surgeries were performed by different surgeons with varied surgical experience and skills. These differences might influence the result.

Conclusion
Based on our results, it can be concluded that while there was no significant benefit on pain after surgery in patients with ST compared to UC after RARP, an obvious advantage was observed in favor of ST on bother and discomfort caused by the catheter, especially in short term (1–5 days). Patients with ST and those with UC reported a comparable high rate of continence recovery. Safety outcomes including BNC, emergency department visit and urinary retention were also not significantly different between the two methods. Thus, it may be a good choice to choose ST instead of UT in postoperative management of RARP patients.

Abbreviations
BNC: Bladder neck contracture; POD: Postoperative day; RARP: Radical prostatectomy; RR: Risk ratio; RRP: Retropubic radical prostatectomy; ST: Suprapubic tube; UC: Urethral catheter; VAS: Visual analog scale; WMD: Weighted mean difference

Acknowledgements
None.

Funding
This study was funded by grants from the Technology Support Program of Science and Technology Department of Sichuan Province(Nos. 2014SZ0028).

Authors' contributions
ZYJ and SJF: project development, data collection and management, manuscript writing and revising; YTC: data collection, data analysis; XW, DYL: data analysis and interpretation, manuscript editing and revising; H L: project design; manuscript editing and revising; KJ W: project design and development, data interpretation, manuscript editing and revising. All authors read and approved the final manuscript.

Competing interests
The authors declare that they have no competing interests.

References
1. Siegel R, Desantis C, Jemal A. Colorectal cancer statistics, 2014. CA Cancer J Clin. 2014;64(2):104–17.
2. Heidenreich A, Bastian PJ, Bellmunt J, Bolla M, Joniau S, van der Kwast T, Mason M, Matveev V, Wiegel T, Zattoni F, et al. EAU guidelines on prostate cancer. Part 1: screening, diagnosis, and local treatment with curative intent-update 2013. European urology. 2014;65(1):124–37.
3. Webb DR, Sethi K, Gee K. An analysis of the causes of bladder neck contracture after open and robot-assisted laparoscopic radical prostatectomy. BJU Int. 2009;103(7):957 63.

4. Albani JM, Zippe CD. Urethral catheter removal 3 days after radical retropubic prostatectomy is feasible and desirable. Prostate Cancer Prostatic Dis. 2002;5(4):291–5.

5. Lepor H, Nieder AM, Fraiman MC. Early removal of urinary catheter after radical retropubic prostatectomy is both feasible and desirable. Urology. 2001;58(3):425–9.

6. Tewari A, Rao S, Mandhani A. Catheter-less robotic radical prostatectomy using a custom-made synchronous anastomotic splint and vesical urinary diversion device: report of the initial series and perioperative outcomes. BJU Int. 2008;102(8):1000–4.

7. Krane LS, Bhandari M, Peabody JO, Menon M. Impact of percutaneous suprapubic tube drainage on patient discomfort after radical prostatectomy. Eur Urol. 2009;56(2):325–30.

8. Prasad SM, Large MC, Patel AR, Famakinwa O, Galocy RM, Karrison T, Shalhav AL, Zagaja GP. Early removal of urethral catheter with suprapubic tube drainage versus urethral catheter drainage alone after robot-assisted laparoscopic radical prostatectomy. J Urol. 2014;192(1):89–95.

9. Afzal MZ, Tobert CM, Bulica E, Noyes SL, Lane BR. Modification of technique for suprapubic catheter placement after robot-assisted radical prostatectomy reduces catheter-associated complications. Urology. 2015;86(2):401–6.

10. Morgan MS, Ozayar A, Friedlander JI, Shakir N, Antonelli JA, Bedir S, Roehrborn CG, Cadeddu JA. An assessment of patient comfort and morbidity after robot-assisted radical prostatectomy with suprapubic tube versus urethral catheter drainage. J Endourol. 2016;30(3):300–5.

11. Martinschek A, Pfalzgraf D, Rafail B, Ritter M, Heinrich E, Trojan L. Transurethral versus suprapubic catheter at robot-assisted radical prostatectomy: a prospective randomized trial with 1-year follow-up. World J Urol. 2016;34(3):407–11.

12. Harke N, Godes M, Habibzada J, Urbanova K, Wagner C, Zecha H, Addali M, Witt JH. Postoperative patient comfort in suprapubic drainage versus transurethral catheterization following robot-assisted radical prostatectomy: a prospective randomized clinical trial. World J Urol. 2017;35(3):389–94.

13. Kidd EA, Stewart F, Kassis NC, Hom E, Omar MI. Urethral (indwelling or intermittent) or suprapubic routes for short-term catheterisation in hospitalised adults. The Cochrane database of systematic reviews. 2015;12:CD004203.

14. Prasad SM, Smith ND, Catalona WJ, Sammon J, Menon M. Suprapubic tube after radical prostatectomy. J Urol. 2013;189(6):2028–30.

15. Sammon JD, Sharma P, Trinh QD, Ghani KR, Sukumar S, Menon M. Predictors of immediate continence following robot-assisted radical prostatectomy. J Endourol. 2013;27(4):442–6.

16. Sammon JD, Trinh QD, Sukumar S, Diaz M, Simone A, Kaul S, Menon M. Long-term follow-up of patients undergoing percutaneous suprapubic tube drainage after robot-assisted radical prostatectomy (RARP). BJU Int. 2012;110(4):580–5.

17. Koch MO, Nayee AH, Sloan J, Gardner T, Wahle GR, Bihrle R, Foster RS. Early catheter removal after radical retropubic prostatectomy: long-term followup. J Urol. 2003;169(6):2170–2.

Penile cancer in Maranhão, Northeast Brazil: the highest incidence globally?

Ronald Wagner Pereira Coelho[1], Jaqueline Diniz Pinho[2], Janise Silva Moreno[1], Dimitrius Vidal e Oliveira Garbis[3], Athiene Maniva Teixeira do Nascimento[3], Joyce Santos Larges[4], José Ribamar Rodrigues Calixto[3,4], Leandra Naira Zambelli Ramalho[5], Antônio Augusto Moura da Silva[6], Leudivan Ribeiro Nogueira[1], Laisson de Moura Feitoza[3] and Gyl Eanes Barros Silva[4,5,7*]

Abstract

Background: The objectives of this study were to determine the minimum incidence of penile cancer in the poorest Brazilian state, and to describe the epidemiologic and clinical characteristics of patients diagnosed with the disease.

Methods: A retrospective study of 392 patients diagnosed with penile cancer in the three most important referral center in the state was conducted during 2004–2014.

Results: The age-standardized incidence was 6.15 per 100,000 and the crude annual incidence was 1.18 per 100,000. More than half (61.1%) of the tumors were histological grades 2 and 3, and 66.4% of tumors were classified as at least stage T2. The average age of patients was 58.6 ± 15.7 years (range, 18 to 103 years), with 20.8% of patients ≤40 years of age at diagnosis. The vast majority underwent penectomy (93%). Only 41.8% underwent lymphadenectomy, 58 patients (14.8%) received chemotherapy, and 54 patients (13.8%) received radiotherapy. Stage 3/4 and vascular invasion were statically significant at disease-free survival analysis.

Conclusion: The state of Maranhão has the highest incidence of penile cancer in Brazil and globally. Tumors are locally advanced and at the time of diagnosis, and there is a high frequency among young individuals. Patients have a low socioeconomic status, making it difficult to complete treatment and receive appropriate follow-up.

Keywords: Carcinoma, Penis cancer, Age-standardized incidence, Penectomy, Squamous cell carcinoma

Background

Penile cancer is a rare neoplasm in developed countries. However, the incidence in developing countries in Asia, Africa, and Latin America is high, accounting for up to 10% of malignant neoplasms in men [1–3]. Brazil stands out among the countries with the highest incidences of penile cancer in the world, although no reliable data exist [4, 5]. In Brazil, the condition may account for 2.1% of all neoplasias in men, and affects mainly inhabitants of the North and Northeast regions [6]. Among the known risk factors for the development of penile cancer, poor hygiene, phimosis, human papillomavirus (HPV) infection, use of tobacco, and risky sexual behavior, are the most highlighted [7–10]. The disease mainly affects individuals with low socioeconomic levels and low levels of education [11–15].

Maranhão is the most rural state in Brazil, being historically marked by great social inequality and extreme poverty. Access to health care in the rural parts is poor, which leads the male population to seek medical attention in the capital city only when the disease is at an advanced stage. According to the Ministry of Health, during the period 1992–2007, 6716 penectomies were performed in Brazil, out of which 419 (6.2%) in the state of Maranhão. These data, albeit alarming, are underestimated and insufficient for understanding the reality of penile cancer in Maranhão. Hence, the objectives of this study were to estimate the minimum incidence of penile

* Correspondence: gyleanes@fmrp.usp.br
[4]University Hospital of Federal University of Maranhão, Barão de Itapari Street, Centro, São Luís, Brazil
[5]Department of Radiology and Pathology, Ribeirão Preto Medical School of University of São Paulo, Bandeirantes Avenue, Monte Alegre, Ribeirão Preto 14049-900, Brazil
Full list of author information is available at the end of the article

cancer in the state of Maranhão, and to describe the epidemiologic and clinical characteristics of patients diagnosed with the disease, in order to provide the basis for the development of measures to confront this disease and to act as an impetus for future studies.

Methods

A retrospective cohort study was conducted. The studied sample was of composed of 286 patients newly diagnosed with penile cancer from January 2004 to December 2014 at the Cancer Hospital Aldenora Bello (HCAB). HCAB is a high complexity oncology center in Maranhão and the main referral center for the treatment of penile cancer in the state, which has an estimated population of 6,680,884 inhabitants, according to data from the Brazilian Institute of Geography and Statistics (IBGE).

Data were collected from physical and electronic records of all patients classified by the Hospital Cancer Record of HCAB as having penile cancer. The studied variables were age, marital status, education, occupation, home town, tumor location, histological type and grade, tumor size, type of surgery, lymphadenectomy, staging (TNM system, 2010), chemotherapy, and radiotherapy. Data were stored in Microsoft Excel spreadsheet editor and analyzed using Stata statistical software (Version 7.0, StataCorp, College Station, Texas).

Frequencies and percentages were used to express categorical variables, while numerical variables were presented as means and standard deviations. Age-standardized incidence rate (ASR) were calculated using the standard world population proposed by Segi and modified by Doll et al. [16] This method was also applied in the *Cancer Incidence in Five Continents* series of the International Agency for Research on Cancer (IARC), wherein the number of cases, in each 5-year age-stratum was divided by the population size in each age group [16]. In addition, due to the unavailability of ASR data in studies conducted in Brazil, we calculated an estimated annual crude incidence rate in our sample, in order to compare with data from previous Brazilian studies. Since there are others small centers that receive patients with penile cancer in Maranhão, the incidence estimated from the data herein therefore provides only a minimum estimate.

Survival analysis was performed using the Kaplan-Meier method to determine disease-free survival. The Log Rank test was used to compare survival curves. The significance threshold use was $p \leq 0.05$. This work was in accordance with the principles of the Declaration of Helsinki and approved by the Research Ethics Committee of the Universidade Federal do Maranhão [process no. 43774215.7.0000.5086] and informed consent was waived.

Results

From 2004 to 2014, 392 patients were diagnosed with penile cancer, resulting in an average of 36 cases per year. This translates to an ASR of 13.89 per 100,000 men over an 11-year period, corresponding to an average ASR of 6.15 per 100,000 men over a 5-year period. The crude incidence rate was 1.18 per 100,000 men per year. Patients from rural areas comprised 82.1% of the sample (322/392). Most were farmers (71%) and most (66,3%) reported being married. The average age of the studied sample was 58.6 ± 15.7 years (range 18 to 103 years), with 19.7% of patients aged ≤40 years at diagnosis. The majority of our patients 29% (72/248) were non-swokers.

All patients were diagnosed with squamous cell carcinoma. Among 136 the cases with reviewed histological subtype, according to most recent WHO classification (2016), 91 (66.9%) were of the subtypes of cancer that are associated with the presence of HPV, which include warty, basaloid, or mixed carcinomas with warty or basaloid components. More aggressive subtypes such as basaloid or sarcomatoid carcinoma was observed in 13 cases (9.6%) and 01 case (0.7%), respectively. The primary location of the tumor was the glans in 74.0% (158/212216/292) of cases. More than half (66.1%) of the tumors were histological grades 2 and 3. Using the TNM classification system, 66.4% (157/246) of tumors were classified as ≥T2. Lymph node involvement was present in 54% (93/175) of patients, and was distributed as follows: N1 in 8.6%, N2 in 28.7%, and N3 in 16.7%. Distant metastases were detected in 9 of the 138 patients for whom it was possible to search for metastatic disease (Table 1).

In terms of surgical procedures performed, the vast majority of patients (93%) underwent penectomy (210/279): 74.7% partial, 17.3% total, and 1% complete emasculation. Lymphadenectomy was performed in 41.8% (164/392) of patients overall; 64.2% underwent bilateral lymphadenectomy and 34.8% underwent unilateral lymphadenectomy. Chemotherapy was administered to 21.9% (54/246) of patients. Of these, 65% received chemotherapy as palliative therapy, and 3.6% as adjuvant therapy. Almost all (92.3%) patients who received chemotherapy had presented with advanced disease. Cisplatin and 5-fluorouracil were the most frequently used chemotherapeutic agents. Radiotherapy was used in the treatment of 27.1% (54/199) of patients, being adjuvant in 10 cases and palliative in the others. The radiation dose ranged from 20.2–60 Gy, with a dose of 50 Gy being most common (Table 2).

As shown in Figs. 1 and 2, Kaplan-Meier curves demonstrated that stage 3/4 and vascular invasion were associated with decreased disease-free survival (recurrence, Lymph node or systemic metastasis). Histological grade, tumor thickness, perineural invasion and tumor subtype were not significant predictors for disease-free disease. Due to great number of patients without follow-up, only

Table 1 Histologic features and staging of patients with penile cancer

	% (N)
Histological subtype	
Epidermoid carcinoma	100 (392/392)
Initial anatomic site	
Glans	74.0(216/392)
Undetermined[a]	15.0 (44/392)
Foreskin	11.0 (32/392)
Histologic grade	
Grade 1	38.9 (123/316)
Grade 2	54.1 (171/316)
Grade 3	7.0 (22/316)
Primary tumor (T stage)	
Tis	0.6 (2/335)
T1(a, b)	33.0 (107/335)
T2	44.6 (145/335)
T3	17.5 (57/335)
T4	4.3 (14/335)
Regional lymph nodes (N stage)	
N0	46.0 (107/233)
N1	8.6 (20/233)
N2	28.7 (67/233)
N3	16.7 (39/233)
Distant metástasis	
M0	45.9 (180/392)
M1	2.3 (9/392)
Mx	51.8 (203/392)
Staging	
Stage 0	26.0 (95/366)
Stage 1	30.0 (110/366)
Stage 2	26.5 (97/366)
Stage 3	15.3 (56/366)
Stage 4	2.2 (8/366)

[a]advanced destructive lesions

Table 2 Treatment modalities in patients with penile cancer

	% (N)
Type of surgery	
Partial penectomy	74.7 (286/383)
Total penectomy	17.3 (66/383)
Emasculation	1.0 (4/383)
Others (postectomy, glansectomy and excision)	7.0 (27/383)
Lymphadenectomy	
Yes	41.8 (164/392)
No	58.2 (228/392)
Chemotherapy	
Yes	23.6 (58/246)
No	76.4 (334/246)
Radiotherapy	
Yes	21.9 (54/246)
No	78.1 (145/246)

111 cases were included in this analysis. Follow-up ranged from 01 to 39 months (median 13,4 months). There was insufficient data on mortality for overall survival analysis.

Discussion

The ASR of 6.1 per 100,000 men (5-year interval) recorded in this study exceeds the highest international rates reported by IARC (Table 3) [16]. No previous Brazilian study used age-adjusted or age-standardized incidence rates. In these prior studies, only the cumulative incidence rates were reported for different time intervals, making it necessary to calculate the annual average for comparison. The annual crude incidence rate in the present study was 1.18 per 100,000 men, far higher than any previously reported national annual crude incidence rate (Table 4) [6, 12, 17, 18].

It is believed that incidence of penile cancer is even higher in the state of Maranhão, because a proportion of the affected population seek treatment in the Southeast states, as reported by Favorito et al. [19], where 53.2% of their study participants were from the Northeast, particularly from Maranhão. Maranhão has a geographically isolated capital. Thus, the demand for health services in neighboring states, that are more accessible, is high. Moreover, there are other small care centers for patients with penile cancer in the state of Maranhão; these were not included in our study. Thus, the calculated cumulative incidence in this study is a lower range estimate of the true incidence. Furthermore, the age-standardized estimate of incidence was higher than the crude estimate. This was due to the fact that the population of Maranhão is younger than the standard world population of Segi modified by Doll [16].

A likely explanation for high penile cancer incidence in the state of Maranhão is the high HPV infection rate. An unpublished prospective study (with 57 penile cancer cases from Maranhão) reported an HPV infection rate of over 75% [20]. These data are corroborated by the fact that Maranhão has the highest cervical cancer incidence

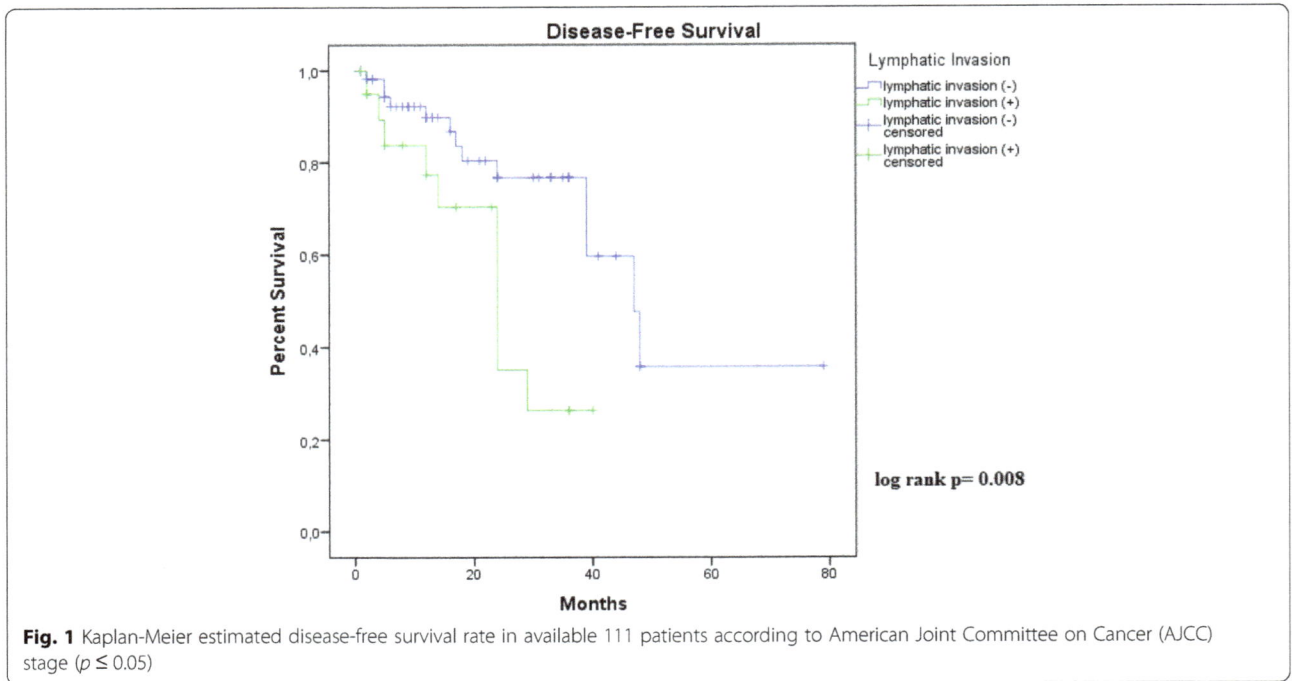

Fig. 1 Kaplan-Meier estimated disease-free survival rate in available 111 patients according to American Joint Committee on Cancer (AJCC) stage ($p \leq 0.05$)

in Brazil [21], and the pathogenesis of cervical cancer is directly related to HPV infection. Therefore, immunization of male adolescents is pivotal for disrupting the HPV transmission trail. Surprisingly, only three patients were diagnosed with HIV/AIDS (human immunodeficiency virus, acquired immune deficiency syndrome).

The epidemiological and clinical characteristics of the patients in this study were similar to those reported in other studies, particularly those from developing regions whose socioeconomic reality is similar to that of Maranhão [1, 3, 6, 12, 17, 18]. The state of Maranhão has a Human Development Index (HDI) of 0.639, considered the lowest in Brazil. According to IBGE, 71.7% of the families in Maranhão earn less than USD 220.00 a month. In this study, 71% of patients reported being farmers, and 82.1% were from rural areas. When compared with other studies [3, 12], our patients have pretty

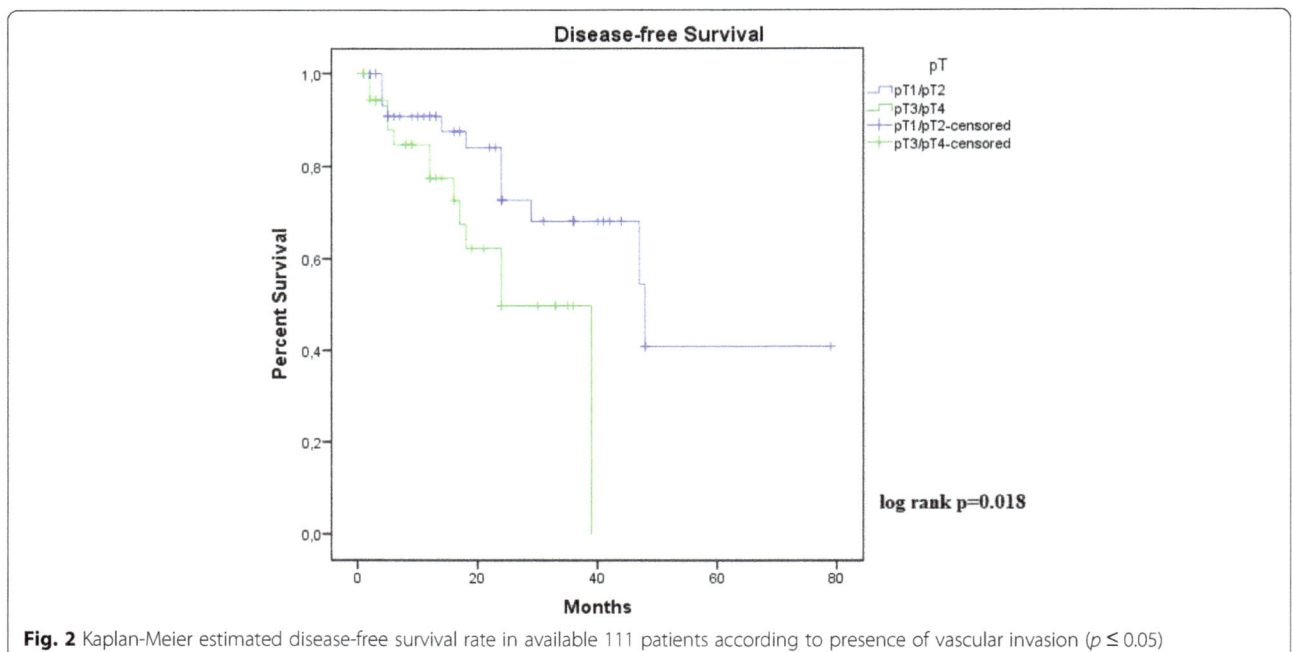

Fig. 2 Kaplan-Meier estimated disease-free survival rate in available 111 patients according to presence of vascular invasion ($p \leq 0.05$)

Table 3 Highest age-standardized incidence rates of penile cancer in geographical areas of the world

Population	Age-standardized incidence (per 100,000)
Brazil, Maranhão	6.1
Brazil, Goiania	3.3
USA, Montana: American Indian	2.8
Brazil, Aracaju	2.7
Malawi, Blantyre	2.7
Brazil, Cuiaba	2.5
Uganda, Kyadondo County	2.4
Colombia, Manizales	2.4
India, Barshi	2.2
Spain, Cuenca	2.1
Brazil, Sao Paulo	2.0
Thailand, Songkhla	1.9
USA, Puerto Rico	1.9
Chile, Region of Antofagasta	1.8
India, Chennai (Madras)	1.8
Brazil, Fortaleza	1.8

Adapted from Forman et al. [16]

low smoking rates in the overall population. This would be consistent with the relatively low smoking rates in Maranhão State. Although the average age of 58.5 years is similar to the majority of studies reported in the literature, the Brazil series show a higher frequency of cases in young individuals [18, 19, 22, 23]. This study showed that 19.7% of patients diagnosed with penile cancer were ≤ 40 years of age (Fig. 3). In young people with squamous cell carcinomas, tumor infiltrative growth pattern perineural invasion, and recurrence are more likely [18]. However, the literature and current prognostic indicators do not include the age at diagnosis as an important prognostic marker [8, 18, 24–26].

In terms of the characteristics of the primary tumor, the majority of patients presented with an advanced stage of disease. Approximately 66.4% of tumors were classified as TNM stage T2 or higher. These data are similar to those presented by Couto et al. (63.6%) [6], and slightly higher than those described by Favorito et al. (57.9%) [19]. However, these frequencies are higher

than those found in studies conducted in developed countries, such as the United States (45.9 and 50.6%) [26, 27] and Canada (36.4%) [14].

In this case series, penectomy was performed in 93% of patients. Penectomy was partial, total, or involved complete emasculation in 74.7, 17.3, and 1% of cases, respectively. The frequency of penectomy in this series is higher than that reported by Paiva et al. (82%) [18], Koifman et al. (80.9%) [12], Zhu et al. (75.8%) [27], and Chalya et al. (73.9%) [28]. These data demonstrate that patients from Maranhão seek treatment late; hence, they require mutilating treatments. Treatment of penile cancer has a negative impact on welfare in up to 40% of patients and results in psychiatric symptoms in about 50% [29]. The high frequency of more aggressive treatments in this study may contribute to a greater occurrence of psychological and sexual dysfunction.

Among patients who received chemotherapy, 92.3% had advanced, unresectable disease and chemotherapy was palliative. Only two patients received chemotherapy with adjuvant intent and, despite the large proportion of patients with lymph node status N3, only one patient received chemotherapy with neoadjuvant intent. Cisplatin—alone as a radiosensitizing agent or in combination with 5-fluorouracil—and 5-fluorouracil were the most frequently used drugs. The addition of a taxane or ifosfamide was not used as currently recommended [30].

Despite 34.2% of patients having lymph node involvement at the time of undergoing surgical treatment, only 19% of patients treated with radiotherapy were treated with adjuvant intent. The vast majority, 81%, received radiotherapy because of local or regional recurrence and/or ineligibility for surgical rescue. Despite the poor level of evidence for adjuvant radiotherapy, European and American guidelines recommend performing prophylactic radiotherapy for patients at high risk of relapse [31, 32].

The number of patients undergoing lymphadenectomy (41.8%) is much lower than that of patients with tumors classified as ≥ T2 (66.4%) who should, in theory, be submitted to lymph node staging. The lower than expected number of lymphadenectomies is justified by the fact that many patients returned for evaluation only when there was local or regional recurrence.

The presence of recurrences, mainly lymph-node involvement, is the most important prognostic factor for

Table 4 Comparison of the incidence of previous studies in other states of Brazil and Maranhão

State	Number of cases	Period	Crude incidence rate (100.000 homens/ano)
Maranhão	392	2004-2014	1,18
Bahia [18]	378	1997-2007	0,72
Pará [17]	208	1996-2006	0,46
Pernambuco [6]	88	2007-2012	0,34
Rio de Janeiro [12]	230	2002-2008	0,43

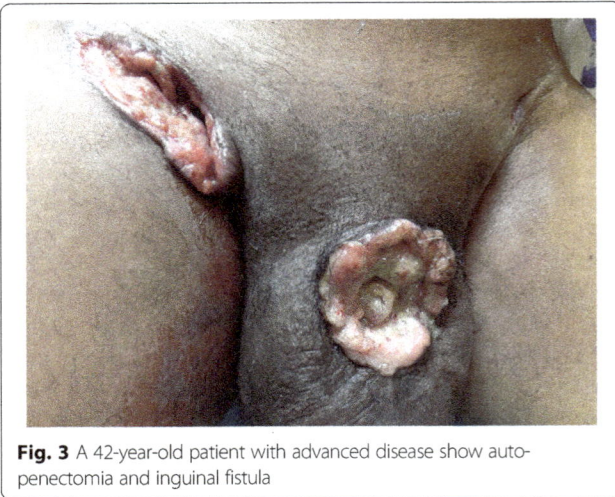

Fig. 3 A 42-year-old patient with advanced disease show auto-penectomia and inguinal fistula

survival in penile cancer [33]. Several possible histological parameters have been associated with recurrences and penile cancer prognosis. These include, histological grade, tumor thickness, vascular embolization, perineural invasion, tumor subtype and, clinical stage [18, 24–26]. In our study, only tumor stage and vascular invasion were significant predictors for disease-free survival. Although, perineural invasion is an important predictor of nodal metastasis [24], our data show no significant increase in risk of disease recurrence.

This study has some limitations, mainly owing to missing data from medical records and the abandonment of treatment by patients. Many patients were rural residents, who had difficulty returning to the capital city to continue treatment. When they again sought medical care, the presence of bulky local and/or regional recurrence—amenable only to palliative treatment—was common. Still, due to the limited patient follow-up, only the deaths of those who died at HCAB were recorded. Finally, the specimens were evaluated by different pathologists, which may be considered as an inherent limitation of multicenter studies.

Conclusion

With a minimum ASR of 6.1 per 100,000 men and a minimum crude annual incidence rate of 1.18 per 100,000 men, Maranhão has the highest incidence of penile cancer registered in Brazil, and globally, considering data from a single treatment center. The tumors are locally advanced and there is a high frequency among young individuals at the time of diagnosis. Patients generally have low socioeconomic status, making it difficult to complete treatment and attend appropriate follow-up. Therefore, it is necessary to implement measures to enable prevention, early diagnosis, and treatment in order to change this disastrous scenario.

Abbreviations
ASR: Age-standardized incidence rate; HCAB: Cancer Hospital Aldenora Bello; HDI: Human Development Index; HPV: Human papillomavirus; IARC: International Agency for Research on Cancer; IBGE: Brazilian Institute of Geography and Statistics

Funding
This article was funded by the Research Support Foundation of Maranhão (Fundação de Amparo a Pesquisa do Maranhão – FAPEMA [grant number 00696/14]), Ministry of Education (grant number ProEXT 4482.2.6549.09042014) and the Study Group on Penile Cancer (Grupo de Estudos com Câncer de Pênis – GECAP).

Authors' contributions
RWPC, LMF and GEBS are the principal investigators and wrote the first version of the manuscript. JDP, JSM, DVOG, JSL, LRN and AMTN participated in the care and management of the patient and preparation of the manuscript. LNZR and GEBS performed pathological analysis and interpretation. AAMS, JRRC contributed to critical revision of important intellectual content of the manuscript. All authors contributed to the writing process and read and approved the final manuscript. All authors read and approved the final manuscript.

Competing interests
The authors declare that they have no competing interests.

Author details
[1]Aldenora Bello Cancer Hospital, Seroa da Mota Street, Apeadouro, São Luís 65031-630, Brazil. [2]Federal University of Pará, Brazil, Gov. José Malcher Avenue, Belém 66055-260, Brazil. [3]Federal University of Maranhão, São Luís, Brazil, dos Portugueses Avenue, Bacanga, São Luís 65080-805, Brazil. [4]University Hospital of Federal University of Maranhão, Barão de Itapari Street, Centro, São Luís, Brazil. [5]Department of Radiology and Pathology, Ribeirão Preto Medical School of University of São Paulo, Bandeirantes Avenue, Monte Alegre, Ribeirão Preto 14049-900, Brazil. [6]Public Heath Departament, Federal University of Maranhão, São Luís, Brazil, dos Portugueses Avenue, Bacanga, São Luís 65080-805, Brazil. [7]Ribeirão Preto Medical School - USP, Av. Bandeirantes, 3900, Ribeirão Preto, SP 14048-900, Brazil.

References
1. Christodoulidou M, Sahdev V, Houssein S, Muneer A. Epidemiology of penile cancer. Curr Probl Cancer. 2015;39:126–36.
2. Culkin DJ, Beer TM. Advanced penile carcinoma. J Urol. 2003;170:359–65.
3. Chaux A, Netto GJ, Rodríguez IM, Barreto JE, Oertell J, Ocampos S, et al. Epidemiologic profile, sexual history, pathologic features, and human papillomavirus status of 103 patients with penile carcinoma. World J Urol. 2013;31:861–7.
4. Pow-Sang MR, Ferreira U, Pow-Sang JM, Nardi AC, Destefano V. Epidemiology and natural history of penile cancer. Urology. 2010;76:S2–6.
5. Reis AA da S, Paula LB de, Paula AAP de, Saddi VA, Cruz AD da. Clinico-epidemiological aspects associated with penile cancer. Cien Saude Colet. 2010;15:1105–11.
6. do Couto TC, Barbosa Arruda RM, do Couto MC, Barros FD. Epidemiological study of penile cancer in Pernambuco: Experience of two reference centers. Int Braz J Urol. 2014;40:738–44.
7. Ferrándiz-Pulido C, de Torres I, García-Patos V. [Penile squamous cell carcinoma]. Actas dermo-sifiliográficas. 2012;103:478–87.
8. Flaherty A, Kim T, Giuliano A, Magliocco A, Hakky TS, Pagliaro LC, et al. Implications for human papillomavirus in penile cancer. Urol Oncol. 2014;32:53.e1-8.
9. Kayes O, Ahmed HU, Arya M, Minhas S. Molecular and genetic pathways in penile cancer. Lancet Oncol. 2007;8:420–9.
10. Madsen BS, van den Brule AJC, Jensen HL, Wohlfahrt J, Frisch M. Risk factors for squamous cell carcinoma of the penis–population-based case-control study in Denmark. Cancer Epidemiol Biomarkers Prev. 2008;17:2683–91.

11. Hakenberg OW, Compérat E, Minhas S, Necchi A, Protzel C, Watkin N. Guidelines on Penile Cancer. Uroweb Org. 2015;67:142–50.

12. Koifman L, Vides AJ, Koifman N, Carvalho JP, Ornellas AA. Epidemiological aspects of penile cancer in Rio de Janeiro: Evaluation of 230 cases. Int Braz J Urol. 2011;37:231–40.

13. Thuret R, Sun M, Budaus L, Abdollah F, Liberman D, Shariat SF, et al. A population-based analysis of the effect of marital status on overall and cancer-specific mortality in patients with squamous cell carcinoma of the penis. Cancer Causes Control. 2013;24:71–9.

14. McIntyre M, Weiss A, Wahlquist A, Keane T, Clarke H, Savage S. Penile cancer: an analysis of socioeconomic factors at a southeastern tertiary referral center. Can J Urol. 2011;18:5524–8.

15. Benard VB, Johnson CJ, Thompson TD, Roland KB, Sue ML, Cokkinides V, et al. Examining the association between socioeconomic status and potential human papillomavirus-associated cancers. Cancer. 2008;113:2910–8.

16. Bray F, Ferlay J. Age standardization. In: Forman D, Bray F, Brewster DH, et al., editors. Cancer Incidence in Five Continents, vol X. Lyon: IARC Scientific Publication No. 164, International Agency for Research on Cancer; 2014.

17. Fonseca AG da, Pinto JAS de A, Marques MC, Drosdoski FS, Fonseca Neto LOR da. Estudo epidemiológico do câncer de pênis no Estado do Pará, Brasil. Rev. Pan-Amazônica Saúde. Instituto Evandro Chagas / Secretaria de Vigilância em Saúde / Ministério da Saúde. 2010;1:85–90.

18. Paiva GR, de Oliveira Araujo IB, Athanazio DA, Rodrigues de Freitas LA. Penile cancer: impact of age at diagnosis on morphology and prognosis. Int Urol Nephrol. 2015. p. 295–9.

19. Favorito LA, Nardi AC, Ronalsa M, Zequi SC, Sampio FJB, Glina S. Epidemiologic study on penile cancer in Brazil. Int Braz J Urol. 2008;34:587–91.

20. Silva GEB, Pinho JD, Pereira SRF, Khaya AS, Nogueira LR, Calixto JR, et al. NF-kB expression in HPV-and non-HPV-related subtypes of penile squamous cell.

21. De J, Pinho-França R, Da MB, Chein C, Santos Thuler LC. Patterns of cervical cytological abnormalities according to the Human Development Index in the northeast region of Brazil. BMC Women's Health. 2016;16:54.

22. Rippentrop JM, Joslyn SA, Konety BR. Squamous cell carcinoma of the penis: Evaluation of data from the surveillance, epidemiology, and end results program. Cancer. 2004;101:1357–63.

23. Tsen HF, Morgenstern H, Mack T, Peters RK. Risk factors for penile cancer: results of a population-based case-control study in Los Angeles County (United States). Cancer Causes Control. 2001;12:267–77.

24. Chaux A, Caballero C, Soares F, Guimaraes GC, Cunha IW, Reuter V, et al. The prognostic index: a useful pathologic guide for prediction of nodal metastases and survival in penile squamous cell carcinoma. Am J Surg Pathol. 2009;33:1049–57.

25. Pond GR, Di Lorenzo G, Necchi A, Eigl BJ, Kolinsky MP, Chacko RT, et al. Prognostic risk stratification derived from individual patient level data for men with advanced penile squamous cell carcinoma receiving first-line systemic therapy. Urol Oncol Semin Orig Investig. 2014;32:501–8.

26. Jayaratna IS, Mitra AP, Schwartz RL, Dorff TB, Schuckman AK. Clinicopathologic characteristics and outcomes of penile cancer treated at tertiary care centers in the Western United States. Clin Genitourin Cancer. 2014;12:138–42.

27. Zhu Y, Gu W-J, Wang H-K, Gu C-Y, Ye D-W. Surgical treatment of primary disease for penile squamous cell carcinoma: A Surveillance, Epidemiology, and End Results database analysis. Oncol Lett. 2015;10:85–92.

28. Chalya PL, Rambau PF, Masalu N, Simbila S. Ten-year surgical experiences with penile cancer at a tertiary care hospital in northwestern Tanzania: a retrospective study of 236 patients. World J Surg Oncol. 2015;13:71.

29. Maddineni SB, Lau MM, Sangar VK. Identifying the needs of penile cancer sufferers: a systematic review of the quality of life, psychosexual and psychosocial literature in penile cancer. BMC Urol. 2009;9:8.

30. Pagliaro LC. Role of chemotherapy in treatment of squamous cell carcinoma of the penis. Curr Probl Cancer. 2015;39:166–72.

31. Crook J. The role of radiotherapy in the management of penile cancer. Curr Probl Cancer. 2015;39:158–65.

32. Li F, Xu Y, Wang H, Chen B, Wang Z, Zhao Y, et al. Diagnosis and treatment of penile verrucous carcinoma. Oncol Lett. 2015;9:1687–90.

33. Chipollini J, Tang DH, Gilbert SM, Poch MA, Pow-Sang JM, Sexton WJ, et al. Delay to Inguinal Lymph Node Dissection Greater than 3 Months Predicts Poorer Recurrence-Free Survival for Patients with Penile Cancer. J Urol. 2017; 198:1346–52.

Unilateral pedal lymphangiography plus computed tomography angiography for location of persistent idiopathic chyle leakage not detectable by ordinary contrast computed tomography

Dingyi Liu[1†], Boke Liu[2†], Weimu Xia[3], Qi Tang[1], Haidong Wang[1], Jian Wang[1], Yanfeng Zhou[1], Jiashun Yu[1], Wenmin Li[1], Mingwei Wang[2], Wenlong Zhou[2], Sang Hu[4] and Yuan Shao[2,5*]

Abstract

Background: To identify the value of unilateral pedal lymphangiography (LPG) plus computed tomography angiography (CTA) in accurate depiction of persistent idiopathic chyluria undetectable by ordinary contrast CT.

Methods: Eighteen patients 44–63 years of age with persistent idiopathic chyluria who failed conservative management were included. Ordinary CT had not revealed a chyle leak. Cystoscopy, unilateral LPG, and post-LPG CT angiography (CTA) were sequentially performed. Ligation and stripping of the perirenal lymphatics were subsequently performed guided by lymphangiography and CTA.

Results: LPG and post-LPG CTA detected 17 unilateral and one bilateral chyle leaks in the 18 patients, with clear images of the communication of lymphatic vessels and the renal collecting or vascular system. The success rate was significantly better than cystoscopy (100% vs 50.0%, $P = 0.005$) or LPG alone (100% vs. 72.2%, $P = 0.016$). Chyluria resolved after surgery in all patients; no relapses were found.

Conclusions: LPG plus post-LPG CTA accurately characterized perirenal lymphangiectasia that was not demonstrated by routine contrast-enhanced CT or not suitable for magnetic resonance imaging. Despite of its invasiveness, this method is a good diagnostic alternative to LPG in patients with persistent chyluria requiring surgery.

Keywords: Lymphangiography, Chyluria, Computerized tomographic angiography, Precise location

Background

Chyluria is the passage of chyle in the urine caused by the rupture of retroperitoneal lymphatics with leakage into the pyelocaliceal system, giving urine a milky appearance. The etiologies include thoracic duct stenosis, tuberculosis, cancer, trauma, pregnancy, filariasis,

* Correspondence: shaoyuan15@hotmail.com
†Equal contributors
2Department of Urology, Shanghai Jiao Tong University Medical School Affiliated Ruijin Hospital, 197 Ruijin Er Road, Shanghai 200025, People's Republic of China
5Department of Urology, Shanghai Jiao Tong University Medical School Affiliated Ruijin Hospital North, 999 Xiwang Road, Shanghai 201801, People's Republic of China
Full list of author information is available at the end of the article

or the cause may not be clear. The result is dilatation of distal lymphatics and the eventual rupture of lymphatic vessels into the urinary collecting system [1, 2]. Although rare, severe fluid and protein loss may cause hypovolemia and hypoproteinemia in some patients. Cystoscopy, lymphangiography (LPG), computed tomography (CT), magnetic resonance imaging (MRI) and lymphoscintigraphy are used to diagnose and locate the origin of chyluria [2–4]. Combining LPG with post-LPG CT imaging may increase the ability to locate chyle leaks [2, 5, 6]., MRI is contraindicated in patients with implanted metal devices. Some patients fail conservative management because their chyle leaks are not visualized by routine contrast CT, and require additional evaluation of the lymphatic system before treatment can be started. The aim of this study was to evaluate the value of unilateral LPG with post-LPG CT angiography (CTA) in chyluria patients who failed to conservative management with chyle leaks undetectable by ordinary contrast CT.

Methods

Patients

Eighteen patients diagnosed with persistent idiopathic chyluria between January 2013 and March 2017 were included. Ten were men and eight were women. Their median age was 51.5 (range 44–63) years, and the duration of chyluria ranged from 3 to 30 years. No patient had a history of tuberculosis or trauma. The main clinical manifestations were recurrent milky urine and asthenia. Seven patients experienced edema, one experienced severe anemia, 16 had intermittent recurrent chyluria, and two had persistent chyluria. All patients had test-confirmed chyluria; three had chylous hematuria. All were negative for filariasis antibody, urinalysis showed no urinary tract infections, other diseases cancer, and trauma were excluded. Conservative treatments such as bed rest, plenty of water with limited fat intake, and renal pelvic instillation via retrograde ureteral perfusion, had all failed in these patients. Renal pelvic sclerotherapy with povidone iodine or dextrose was performed one or two times in 11 patients without effect. The sites of chyle leaks could not be visualized with routine contrast CT. Cystoscopy including at least 5 min of observations of both ureteric orifices found unilateral urinary excretion of chyle in only nine patients (six left and three right). LPG CTA was subsequently performed.

LPG

The lymphatics were stained by injecting 2 ml methylene blue into the web space between the first and second toes of one foot. A linear cut-down was performed on the dorsum of the foot below the ankle 30 min later to isolate a lymphatic vessel. After cannulation of the lymphatic vessel with a 30 gauge needle, iodized oil (Lipiodol; Laboratoire Guerbet, Roissy, France), a contrast agent for LPG, was injected at a rate of 0.1 ml/min, not exceeding a total volume of 14 ml. CTA was performed immediately to assess apparent chyle leaks and to document the filling phase of the LPG.

CTA

CTA was performed with a 320 × 0.5 mm detector row CT unit (Aquilion ONE, Toshiba, Japan). A 40 ml volume of Iobitridol or Omnipaque nonionic contrast medium, 350 mg/ml was administered via an antecubital vein by bolus injection at rate 3–4 mL/s using a power injector. Renal artery imaging scans were performed

20–30 s after injection, and scans of the urinary collecting system were performed after 3–5 min. Volume rendering (VR), maximum intensity projection (MIP) and multiplanar reformation (MPR) of the CT scans allowed accurate visualization of abdominal or retroperitoneal lymphatic vessels, lymphatic leakage, the kidney, renal artery, and the collecting system.

Surgical treatment

Renal lymphatic stripping and ligation were performed in all patients based on the anatomic location indicated by the LPG and post-LPG CTA. Surgical approach was decided according to the patient's condition, and both laparoscopy (4 cases) and open surgery (14 cases) were performed. A urine chyle test verified the therapeutic effect.

Statistical analysis

Qualitative variables were compared using the χ^2 test. P-values < 0.05 considered statistically significant. The statistical analysis was performed with SPSS 20.0 (SPSS Inc., Chicago, IL, USA).

Results

LPG and post-LPG CTA succeeded in delineating the thoracic ducts and confirming the absence of obvious obstructions. Ten of the 18 patients had lympho-urinary fistulas on the left side, seven were on the right side, nine of which were consistent with the cystoscopy results. The remaining patient was diagnosed with unilateral chyluria by cystoscopy, LPG found bilateral lesions. LPG plus CTA was more successful than cystoscopy in locating the side of chyle leaks (100% vs. 50.0%, $P = 0.005$, Table 1). When combined with post-LPG CTA, VR displayed the lymphatic reticular distribution in the kidney and renal fascia. In nine patients, VR and MIP revealed retroperitoneal lymphatic distortion, with reflux of lymphangiography contrast into the region of the contralateral iliac artery as well as showing the lymphatics adjacent to the renal arteries and veins (Fig. 1). LPG CTA provided detailed imaging information in all 18 patients. LPG alone provided imaging of equivalent value in only 13 patients. Accuracy of chyle leak location was better with LPG CTA than with LPG alone (100% vs. 72.2%, $P = 0.016$; Table 2). The

Table 1 The location of chyluria shown by cystoscopy and LPG CTA

Location of chyluria	Patient number	Cystoscopy	LPG + CTA	LPG	p-value*
Unilateral	17	9(52.9%)	17(100%)	17	0.0004
Left	10	6	10(58.8%)	10	
Right	7	3	7(41.2%)	7	
Bilateral	1	0	1	1	
Overall	18	9(50.0%)	18(100%)	18	0.005

LPG lymphangiography, *CTA* computerized tomographic angiography
*χ^2 test

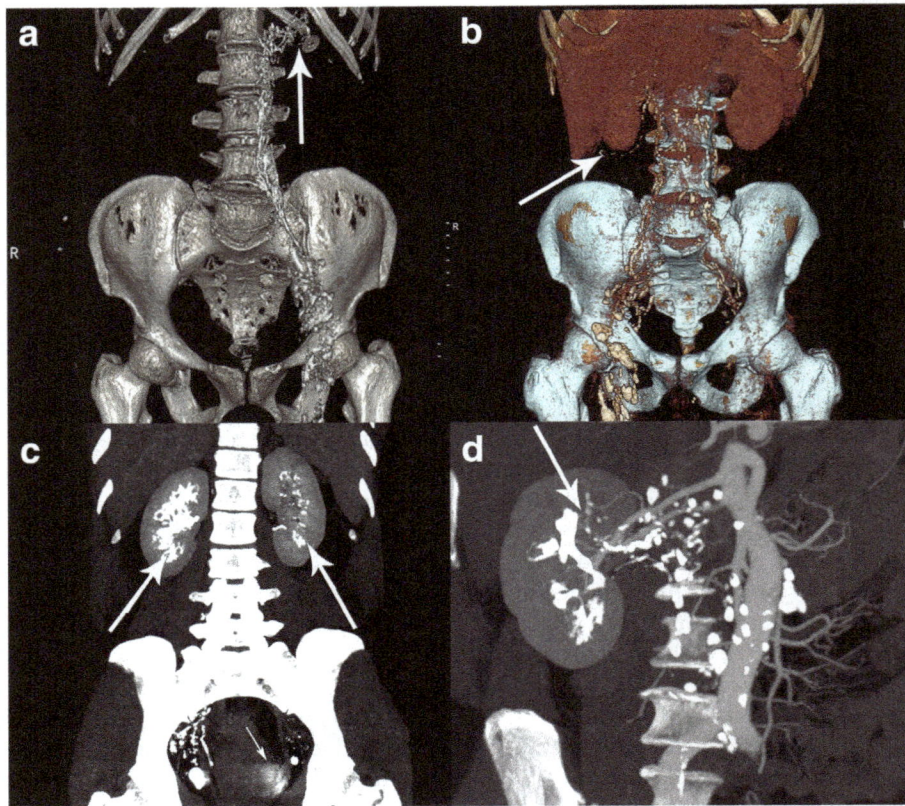

Fig. 1 VR of CT data showing (**a**) the distribution of lymphatic vessels around the left renal artery and vein. **b** Chyle leaks in right renal fascia. MIP of CT data showing (**c**) Bilateral lymphatic leakage of the renal pelvis, and reflux of contrast agent into the bladder and (**d**) right renal lymphatic leakage and lymphatic vessel lesions adjacent to the renal vein

results obtained with LPG CTA were sufficient to allow performing renal lymphatic stripping and ligation in all patients. Chyluria resolved immediately after surgery in 17 unilateral chyle leakage patients, with negative urine chyle tests. The remaining patient with bilateral lympho-urinary fistulas received renal lymphatic stripping on right side, which was the more severe side. His milky urine disappeared within 7 days after surgery, and a urine chyle test was negative. No recurrences were observed over a median follow-up 31 (range 8–52) months after surgery.

Table 2 Successful location of chyluria by cystoscopy, CT, LPG, and LPG CTA

	Cystoscopy	CT	LPG	LPG + CTA
Invasive	Y	N	Y	Y
Sides	Y/N	Y/N	Y	Y
Sites	N	Y/N	Y/N	Y
precise location	N	N	13/18	18/18*
Radiation	N	N	Y	Y**

LPG lymphangiography, *CTA* computerized tomographic angiography, *Y* Yes, *N* No
* *P* = 0.016 (LPG CTA vs. LPG)
** more radiation exposure than LPG or CT alone

Discussion

Chyluria can be confirmed by a urine chyle test. About 80% of patients respond to conservative management with a low-fat, high-protein diet or intraperitoneal injection of sclerotherapy such as silver nitrate, povidone iodine or dextrose, about 22% relapse within 2 years [7, 8]. Surgical intervention is needed for patients with severe chyluria patients who fail to respond to conservative management or have short-term relapses. Successful surgery requires clear identification and accurate location of the site of chyle leakage, especially the relationship between lymphatic vessels and the renal collection system or vascular system.

Imaging studies in patients with severe chyluria generally include cystoscopy and LPG. LPG is more successful than cystoscopy in detecting bilateral lymphatic renal pelvis fistulas than cystoscopy [2]. The appearance of LPG images in these chyluria patients was wire-like, with semicircular or coralline-shaped shadows that were primarily distributed in the renal pelvis and parenchyma (Fig. 2a). The renal hilus was distorted and dilated, lumbar or iliac lymph vessels could be seen, and obviously dilated truncus lumbalis

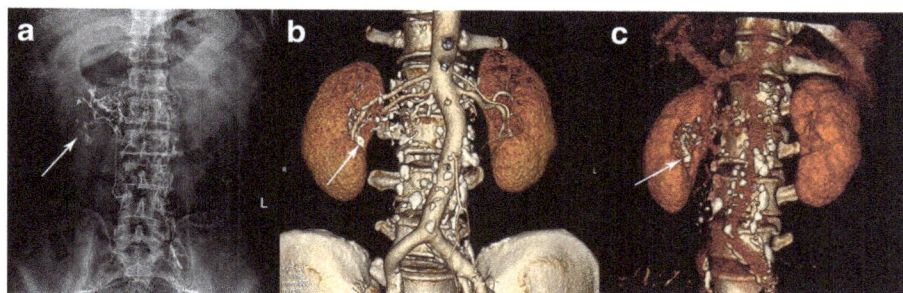

Fig. 2 A 60-year-old man with persistent idiopathic chyluria. **a** Pre-CTA LPG showing wire-like, semicircular shadow at the renal pelvis area and parenchyma in LPG (KUB) indicated right renal lymphatic leakage. **b**, **c** LPG CTA showing accumulation of contrast agent in right renal hilus

lymph vessels were occasionally observed. Single photon emission computed tomography (SPECT)/CT or MRI may be useful in the location of lymphatic ducts and chyle leakage sites [9–11], but LPG remains the most widely used method [12]. Evaluation of abdominal and retroperitoneal lymphatic abnormalities, including lymphatic leaks, using MRI lymphography with heavily T2-weighted fast spin echo sequences [10]. Nonenhanced MRI lymphangiography is a safe and effective method for imaging the central lymphatic system, and can contribute to differential diagnosis and appropriate preoperative evaluation of chylothorax or lymphangioma [13]. However there been few reports have described its use in chyluria patients [14].

We previously reported the successful use of LPG in diagnosing chyluria and LPG followed by a CT scan to directly show fistulae between the perinephric collection and lymphatic systems in either a plain scan or reconstructed image [2]. It is not clear whether a CT scan is of help after LPG. The CT increases the radiation exposure, and may not provide the information needed to perform the required surgery. It cannot show the details of the connections between lymphatic vessels and renal blood vessels, which may result in surgical failure because of incomplete ligation of all the lymphatic branches surrounding the renal arteries or veins. LPG combined with post-LPG CTA clearly show such structures and the relation of the lymphatic vessels and the renal collecting or vascular systems. In this study, the lymphatic lesions were well visualized by LPG with post-LPG CTA in all patients (Figs. 2 and 3), providing a reliable basis for renal pedicle lymphatic ligation and stripping.

Cystoscopy correctly found the side of the chyle leak in only about half the patients. LPG, the classic diagnostic tool [12], revealed not only the side of the lymphatic leaks, but also the approximate sites of reflux of contrast agent reflux into the renal collecting system (see Fig. 2a). However, LPG was unsatisfactory in some complicated cases, and it was difficult to obtain more information on the chyle leak in addition to the side of chyluria. LPG combined with post-LPG CTA clearly showed additional detail including the course of renal blood vessels, lymphatic vessels, the collection system, and their interlaced

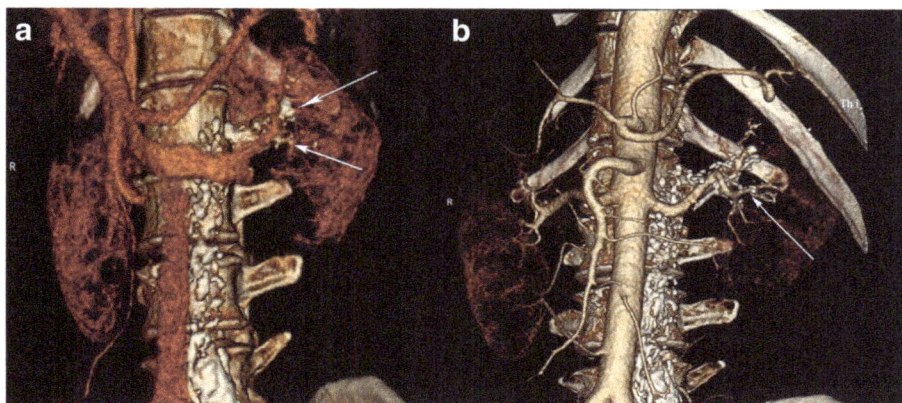

Fig. 3 A 61-year-old woman with persistent idiopathic chyluria. **a**, **b** LPG CTA showing contrast agent adjacent to the left renal artery and its branches into the kidney

connections. The radiation exposure was more with LPG CTA than with LPG alone (Table 2), but in complicated cases in which CT or LPG alone were not satisfactory, LPG combined with post-LPG CTA provided precise location and clear imaging information, especially in cases not suitable for use of MRI. Despite its level of invasiveness, this method is a good option in the diagnosis of persistent chyluria requiring surgery. Fever and pain are the most frequent complications after LPG. Severe complications such as hemoptysis, wound infection, and embolism of blood vessels have been reported [12, 15, 16], but did not occur in this patient series.

The study was limited by a small number of patients because of the rarity of persistent idiopathic chyluria and by the absence of a randomized control group. A multicenter, randomized control study with large number of patients is necessary to further investigate the advantages of LPG with CTA in the accurate location of chyle leaks and the management of chyluria.

Conclusions

LPG combine with post-LPG CTA could provide precise location and clear imaging information for chyluria patients which cannot be detected by routine contrast CT or not suitable for MR examination. Despite of its mild invasiveness, this method could be better than LPG alone and be a good option in the diagnosis of persistent chyluria requiring surgery.

Abbreviations
CT: Computed tomography; CTA: Computerized tomographic angiography; LPG: Unilateral pedal lymphangiography; MIP: Maximum intensity projection; MPR: Multiplanar reformation; MRI: Magnetic resonance imaging; SPECT/CT: Single photon emission computed tomography/computed tomography; VR: Volume rendering

Acknowledgements
The authors thank all the patients and their families for their cooperation during regular follow-up.

Funding
This article is supported by Major Subjects Project of Health and Med system, Pudong New District, Shanghai (PWZX2014–19); Science and Technology Innovation Project of Pudong New District, Shanghai (PKJ 2013-y33).

Authors' contributions
DL, YS, and SH conceived and designed the study. DL, QT, WL, WZ, WX, and MW performed the surgery and the case follow-up. JW, YZ, and JY performed data acquisition. HW performed LPG and CTA, provided the figs. BL performed the data analysis and wrote the manuscript. DL and YS edited the manuscript. All authors reviewed the manuscript. All authors read and approved the final manuscript.

Competing interests
The authors declare that they have no competing interests.

Author details
[1]Department of Urology, Department of Radiology, Shanghai Punan Hospital, Shanghai, People's Republic of China. [2]Department of Urology, Shanghai Jiao Tong University Medical School Affiliated Ruijin Hospital, 197 Ruijin Er Road, Shanghai 200025, People's Republic of China. [3]Department of Urology, Chinese People's Liberation Army Hospital 184, Yingtan, People's Republic of China. [4]Department of Urology, Shanghai Post and Telecommunication Hospital, 666 Changle Road, Shanghai 200040, People's Republic of China. [5]Department of Urology, Shanghai Jiao Tong University Medical School Affiliated Ruijin Hospital North, 999 Xiwang Road, Shanghai 201801, People's Republic of China.

References
1. Nandy PR, Dwivedi US, Vyas N, Prasad M, Dutta B, Singh PB. Povidone iodine and dextrose solution combination sclerotherapy in chyluria. Urology. 2004;64:1107–9. 1110
2. Liu DY, He HC, Zhou WL, et al. The advantages of unilateral pedal lymphography in the diagnosis of chyluria. Urol Int. 2015;94:215–9.
3. Kos S, Haueisen H, Lachmund U, Roeren T. Lymphangiography: forgotten tool or rising star in the diagnosis and therapy of postoperative lymphatic vessel leakage. Cardiovasc Intervent Radiol. 2007;30:968–73.
4. Matsumoto T, Yamagami T, Kato T, et al. The effectiveness of lymphangiography as a treatment method for various chyle leakages. Br J Radiol. 2009;82:286–90.
5. Liu DY, Shao Y, Shi JX. Unilateral pedal lymphangiography with non-contrast computerized tomography is valuable in the location and treatment decision of idiopathic chylothorax. J Cardiothorac Surg. 2014;9:8.
6. Yoshimatsu R, Yamagami T, Miura H, Matsumoto T. Prediction of therapeutic effectiveness according to CT findings after therapeutic lymphangiography for lymphatic leakage. Jpn J Radiol. 2013;31:797–802.
7. Koga S, Nagata Y, Arakaki Y, Matsuoka M, Ohyama C. Unilateral pedal lymphography in patients with filarial chyluria. BJU Int. 2000;85:222–3.
8. Seleem MM, Eliwa AM, Elsayed ER, et al. Single versus multiple instillation of povidone iodine and urographin in the treatment of chyluria: a prospective randomised study. Arab J Urol. 2016;14:131–5.
9. Suh M, Cheon GJ, Seo HJ, Kim HH, Lee DS. Usefulness of additional SPECT/CT identifying Lymphatico-renal shunt in a patient with Chyluria. Nucl Med Mol Imaging. 2015;49:61–4.
10. Arrive L, Azizi L, Lewin M, et al. MR lymphography of abdominal and retroperitoneal lymphatic vessels. AJR Am J Roentgenol. 2007;189: 1051–8.
11. Zelmanovitz F. Location of regional intestinal lymphangiectasia using Tc-99m dextran lymphoscintigraphy. Clin Nucl Med. 1999;24:210–1.
12. Guermazi A, Brice P, Hennequin C, Sarfati E. Lymphography: an old technique retains its usefulness. Radiographics. 2003;23:1541–58. 1559-1560
13. Kim EY, Hwang HS, Lee HY, et al. Anatomic and functional evaluation of central Lymphatics with noninvasive magnetic resonance lymphangiography. Medicine (Baltimore). 2016;95:e3109.
14. El MS, Arrive L. Magnetic resonance lymphography of chyluria. Kidney Int. 2010;78:712.
15. Deso S, Kabutey NK, Vilvendhan R, Kim D, Guermazi A. Lymphangiography in the diagnosis, localization, and treatment of a lymphaticopelvic fistula causing chyluria: a case report. Vasc Endovasc Surg. 2010;44:710–3.
16. Kusumoto S, Imamura A, Watanabe K. Case report: the incidental lipid embolization to the brain and kidney after lymphography in a patient with malignant lymphoma: CT findings. Clin Radiol. 1991;44:279–80.

Cost implications of PSA screening differ by age

Karthik Rao[1], Stella Liang[2], Michael Cardamone[2], Corinne E. Joshu[3,4], Kyle Marmen[5], Nrupen Bhavsar[3], William G. Nelson[4,6,7], H. Ballentine Carter[6], Michael C. Albert[8], Elizabeth A. Platz[3,4,6] and Craig E. Pollack[9*]

Abstract

Background: Multiple guidelines seek to alter rates of prostate-specific antigen (PSA)-based prostate cancer screening. The costs borne by payers associated with PSA-based screening for men of different age groups—including the costs of screening and subsequent diagnosis, treatment, and adverse events—remain uncertain. We sought to develop a model of PSA costs that could be used by payers and health care systems to inform cost considerations under a range of different scenarios.

Methods: We determined the prevalence of PSA screening among men aged 50 and higher using 2013-2014 data from a large, multispecialty group, obtained reimbursed costs associated with screening, diagnosis, and treatment from a commercial health plan, and identified transition probabilities for biopsy, diagnosis, treatment, and complications from the literature to generate a cost model. We estimated annual total costs for groups of men ages 50-54, 55-69, and 70+ years, and varied annual prostate cancer screening prevalence in each group from 5 to 50% and tested hypothetical examples of different test characteristics (e.g., true/false positive rate).

Results: Under the baseline screening patterns, costs of the PSA screening represented 10.1% of the total costs; costs of biopsies and associated complications were 23.3% of total costs; and, although only 0.3% of all screen eligible patients were treated, they accounted for 66.7% of total costs. For each 5-percentage point decrease in PSA screening among men aged 70 and older for a single calendar year, total costs associated with prostate cancer screening decreased by 13.8%. For each 5-percentage point decrease in PSA screening among men 50-54 and 55-69 years old, costs were 2.3% and 7.3% lower respectively.

Conclusions: With constrained financial resources and with national pressure to decrease use of clinically unnecessary PSA-based prostate cancer screening, there is an opportunity for cost savings, especially by focusing on the downstream costs disproportionately associated with screening men 70 and older.

Keywords: Prostate cancer, Screening, Costs

Background

Increasingly, health care systems are adopting risk-based payment strategies in which they are responsible for the health care costs incurred by their patients [1]. In this setting, health care systems are under pressure to provide evidence-based and efficient care for their beneficiaries. One area in which health systems may better align practice with evidence-based guidelines is cancer screening. Research suggests that many patients, including elderly patients and those with limited life expectancies, routinely receive cancer screening when they are unlikely to benefit [2]. The downstream costs of screening and subsequent treatment are substantial [3].

Recent guidelines for prostate specific antigen (PSA)-based prostate cancer screening have called for a reduction in the number of men who receive screening. The United States Preventive Services Task Force (USPTF) recommends against routine screening in all men (though draft guidelines may modify this) whereas the American Urological Association (AUA) advises against screening in men aged 70 or higher, except in those in the best health after shared decision making [4–6]. Early

---

* Correspondence: Cpollac2@jhmi.edu
[9]Department of Medicine, Johns Hopkins University School of Medicine, 2024 E. Monument Street, Suite 2-519, Baltimore, MD 21287, USA
Full list of author information is available at the end of the article

evidence suggests that the rate of PSA screening has decreased with a corresponding decline in prostate cancer incidence [7–9]. Nonetheless, many men aged 70 and higher continue to receive screening [10, 11]. While health systems may have an incentive to reduce clinically unnecessary PSA screening among their beneficiaries, the financial costs—from a health care system perspective—have not, to our knowledge, been quantified.

In this study, we tested how varying the rates of PSA screening among men of different age groups may influence associated health care expenditures. To do so, we generated a model using data from a large network of primary care providers in Maryland and Washington D.C. along with insurance claim data and estimates from the medical literature. These data were used to calculate the costs borne by payers associated with screening, subsequent diagnosis, treatment, and adverse events of prostate cancer. We then used our model to test how a number of different scenarios may impact costs including changing the prevalence of PSA screening among men in different age groups, increasing the proportion of men with low risk disease who undergo active surveillance, and changing the positive and negative predictive value of the screening test itself. By altering the rates of PSA screening or unit costs, our model is adaptable to different healthcare systems and with institution specific data, could be used to make cost conscientious decisions for system, provider, and patient interventions that seek to alter current patterns of PSA screening.

Methods

We conducted a retrospective study to create a model of prostate cancer screening costs using data on (1) the prevalence of prostate cancer screening; (2) the reimbursed costs using procedure and complication reimbursement claims; and (3) the probabilities of screened patients developing and being treated for prostate cancer, and experiencing adverse events.

Prostate cancer screening

We determined the annual prevalence of PSA screening among men aged 50 and higher who received primary care from a large, multispecialty group of ambulatory practices from April 1, 2013 to March 31, 2014 using electronic medical record data. Men with a known history of prostate cancer based on Internal Classification of Diseases (ICD)-9 code were excluded. The multispecialty group encompasses urban, suburban, and rural settings from an academic healthcare network in Maryland and Washington DC with over 39 clinic locations and 240,000 patients seen in the past year.

Identification of procedure and complication costs

We estimated costs associated with screening and subsequent diagnosis, treatment, and complications using reimbursement claims data from a large, self-insured health plan in the mid-Atlantic region. Events of PSA screening, prostate biopsy, and treatment (radical prostatectomy and radiation) were identified by Current Procedural Terminology (CPT) codes (Additional file 1) in the claims database. The cost associated with each claim was the payment from the insurance carrier to the healthcare provider and does not include patients' out-of-pocket, co-pay and secondary insurance payments. Data from 2004-2013 was employed to ensure enough patients for stable cost estimates; the time period ended in 2013 based on data availability at the time of analysis.

We estimated the costs and rate of short-term complications resulting from prostate biopsy, radical prostatectomy, and prostate-targeted radiation therapy by identifying patients who utilized healthcare resources within 30 days (biopsy, radiation) or 90 days (prostatectomy) of the procedure and had ICD-9 diagnosis codes consistent with a complication for the procedure of interest (Additional file 2). The rates of complication were calculated by dividing the number of patients with a complication by the number of patients who had the procedure. To make our costs of complications less sensitive to outliers, we removed 5 patients whose costs were greater than 2 standard deviations from the mean. After outliers were removed, the average cost of treatment for complications from prostate biopsy, and prostate targeted radiation therapies from 2004-2013 was determined and inflated to 2013 dollars.

Transition probabilities from prostate cancer screening to diagnosis and treatment

A node diagram (Fig. 1) was created to model a patient's experience beginning with prostate cancer screening through treatment. For node 1, PSA screening practice data from patients treated by the multispecialty group on April 1, 2013 to March 31, 2014 was used to model screening prevalence. At each node, literature probabilities were used to determine the proportion of patients, by age group, who moved forward to the next node. The specific nodes that were modeled included the proportion of men who had a PSA greater than 4 ng/dl (node 2) [12], proportion of men who had a biopsy (node 3) [13], proportion of men who had a positive biopsy (node 4) [13], proportion of men classified by prostate cancer risk (node 5) [14], and proportion of men classified by treatment received (node 6) [14].

Table 1 Patient Stratification by Prostate Cancer Risk and Treatment Modality with Treatment and Complication Costs for Radical Prostatectomy and Radiotherapy

	Active Surveillance	Radical Prostatectomy	Radiotherapy	Cryotherapy	Primary Androgen Deprivation Therapy
%					
Low	9.2%	56.8%	23.3%	3.1%	7.6%
Intermediate	4.8%	52.9%	25.8%	4.5%	11.9%
High	3.2%	32.2%	25.6%	6.1%	32.8%
Unknown	9.9%	42.2%	26.3%	2.6%	18.9%
N					
Low	5	28	11	2	4
Intermediate	2	26	13	2	6
High	1	6	5	1	7
Unknown	2	7	4	0	3
Total	10	67	33	5	20
Total cost by treatment as a percentage of total cost of screening and treatment		31.3%	32.0%		
Complication rate		17.0%	1.6%		
Total complication cost by treatment as a percentage of total cost of screening and treatment		10.4%	0.11%		
Total treatment cost as a percentage of total screening and treatment cost	66.6%				

Source of cost estimate is insurance claim data from a commercial health plan in the mid-Atlantic
Active surveillance, cryotherapy, and primary androgen deprivation therapy are not included in total cost amount as they are not primary modalities of active therapy, which we focused our analysis on

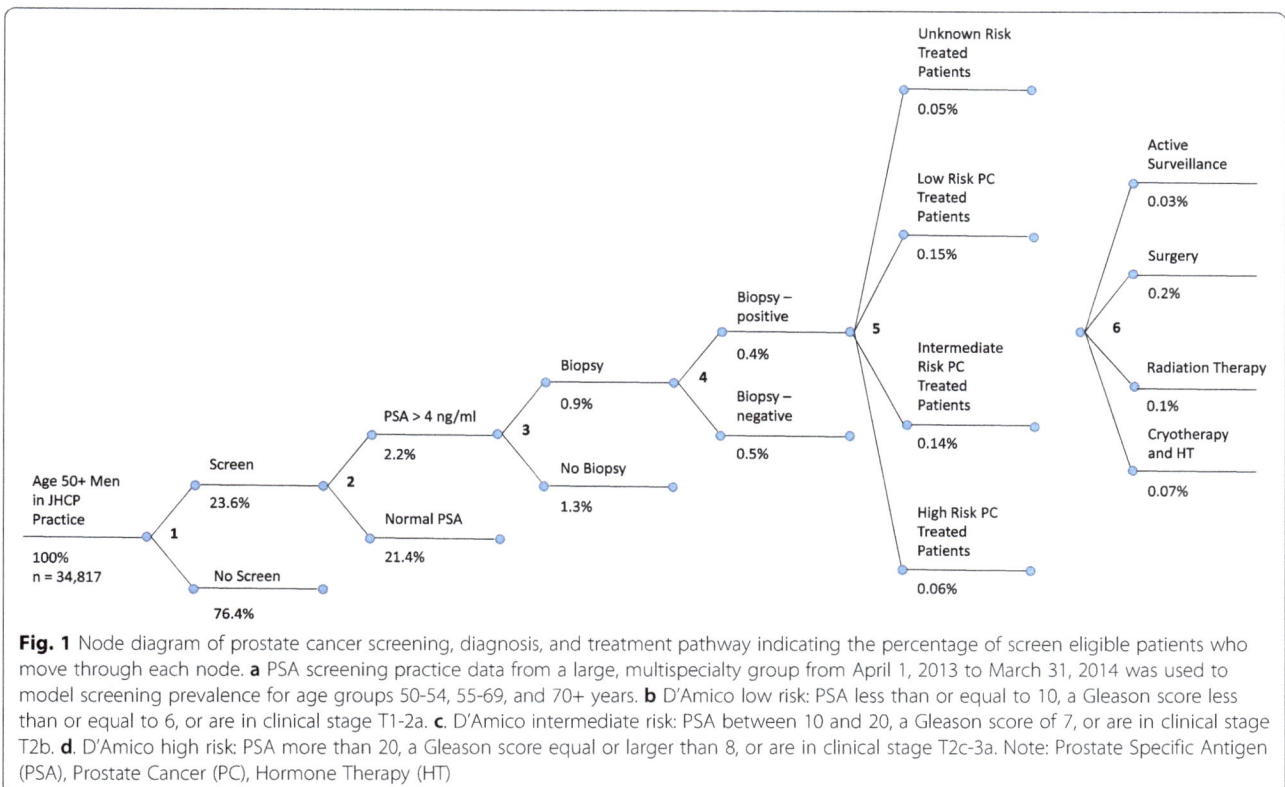

Fig. 1 Node diagram of prostate cancer screening, diagnosis, and treatment pathway indicating the percentage of screen eligible patients who move through each node. **a** PSA screening practice data from a large, multispecialty group from April 1, 2013 to March 31, 2014 was used to model screening prevalence for age groups 50-54, 55-69, and 70+ years. **b** D'Amico low risk: PSA less than or equal to 10, a Gleason score less than or equal to 6, or are in clinical stage T1-2a. **c**. D'Amico intermediate risk: PSA between 10 and 20, a Gleason score of 7, or are in clinical stage T2b. **d**. D'Amico high risk: PSA more than 20, a Gleason score equal or larger than 8, or are in clinical stage T2c-3a. Note: Prostate Specific Antigen (PSA), Prostate Cancer (PC), Hormone Therapy (HT)

Statistical analysis

For men who underwent screening during the 12-month period, we calculated the number of men who would be expected to progress through each node of the diagram. For each node, the per patient costs were multiplied by the total number of patients to determine the final costs of prostate cancer screening and treatment in the current scenario. We report the costs of the different lines of service/nodes as percentages of the total costs.

To understand the cost impact of changes in the prevalence of PSA-based prostate cancer screening, we developed scenarios in which we changed the screening prevalence during the 12 months among men of different age groups. In particular, we assessed PSA screening prevalences ranging between 5-50% in each age group (50-54, 55-69, 70+ years). We next sought to evaluate the impact of changing current patterns of treatment. With studies suggesting that older men with low risk disease frequently do well without active treatment [15], we modeled the cost implications of having more men 70+ with low risk disease (defined as PSA less than or equal to 10, a Gleason score less than or equal to 6, or are in clinical stage T1-2a by D'Amico criteria [16] and as modeled in node 5) move from radical prostatectomy to active surveillance.

Finally, new tools for prostate cancer screening are on the horizon which have the potential to (a) reduce the number of men without prostate cancer who undergo prostate biopsies (e.g., reduce the false positive rate of the screening test) and (b) increase the number of men with prostate cancer who screen positive (e.g., increase the true positive rate of the screening test). We modeled the potential cost implications of each scenario using a 10% reduction in the false positive rate and a 10% increase in the true positive rate as estimates of what a novel test may achieve. To estimate the total number of patients with prostate cancer for this analysis, we used literature estimates to determine the percentage of PSA screen positive patients with prostate cancer that may be missed by biopsy and also the percentage of patients with a negative PSA screen that may have prostate cancer. We assume that first biopsy misses 25% of positive prostate cancers [17] and that 15.2% of men with a negative PSA screen have prostate cancer [18].

Results

We identified 34,817 men treated by the multispecialty group who were eligible for PSA-based prostate cancer screening; approximately 18% were ages 50-54, 52% were ages 55-69, and 30% were ages 70 and older. Of these, 8,213 (23.6%) were screened. The prevalence of screening varied by age group with men between the ages of 55-69 being the most likely to be screened (28.5%). In comparison, 17.8% of men ages 50-54 and 18.4% ages 70 and older were screened.

Based on current patterns of screening, we estimated that the costs of the PSA screening represented 10.1% of the total costs of screening, diagnosis, treatment, and complications for eligible patients. The costs of biopsies and associated complications were 23.3% of the total costs whereas the cost of treatment and associated complications were 66.6% of the total costs (Table 1). Although only 0.3% of all screen eligible patients were treated, they accounted for two thirds of all costs in the screening, diagnosis, treatment, and associated complications pathway. Complications from radical prostatectomy accounted for 10.4% of the treatment costs, whereas radiotherapy complications accounted for 0.1% and biopsy complications accounted for 5.4% of treatment costs. In the Additional file 3, we present the model we generated for the above analysis, which other health systems can use to estimate and partition costs. The following parameters can be modified: population size, screening rate among men of different age groups, and costs of treatment and associated complications.

In Fig. 2, we show how different screening prevalences among men from different age groups influence costs. Increasing the prevalence of screening from the observed baseline in the multispecialty group (where the baseline prevalence is represented by the point each line intersects with the x-axis) is associated with increased costs from the current scenario. As the groups increased in age, there was a greater effect on overall cost from varying screening rate with the highest costs associated with changing screening amongst the oldest men. For each 5-percentage point increase in PSA screening among men 70 years and older, the total costs to the health care system increased by 13.8%. A 5-percentage point increase in PSA screening among men age 50-54 and 55-69 resulted in a smaller increase in total costs: 2.3% and 7.3% increase in total costs from the current scenario, respectively.

In assessing the cost impact of men age 70 and older with low risk prostate cancer choosing active surveillance instead of radical prostatectomy, we used $3,782 [19] as the cost of active surveillance over a 1-year time frame in contrast to the 30 day-time frame (radiation) and 90-day time frame (prostatectomy) used to determine the costs of active treatment. In our initial scenario, only 7.7% of the 26 men over 70 diagnosed with low risk disease were estimated to receive active surveillance. For every 10-percentage point increase in the proportion of low risk men 70+ who elect active surveillance, there would be a resulting 2.1% reduction in costs treating men in this age group and a more modest 1.1% reduction in total costs compared to the current scenario.

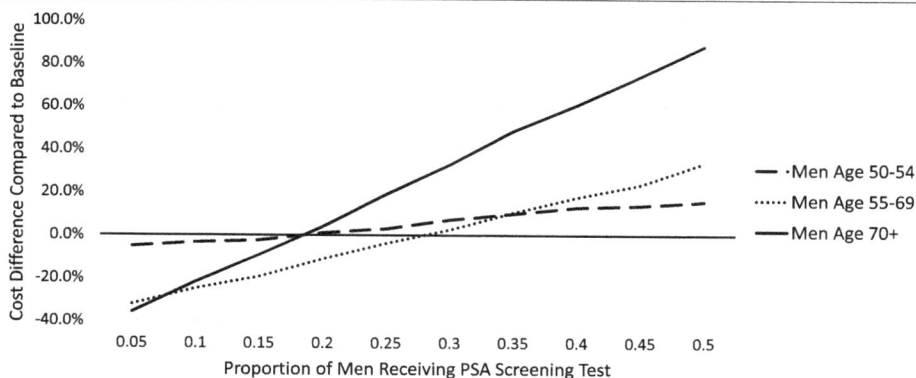

Fig. 2 Change in the percentage of total costs of prostate cancer screening, diagnosis, treatment, and associated complications as a function of PSA screening prevalence among eligible men. Observed screening prevalence at the multispecialty group is represented by the point each line intersects with the x-axis

To determine the cost implications of a reduction in the false positive rate for a new theoretical prostate cancer screening test, we used a false positive proportion of 42.1% for PSA screening (assuming a cutoff of 4 ng/ml is used to determine patients who receive biopsy) [20]. For a 10-percentage point reduction in the false positive proportion, we would expect savings that equate to 14.7% of the overall cost of biopsies and 3.4% of overall screening, diagnosis, treatment and associated complication costs of the population under study, which would be realized by preventing unnecessary diagnostic biopsies and subsequent treatment and complications. These estimates do not include the potential costs of the new screening test and assume the number of true men identified with prostate cancer remain unchanged, irrespective of the screening tool that is used. Conversely, increasing the true positive rate of the screening test would lead to additional costs to the health system. We estimated that the true positive rate for PSA screening is 28% (e.g., 28% of men with prostate cancer are identified by a PSA cutoff of 4 ng/ml). For a 10-percentage point increase in the PSA screen true positive rate for the study sample, we can expect the cost increase to equate to 35.4% of the overall cost of treatment and 23.6% of the overall cost of screening and treatment compared to the current scenario.

Discussion

Screening, diagnosis, treatment and associated complication costs from the payer perspective among men 70 years old or older—the group least likely to benefit from the practice [4]—amounted to nearly two thirds of the overall cost. Notably, men in this age group make up less than one third of the patient population in the multispecialty group. Correspondingly, a decrease in screening rate by 5

percentage points in men 70 years and older would result in the largest percent decrease in cost when compared to other age groups. Given that a significant proportion of men in this age group who are screened and are diagnosed with low risk prostate cancer will receive aggressive therapy with questionable benefit, there may be an opportunity to be more selective in patients that receive screening and aggressive treatment [4, 21].

In light of revised national guidelines from the United States Preventive Services Task Force and the American Urological Association combined with the move towards risk-based payment strategies nationally [22–24], health systems and payers are incentivized to align practice with evidence based guidelines. Inputs from our model—including the age distribution of the population, rates of screening, and unit costs—may be easily adapted to be employed by other health care systems.

The increased overall cost to screen and treat men aged 70 years and older are driven by higher incidence of cancer in this population among men who are screened [12]. Ma et al. also found that screening and biopsy for older age groups, particularly the 75-99-year-old age group, in the Medicare population resulted in higher costs, but were not able to assess the cost implications of treatment across age groups [25]. Additionally, the complication rates for biopsy and prostate cancer treatments are substantial, and although the rates of complication are not well characterized by age group, it is reasonable to expect that they may be higher in older populations given higher rates of complicating comorbidities [26, 27], which could be an additional cost driver for this age group.

Ninety percent of costs were attributable to post-screening diagnosis and treatment. With new tests on the horizon that may reduce false positive screens and increase true positive screens specifically for lethal prostate cancer, we explored their theoretical post screening financial impact. Reducing the false positive proportion of the PSA screen would result in modest savings on clinically unnecessary biopsies, but perhaps more importantly, allow patients to avoid the anxiety from falsely positive results and risk of undergoing procedures. Increasing the true positive proportion of screening tests may increase costs as more patients would move into the treatment pathway for the prostate cancer diagnosis. A number of nomograms, molecular biomarkers, and genetic markers currently under study may prevent the need for clinically unnecessary biopsies and treatments as well as better identify which patients would be most likely to benefit from active treatment and which patients would benefit from active surveillance [28–31]. The development and implementation of screening tests that are able to identify potentially lethal prostate cancer will be important in allowing us to more optimally allocate resources in constrained healthcare systems.

This study was designed to determine the costs associated with PSA-based prostate cancer screening in a primary care practice group associated with a large health system in the United States. However, the model we developed is flexible and can use inputs (age distribution of the screen-eligible population, the prevalence of screening, and screening, diagnosis, treatment and associated complications costs) tailored to other health care systems (see online Additional file 3). So while the costs of changing PSA screening practices are specific to our population, our approach and model may be more broadly applied when making decisions regarding the appropriate use of resources. With rising healthcare costs, this tool may provide the potential to use cost data as one piece of evaluating the value of PSA screening and downstream treatments as part of healthcare system clinical practice guidelines. In line with this trend, national clinical organizations such as the American Society of Clinical Oncologists and the American Heart Association have begun to use cost data as one part of evaluating the value of treatments [32, 33].

This study has several possible limitations that warrant discussion. First, our costs reflect reimbursement costs, and while they are an accurate reflection of costs from the payer perspective, they do not take into account other direct and indirect costs that influence total healthcare costs. These other costs include patient out-of-pocket costs, time off from work, and travel costs. Nonetheless, focusing on the payer perspective is important because it may impact how they consider different financial opportunities for interventions. Additionally, we recognize that there are many aspects to the costs associated with evaluating patients with an elevated PSA and treating patients with diagnosed

cancer that are joint and may include fixed facility fees, salaried staff costs, and the like. We were unable to accurately assess these joint costs and have not included them in our estimates. In future study, we aim to include both a direct assessment of our own systems costs with screening, diagnosis, and treatment and also evaluation of joint costs. Second, we included costs associated with active treatment for prostate cancer, specifically radiation therapy and radical prostatectomy; in our main scenario, we did not include costs of active surveillance, cryotherapy, or hormone therapy in this analysis due to insufficient claims data to obtain precise cost estimates. With nearly three quarters of patients receiving radiation and/or radical prostatectomy, it is unlikely that excluding these treatments would significantly impact cost projections. Third, the cost of complications was limited to those that occurred shortly after treatment and did not include costs of follow-up visits outside this time frame and intermediate and long-term complications (e.g., erectile dysfunction and urinary incontinence). Given that surgical therapies have higher upfront complications and radiotherapy higher delayed complications, our 90- and 30-day complication windows for surgery and radiotherapy respectively likely under reports overall costs for radiotherapy. Fourth, the 2013-2014 prevalence of PSA screening in screen-eligible men seeking primary care at the physician group were lower than national averages and the rate of PSA screening has changed in recent years following new guidelines [8, 9]. Our model is adaptable to other health care settings and inputs can be adjusted based on institution specific data [34]. In addition, we do not have data on whether men in the sample had been previously screened for prostate cancer, which may impact their likelihood of having a positive/negative test and interval of next screen. Expanding our timeline of analysis may have accounted for these variations in screening but we did not have available data to do so. We also lack data to accurately assess transition probabilities of our sample by racial group and co-morbidity but in future studies hope to include sensitivity analysis across racial groups and different co-morbidity groups [35]. Fifth, in the analysis in which we varied the accuracy of theoretical new prostate cancer screening tests, we did not know the number of patients with true prostate cancer and thus used literature estimates to determine the number of patients undergoing a PSA screen (positive or negative) with true prostate cancer. Though we changed the sensitivity and specificity of theoretical tests, we did not test scenarios in which new tests preferentially identified potentially lethal prostate cancer which may improve the value of screening and subsequent treatment. Lastly, it should be noted that the decision to screen and treat a man for prostate cancer, particularly a man aged 70 years or older, is an individual patient- and provider-level decision and that the assertions from our study cannot be blindly applied without thorough decision-making conversations regarding the pros and cons of PSA screening.

Conclusions

In a healthcare system with constrained financial resources and national pressure to decrease the rate of PSA screening, there is an opportunity for cost savings by more appropriately identifying patients that will most benefit. To move towards this opportunity, we highlight the importance that targeting men of different age ranges can have on overall costs, in particular by focusing on the downstream costs of potential diagnosis, complications and procedures that may be disproportionately associated with screening older patients.

Abbreviations

AUA: American Urological Association; CPT: Current Procedural Terminology; ICD: Internal Classification of Diseases; PSA: Prostate specific antigen; USPTF: United States Preventative Task Force

Acknowledgments

We thank the members of the Optimizing Cancer Screening in Hopkins Covered Lives Working Group.

Funding

Dr. Rao's effort was supported by the Johns Hopkins Dean's Research Fellowship. Dr. Pollack's salary is supported by the National Cancer Institute and Office of Behavioral and Social Sciences (K07 CA151910). Cancer Center Support Grant (P30 CA006973, Nelson WG). Pilot funding was from the Johns Hopkins Individualized Health Initiative (Platz EA).

Authors' contributions

HBC, KR, EAP, CEP, and NB conceived of and designed the study. SL, MC, KM, NB, MCA, and KR acquired the data. KR, SL, MC, CEJ, KM, NB, WGN, HBC, MCA, EAP, and CEP were involved in analysis and interpretation of data. KR drafted the initial manuscript. KR, SL, MC, CEJ, KM, NB, WGN, HBC, MCA, EAP, and CEP critically revised the manuscript draft. All authors have read and approved the final manuscript.

Competing interests

The authors declare that they have no competing interests.

Author details

[1]Johns Hopkins University School of Medicine, Baltimore, MD, USA. [2]Financial Analysis Unit, Johns Hopkins Health System, Baltimore, MD, USA. [3]Department of Epidemiology, Johns Hopkins Bloomberg School of Public Health, Baltimore, MD, USA. [4]Sidney Kimmel Comprehensive Cancer Center at Johns Hopkins, Baltimore, MD, USA. [5]Johns Hopkins Health Care, Glen Burnie, Baltimore, MD, USA. [6]Department of Urology and the James Buchanan Brady Urological Institute, Johns Hopkins University School of Medicine, Baltimore, MD, USA. [7]Department of Environmental Health Sciences, Johns Hopkins Bloomberg School of Public Health, Baltimore, MD, USA. [8]Johns Hopkins Community Physicians, Johns Hopkins Medical Institutions, Baltimore, MD, USA. [9]Department of Medicine, Johns Hopkins University School of Medicine, 2024 E. Monument Street, Suite 2-519, Baltimore, MD 21287, USA.

References

1. The Advisory Board Company. 2013 Accountable Payment Survey.
2. Eckstrom E, Feeny DH, Walter LC, et al. Individualizing cancer screening in older adults: a narrative review and framework for future research. J Gen Intern Med. 2013;28:292–8.
3. Wilson LS, Tesoro R, Elkin EP, et al. Cumulative cost pattern comparison of prostate cancer treatments. Cancer. 2007;109:518–27.
4. Moyer VA, U.S. Preventive Services Task Force. Screening for prostate cancer; U.S. Preventive Services Task Force recommendation statement. Ann Intern Med. 2012;157:120–34.
5. Carter HB, Albertsen PC, Barry MJ, et al. Early detection of prostate cancer: AUA Guideline. J Urol. 2013;190:419–26.
6. Bibbins-Domingo K, Grossman DC, Curry SJ. The US Preventive Services Task Force 2017 Draft Recommendation Statement on Screening for Prostate Cancer. JAMA. 2017;317(19):1949–50.
7. American Cancer Society. Cancer Facts & Figures 2017. Atlanta: American Cancer Society; 2017.
8. Jemal A, Ma J, Siegel R, et al. Prostate Cancer Incidence Rates 2 Years After the US Preventive Services Task Force Recommendations Against Screening. JAMA Oncology. 2016;2(12):1657.
9. Jemal A, Fedewa SA, Ma J, et al. Prostate Cancer Incidence and PSA Testing Patterns in Relation to USPSTF Screening Recommendations. JAMA. 2015;314(19):2054–61.
10. Sammon JD, Abdollah F, Choueiri TK, et al. Prostate-Specific Antigen Screening After 2012 US Preventive Services Task Force Recommendations. JAMA. 2015;315(19):2077–9.
11. Drazer MW, Huo D, Eggener SE. National Prostate Cancer Screening Rates After the 2012 US Preventive Services Task Force Recommendation Discouraging Prostate-Specific Antigen-Based Screening. J Clin Oncol. 2015;33(22):2416–23.
12. Welch HG, Schwartz LM, Woloshin S. Prostate-specific antigen levels in the United States: implications of various definitions for abnormal. J Natl Cancer Inst. 2005;97:1132–7.
13. Andriole GL, Levin DL, Crawford ED, et al. Prostate cancer screening in the prostate, lung, colorectal and ovarian (PLCO) cancer screening trial: findings from the initial screening round of a randomized trial. J Natl Cancer Inst. 2005;97:433–8.
14. Cooperberg MR, Broering JM, Carroll PR. Time trends and local variation in primary treatment of localized prostate cancer. J Clin Oncol. 2010;28:1117–23.
15. Tosoian JJ, Mamawala M, Epstein J, et al. Intermediate and longer-term outcomes from a prospective active-surveillance program for favorable-risk prostate cancer. J Clin Oncol. 2015;33:3379–85.
16. D'Amico AV, Whittington R, Malkowicz SB, et al. Biochemical outcome after radical prostatectomy, external beam radiation therapy, or interstitial radiation therapy for clinically localized prostate cancer. JAMA. 1998;280:969–74.
17. Shariat SF, Roehrborn CG. Using biopsy to detect prostate cancer. Rev Urol. 2008;10:262–80.
18. Thompson IM, Pauler DK, Goodman PJ, et al. Prevalence of prostate cancer among men with a prostate-specific antigen level ≤4.0 ng per milliliter. N Engl J Med. 2004;350:2239–46.
19. Keegan KA, Dall'Era MA, Durbin-Johnson B, et al. Active surveillance for prostate cancer compared with immediate treatment: an economic analysis. Cancer. 2012;118:3512–8.
20. Daneshgari F, Taylor GD, Miller GJ, et al. Computer simulation of the probability of detecting low volume carcinoma of the prostate with six random systematic core biopsies. Urology. 1995;45:604–9.
21. Roth JA, Gulati R, Gore JL, et al. Economic analysis of prostate-specific antigen screening and selective treatment strategies. JAMA Oncol. 2016;2(7):890–8.
22. Emanuel E, Tanden N, Altman S, et al. A systematic approach to containing health care spending. N Engl J Med. 2012;367:949–54.
23. Burwell SM. Setting value-based payment goals – HHS efforts to improve U. S. health care. N Engl J Med. 2015;372:897–9.
24. Press MJ, Rajkumar R, Conway PH. Medicare's new bundled payments: design, strategy, and evolution. JAMA. 2016;315:131–2.
25. Ma X, Wang R, Long JB, et al. The cost implications of prostate cancer screening in the Medicare population. Cancer. 2014;120:96–102.
26. Loeb S, Vellekoop A, Ahmed H, et al. Systematic review of complications of prostate biopsy. Eur Urol. 2013;64:876–92.
27. Simoneau A. Treatment and disease related complications of prostate cancer. Rev Urol. 2006;8(Suppl):56–67.

28. Gurel B, Iwata T, Koh CM, et al. Molecular alterations in prostate cancer as diagnostic, prognostic, and therapeutic targets. Adv Anat Pathol. 2008;15:319–31.
29. Choudury AD, Eeles R, Freedland SJ, et al. The role of genetic markers in the management of prostate cancer. Eur Urol. 2012;62:577–87.
30. Salagierski M, Schalken JA. Molecular diagnosis of prostate cancer: PCA3 and TMPRSS2:ERG gene fusion. J Urol. 2012;187:795–801.
31. Ankerst DP, Xia J, Thompson IM Jr, et al. Precision medicine in active surveillance for prostate cancer: development of the Canary-Early Detection Research Network Active Surveillance Biopsy Risk Calculator. Eur Urol. 2015;68(6):1083–8.
32. Anderson JL, Heidenreich PA, Barnett PG, et al. ACC/AHA statement on cost/value methodology in clinical practice guidelines and performance measures: a report of the American College of Cardiology/American Heart Association Task Force on Performance Measures and Task Force on Practice Guidelines. Circulation. 2014;129:2329–45.
33. Schnipper LE, Davidson NE, Wollins DS, et al. American Society of Clinical Oncology Statement. A conceptual framework to assess the value of cancer treatment options. J Clin Oncol. 2015;33:2563–77.
34. Drazer MW, Huo D, Schonberg MA, et al. Population-based patterns and predictors of prostate-specific antigen screening among older men in the United States. J Clin Oncol. 2011;29:1736–43.
35. Sundi D, Kryvenko ON, Carter HB, et al. Pathological examination of radical prostatectomy specimens in men with very low risk disease at biopsy reveals distinct zonal distribution of cancer in black American men. J Urol. 2014;191:60–7.

Obesity impairs male fertility through long-term effects on spermatogenesis

Yan-Fei Jia[1†], Qian Feng[1†], Zheng-Yan Ge[2], Ying Guo[3,4], Fang Zhou[3,4], Kai-Shu Zhang[3,4], Xiao-Wei Wang[4], Wen-Hong Lu[4], Xiao-Wei Liang[4] and Yi-Qun Gu[3,4*]

Abstract

Objective: This study aimed to investigate the effect and possible underlying mechanisms of high-fat diet-induced obesity on spermatogenesis in male rats.

Methods: A total of 45 male rats were randomly divided into control ($n = 15$, normal diet) and obesity groups ($n = 30$, high-fat diet) and were fed for 16 weeks. Body weight and organ indexes were determined after sacrifice. Indicators of reproductive function, including sperm count, sperm motility, apoptosis of spermatogenic cells, and oxidative stress levels, were measured. Serum metabolic parameters and reproductive hormones were also assayed.

Results: Compared with the control group, epididymal sperm motility in the obese rats was significantly decreased ($P < 0.01$). Morphological analysis of the obesity group showed vacuolar changes in seminiferous tubules, spermatogenic cell dysfunction, and increased apoptosis of spermatogenic cells in testicular tissue ($P < 0.05$). The calculated free testosterone (cFT) concentration in serum was decreased ($P < 0.05$), whereas the serum sex hormone-binding globulin (SHBG) level was significantly increased ($P < 0.01$). The superoxide dismutase (SOD) concentration decreased and the malondialdehyde (MDA) concentration increased in testis tissues; however, neither changes were statistically significant ($P > 0.05$).

Results: Nutritional obesity can damage spermatogenesis in male rats due to long-term effects on spermatogenesis.

Keywords: Obesity, Spermatogenesis, Sex hormone-binding globulin, Testosterone

Background

Obesity refers to excessive accumulation of body fat, which has a negative impact on health. According to the World Health Organization (WHO), a body mass index (BMI) of 25–29.9 kg/m^2 is defined as overweight, while a BMI of 30 kg/m^2 is defined as obesity. The incidence of overweight and obesity has sharply increased [1]. Relevant statistical data show that the obese population has doubled worldwide from 1980 to 2008, and more than 10% of the population is obese [2]. The prevalence of obesity has continued to rise according to subsequent surveys, with the most recent estimate indicating that 35.2% of men and 40.4% of women are obese [3].

Obesity is well documented to be linked to diseases such as type 2 diabetes mellitus, cardiovascular disease, cancers, and sleep apnea syndrome [4, 5]. Recently, the effect of obesity on fertility has been extensively investigated. However, current studies have principally focused on the effects of obesity on the reproductive function of females or female animals, while males or male animals are poorly studied [6]. Additionally, while most reports have examined obesity in relation to reproductive function, the underlying mechanisms have not been elucidated [7, 8]. In addition, conclusions on the effects of obesity on semen parameters and reproductive hormones have differed [9] due to the many factors that may impact male fertility. For example, a meta-analysis performed by MacDonald et al. found no statistically significant association between BMI and semen parameters [10], while a study performed by Sermondade et al. found a significant J-shaped association between BMI and an abnormal sperm count [11]. This study aimed to investigate spermatogenesis in male rats with obesity

* Correspondence: yqgu90@126.com
†Equal contributors
3Graduate School of Peking Union Medical College, No. 9 Dongdansantiao, Dongcheng District, Beijing 100730, People's Republic of China
4National Health and Family Planning Key Laboratory of Male Reproductive Health, Department of Male Clinical Research, National Research Institute for Family Planning, Beijing 100081, People's Republic of China
Full list of author information is available at the end of the article

induced by high-fat diet administration to minimize experimental bias and identify possible mechanisms.

Methods
Animals
Six-week-old male Sprague-Dawley rats were provided by Vital River Laboratory Animal Technology Co., Ltd. (Beijing, China). The rats had a body weight of 130.43 ± 7.15 g. They were maintained on a 12-h day/12-h night schedule (lights on from 19:00 to 07:00 h). Temperature and humidity were maintained at 22 ± 1 °C and 60%, respectively. Food and water were provided ad libitum, and each cage contained 5 rats. We tried our best to minimize animal suffering, and CO_2 inhalation was used for euthanasia.

Experimental design
A total of 45 male rats were enrolled in this study and randomly divided into two groups, namely, the control group ($n = 15$, normal diet) and the obesity group ($n = 30$, high-fat diet), which received a normal diet and a high-fat diet, respectively. The high-fat formula was as follows [12]: 10% lard oil, 10% sucrose, 1.5% cholesterol, 0.5% bile salt, 5% yolk powder, and 73% normal feed. The body weights and lengths of the rats were measured each week for 16 successive weeks. At the 16th week, the rats in the lower quartiles for weight gain ($n = 8$) were excluded from the obesity group. As the rats with body weights in the bottom quartile tended to exhibit obesity resistance, they were also excluded, and 22 obese rats were ultimately analyzed. To ensure appropriate grouping, a comparison of general status was performed between the two groups. The general growth status and metabolic parameters of the two groups were compared at the end of the 16th week.

After being fed with the respective diets for 16 weeks, all rats were anesthetized with CO_2. Blood samples were obtained from the abdominal aorta, centrifuged (2400 rpm for 20 min at 4 °C and frozen at − 70 °C) and were used to measure serum hormone levels [luteinizing hormone (LH), total testosterone TT), estradiol (E_2), and sex hormone-binding globulin (SHBG)]. Testicular histology, apoptosis of spermatogenic cells, and antioxidant status of the testis tissues were analyzed. Sperm suspensions from the cauda epididymis were used to determine sperm counts and motility.

Body index and organ index assessments
Bilateral testes, bilateral epididymides, and visceral fat (surrounding the kidney, testicles and omentum majus) were obtained and weighed. The relevant parameters were determined as follows: Lee index = [weight (g) × 10^3/body length (cm)]$^{1/3}$; fat coefficient = [visceral fat weight (g) × 100%/body weight (g)]; and testicular coefficient = [testicular weight (g) × 100%/weight (g)].

Serum biochemical and hormone assays
Serum SHBG was determined using an enzyme-linked immunosorbent assay (ELISA) kit obtained from Beijing Northern Biological Technology Research Institute (Beijing, China). Serum LH, T, and E_2 were measured with radioimmunoassays (RIAs) using a kit obtained from Beijing Northern Biological Technology Research Institute (Beijing, China). Serum free testosterone (FT) was calculated using the Vermeulen formula:

$$cFT = [T - 23.43FT]/[SHBG - (T - 23.43FT)] \times 10^{-9} mol/L.$$

Histological examination
Small pieces of testis were fixed in Bouin's solution and 70% ethanol, dehydrated in graded ethanol, fixed with 10% formalin solution for 48 h, and treated with mixed decalcifying fluid. After dehydration with alcohol, the femoral heads were embedded with paraffin, cut into 5-μm sections, and stained with HE. Cell morphology was observed under a light microscope and evaluated with Johnsen scoring [13, 14]. The histological criteria for modified Johnsen scoring are as follows: full spermatogenesis (score 10), slightly impaired spermatogenesis, many late spermatids, disorganized epithelium (score 9), less than five spermatozoa per tubule, few late spermatids (score 8), no spermatozoa, no late spermatids, many early spermatids (score 7), no spermatozoa, no late spermatids, few early spermatids (score 6), no spermatozoa or spermatids, many spermatocytes (score 5), no spermatozoa or spermatids, few spermatocytes (score 4), spermatogonia only (score 3), no germinal cells, Sertoli cells only (score 2), and no seminiferous epithelium (score 1).

Sperm count and motility
Sperm from the right cauda epididymis with a length of 1.5 cm were obtained. Internal rinsing with 1.0 ml of modified M199 medium was performed at 37 °C, and the samples were incubated for 30 min in a 37 °C water bath with vibration to induce the sperm to swim. Then, a 15-μl sperm suspension was extracted for sperm count and motility analysis using a Hamilton-Thorne Sperm Analyzer (HTM-IVOS). The sperm count per ml in the suspension from a unilateral epididymis was then calculated.

Assessment of spermatogenic cell apoptosis
The TUNEL method was used to label the 3'-end of fragmented DNA in the apoptotic spermatogenic cells.

The procedure was performed using Roche's TUNEL chemical staining method (Roche, SWISS, Cat. No. 11684817910) [15]. The brownish-orange particles in the cell nucleus observed under a microscope were classified as apoptotic cells. The apoptosis index (AI) was determined as follows: 500 cells were selected from five high-power fields from each section, and AI = apoptotic cell number/500 × 100%.

Antioxidant status evaluation

The kits for assessing testis antioxidation status, including superoxide dismutase (SOD) [16] and malondialdehyde (MDA) [17] concentrations, were purchased from Nanjing Jiancheng Bioengineering Institute (Nanjing, China). Testis tissues were isolated and crushed with liquid nitrogen, a homogenate was prepared, and the remaining procedures were performed following the kit protocols.

Statistical analysis

Statistical analysis was performed using the SPSS 13.0 software package (Chicago, IL, USA). Student's t-tests or Mann-Whitney tests were used to compare the results between the two groups. The results are presented as the mean ± s.e.m. in all cases, and $P < 0.05$ was considered statistically significant.

Results

General growth status and metabolic parameters

The results showed that compared with those in the control group, the Lee index and fat coefficient level of the nutritional obesity rats were significantly increased ($P < 0.05$), whereas the testis coefficient was significantly decreased ($P < 0.05$). No obvious difference was found in body length between the two groups, indicating that the group division was reasonable (Table 1).

Table 1 General growth status and metabolic parameters

	Weight	Length	Lee index	Fat coefficient	Testis coefficient
	(g)	(cm)	(%)	(%)	(%)
Control	552.90	26.50	0.31	4.38	0.63
n = 15)	±7.76	±0.94	±0.01	±0.96	±0.07
Obesity	619.80	26.86	0.32	5.02	0.55
(n = 22)	±7.56	±0.58	±0.01	±0.71	±0.06
P value	0.000**	0.198	0.046*	0.039*	0.001**

The data are presented as the mean ± s.e.m. * $P < 0.05$, ** $P < 0.01$: statistical significance compared with the control group; Weight: body weight; length: body length; Lee index = [weight (g) × 10^3/Body length (cm)]$^{1/3}$; Fat coefficient = [visceral fat weight (g) × 100%/body weight (g)]; Testicular coefficient = [testicular weight (g) × 100%/weight (g)]; and s.e.m.,: standard error of the mean

Sperm concentration and motility

To clarify the effect of obesity on the number and viability of sperm, sperm concentration and motility were detected. The concentrations of sperm extracted from the epididymis were $23.40 ± 9.72 × 10^6$/ml and $24.64 ± 7.16 × 10^6$/ml in the two groups, with no significant difference ($P > 0.05$). As illustrated in Fig. 1, sperm motility [(36.40 ± 9.17)% vs (14.36 ± 7.67)%] was significantly decreased in the obesity group compared with the control group ($P < 0.01$). The results indicated that obesity did not reduce the number of sperm but caused a marked decline in sperm viability.

Histological examination results

To assess the morphology of spermatogenesis and spermatogenic cells, histological examination was performed. HE staining demonstrated vacuolation in the seminiferous tubules and structural dysfunction in the spermatogenic cells or detachment of germ cells from the basement membrane in the obesity group (Fig. 2a, b). No significant difference was found in Johnsen scores [(9.14 ± 0.14) vs (8.86 ± 0.09)] ($P > 0.05$) between the two groups (Fig. 2c). We concluded that the short-term influence of obesity on testicular function may not be very obvious; however, long-term effects may damage spermatogenic function.

Ai

To observe the effects of obesity on spermatogenic cell apoptosis, TUNEL assay was performed. The AI of spermatogenic cells (Fig. 3a, b) was significantly increased in the obesity group compared with the control group [(5.95 ± 0.49)% vs (8.61 ± 1.05)%] ($P < 0.05$) (Fig. 3c). The results suggest that obesity may promote testicular germ cell apoptosis.

Reproductive hormone assays

Regarding the effect of obesity on male reproductive hormones, serum cFT concentrations were decreased, and serum SHBG levels were increased ($P < 0.05$) in the obesity group. Although serum T levels decreased in the obesity group, no statistically significant differences were found between the two groups (Table 2).

Oxidative stress assessment

To determine the effect of obesity on oxidative stress, the concentrations of SOD and MDA in the testis homogenate were determined. The SOD and MDA concentrations of the testicular homogenate were [(64.8 ± 10.2) vs (56.6 ± 14.4) U/ml] and [(3.0 ± 0.7) vs (4.0 ± 0.8) nmol/ml] in the two groups ($P > 0.05$) and ($P > 0.05$), respectively (Fig. 4). The results indicated that the SOD concentration decreased while the MDA concentration

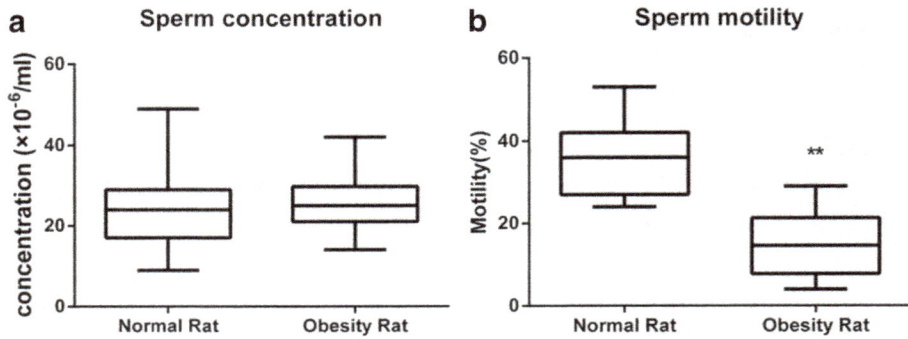

Fig. 1 Comparison of sperm concentration (**a**) and motility (**b**) between the two groups. The data are presented as the mean ± s.e.m.; * P < 0.05 and **P < 0.01

increased; however, neither change was statistically significant.

Discussion

Obesity is a chronic metabolic disease caused by interactions of various genetic and environmental factors. Interestingly, in the past 50 years, along with the annually increasing trend in human obesity, fertility has shown a parallel decreasing trend [18]. Several studies have indicated that a higher BMI is associated with significant decreases in sperm concentration [19–21]. Investigators

have attempted to investigate the relationship between obesity and fertility decline; however, no consensus has been reached.

Currently, no unified standard is available for evaluating obese rats. In 1929, MO Lee [22] proposed the Lee index to evaluate obesity in rats, which is the most commonly used method to evaluate obese rats. In a diet-induced model of obesity reported by Levin, rats became obesity-resistant with high-fat diet administration [23], and differences were found in their energy, endocrine, fat and glutamic acid (GLU) metabolism. Based on the

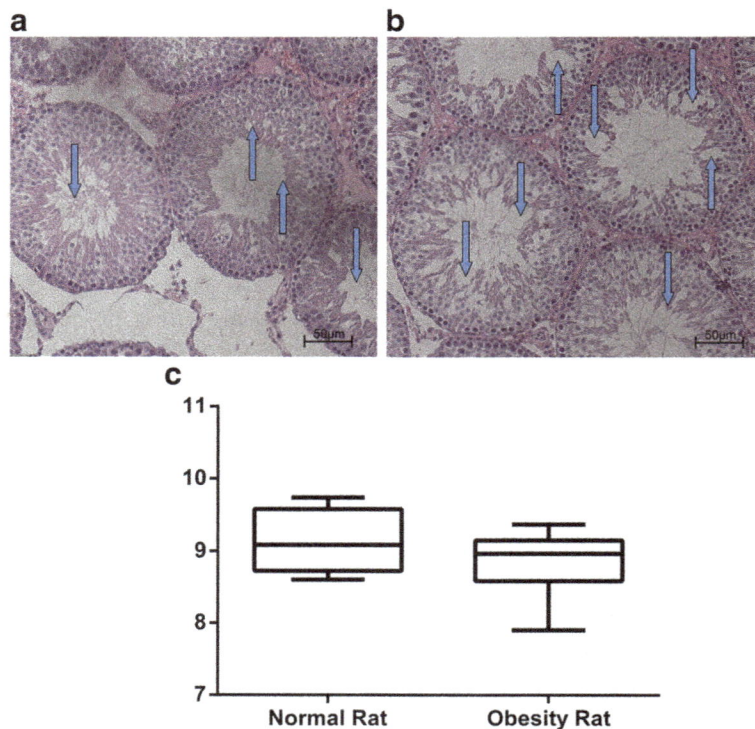

Fig. 2 HE staining of testicular tissues (× 20) and comparison of sperm Johnsen scores between the two groups. **a** control group; **b**, obesity group; **c** the data are presented as the mean ± s.e.m.; * P < 0.05 and **P < 0.01

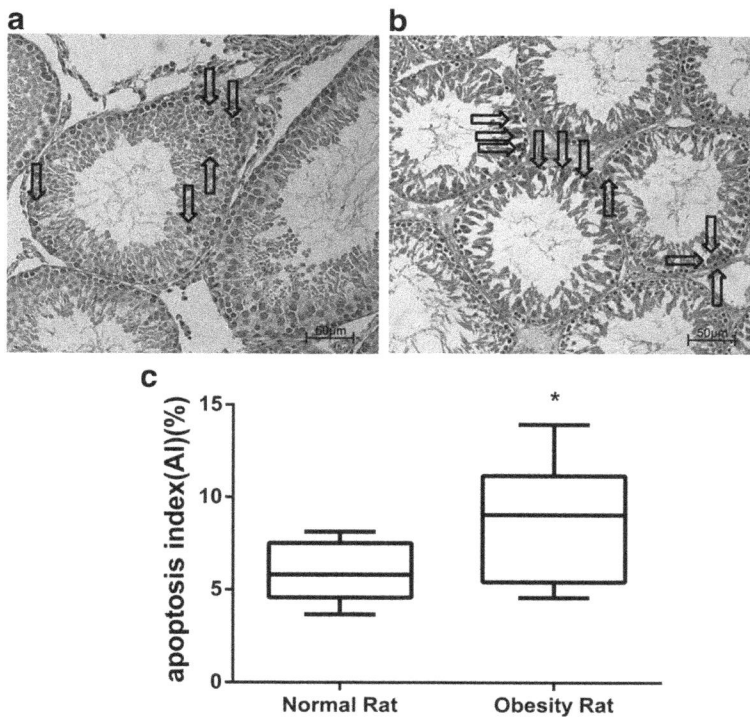

Fig. 3 Apoptosis of spermatogenic cells in testicular tissues and comparison of the apoptosis index between the two groups (× 20, arrows indicate apoptotic cells). **a** control group; **b** obesity group; **c** the data are presented as the mean ± s.e.m.; * $P < 0.05$ and **$P < 0.01$

relevant literature and the Lee index, one-fourth of the rats in the high-fat diet group were excluded in our study because they were obesity-resistant. The remaining three-quarters of the rats were classified as the obesity group [24]. Our results demonstrated successful generation of the obese rat model.

Currently, the effect of male obesity on sperm count, motility, and morphology in humans is controversial. A review found that up to 2015, progressively reduced motility was reported in 13 of 35 articles, while a decreased sperm count with normal morphology was reported in only 9 of 29 papers [6]. However, two recent meta-analyses including 14 and 21 studies demonstrated an increased risk of azoospermia or oligozoospermia in

Table 2 Reproductive hormone levels in the two groups

	LH (mIU/ml)	TT (ng/ml)	E_2 (pg/ml)	SHBG (nmol/L)	cFT (ng/ml)
Control	3.44	0.80	4.49	50.35	0.011
(n = 15)	±2.75	±0.76	±3.60	±6.26	±0.010
Obesity	3.20	0.59	4.39	85.13	0.003
(n = 22)	±2.76	±0.51	±2.45	±9.13	±0.002
P value	0.799	0.356	0.926	0.000**	0.031*

The data are presented as the mean ± s.e.m. * $P < 0.05$, ** $P < 0.01$: statistical significance compared with the control group; *LH* luteinizing hormone, *TT* total testosterone, *E2* estradiol, *SHBG* sex hormone-binding globulin, *cFT* calculated free testosterone, and *s.e.m.* standard error of the mean

overweight or obese males [25, 26]. The results from this study indicated that obesity induced by a high-fat diet can change the histomorphology of seminiferous tubules, which may not have obvious effects on male fertility immediately, but the long-term effects on spermatogenesis induced by obesity may impair male fertility.

Due to gene polymorphisms in the population, many factors (e.g., smoking, alcohol consumption, and medication use) that can affect seminal parameters are often overlooked. In addition, sample selection bias can lead to inconsistent conclusions regarding the impact of obesity on sperm. This study, by controlling various confounding factors, revealed that obesity reduced sperm motility without changing the sperm count, which is consistent with previous reports [25]. The possible mechanism may be damage to the integrity of sperm cell membranes, sperm cell DNA, and sperm mitochondria induced by excessive reactive oxygen species (ROS) [27, 28].

Apoptosis is an autonomous programmed cell death process that is stimulated under specific conditions and is regulated by various genes. We found that the AI of the spermatogenic cells increased significantly in the obesity group. A recent study found that apoptosis of testicular spermatogenic cells is one of the major causes of male subfertility [29]. Cell apoptosis is predominantly regulated and controlled by the

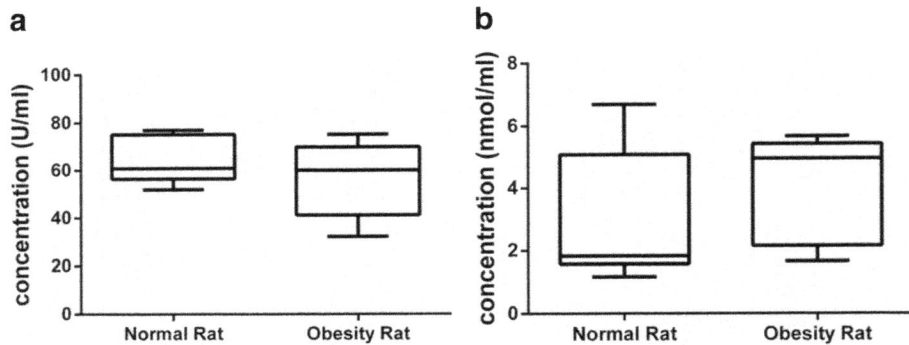

Fig. 4 Comparison of the concentrations of SOD (**a**) and MDA (**b**) in the testis homogenate between the two groups. SOD: superoxide dismutase, MDA: malondialdehyde; the data are presented as the mean ± s.e.m.; * $P < 0.05$ and **$P < 0.01$

homeostasis of Bax and Bcl-2. When the Bcl-2/Bax ratio is disrupted, downstream caspase signaling pathways are activated, resulting in apoptosis. A high-fat diet has been reported to increase Bax and caspase-3 expression but reduce Bcl-2 expression in the testis [30]. Therefore, based on our results, obese rats exhibited increased spermatogenic cell apoptosis due to imbalances of Bcl-2/Bax. Furthermore, obesity resulted in lipid metabolic disorders and hyperlipidemia, which may increase the stress response of the endoplasmic reticulum. Therefore, the incidence of spermatogenic cell apoptosis is further increased [31, 32] via increased GRP78 mRNA and protein expression.

Mammalian reproductive function is predominantly controlled and regulated by the hypothalamus-pituitary-testis (HPT) axis. Male reproductive endocrinology is principally composed of three groups of hormones, including GnRH, GnIH, LH, FSH, and T. T is one of the major sex hormones in males and has an important role in the HPT axis. Hypothalamic hormones are intricately associated with obesity-induced physiological changes, indicating a mutual cause-effect relationship between obesity and gonadal hormone decline [33]. In a study with 3219 European males, Fui and other investigators found that the TT and FT levels in obese males were lower than those in normal-weight males. Another study with 314 Asian males reached the same conclusion [34]. Camacho found that obesity reduces testosterone, low testosterone levels can promote male obesity, and testosterone increases after weight loss [35]. Compared with rats fed a normal diet, rats fed a high-fat diet had lower testosterone levels. When these rats were fed a normal diet, their testosterone levels returned to normal [35]. Although biologically active serum FT only accounts for 2% of TT, it is directly involved in functional activities, such as the development of male secondary sex characteristics, maintenance of spermatogenesis and sexual desire [36]. As a diagnostic marker for male hypogonadism, the

serum cFT level exhibits better sensitivity than the serum TT level [37].

SHBG is a blood transport protein for testosterone and estradiol. Its synthesis and secretion are regulated by androgen and estrogen. Serum SHBG may exert direct or indirect effects on androgen conversion and metabolism, and it regulates GLU homeostasis and fatty acid metabolism. In this experiment, our results confirmed decreases in serum TT and cFT levels and an increase in the serum SHBG concentration in the obese rats. Therefore, we hypothesize that serum SHBG is the key factor in reducing serum cFT levels, and obese rats may develop mild primary hypogonadism (reduced serum TT and cFT, increased SHBG). Primary hypogonadism in the obese rats is likely the initiating factor for alterations in the HPT axis.

Oxidative stress is highly correlated with a wide variety of inflammatory and metabolic disease states, including obesity. Oxidative stress is highly correlated with cumulative damage in the body induced by free radicals that are inadequately neutralized by antioxidants, and oxidative damage is aggravated by decreases in antioxidant enzyme activities, such as those of SOD, catalase (CAT), and glutathione S-transferase (GST) [38]. Evidence suggests that there are many sources of oxidative stress in obesity [39]. In our study, to determine the effect of obesity on oxidative stress, the concentrations of SOD and MDA in testis homogenate were determined.

SOD, which protects cells from free radical damage by ROS, is an important enzyme that protects against injuries caused by internal and external superoxide ions. MDA is an aldehyde generated in the process of lipid peroxidation caused by free radicals. MDA indicates cell membrane damage and reflects the severity of an oxygen radical attack on reactive cells and the levels of free radical metabolism in vivo. Decreased SOD and increased MDA can trigger oxidative stress, causing cell damage and even death. This study found decreased SOD levels and increased MDA levels in the testicular tissues of obese rats, demonstrating that the oxidative stress level of testis tissues in obese rats is increased and may impact sperm motility. Several possible explanations may account for these findings: obesity is associated with elevated serum free fatty acids, and unsaturated fatty acids are susceptible to attacks by ROS, producing peroxidation and subsequently resulting in decreased SOD levels and MDA accumulation, which is ultimately reflected by an increased oxidative stress level [40].

Conclusion

The rats with obesity induced by high-fat diet administration exhibited lipid metabolism dysfunction and altered reproductive hormone levels as well as increased oxidative stress levels in testis tissues, leading to mild primary hypogonadism. Meanwhile, the normal function of the HPT axis is maintained in the short-term through a corresponding feedback mechanism. However, the long-term effects of obesity may cause a decline in male fertility.

Abbreviations

AI: apoptosis index; BMI: body mass index; cFT: Calculated free testosterone; CVD: Cardiovascular disease; DM: Diabetes mellitus; E_2: Estradiol; FT: Free testosterone; HPT: Hypothalamus-pituitary-testis; HTM-IVOS: Hamilton-Thorne Sperm Analyzer; LH: Luteinizing hormone; MDA: Malondialdehyde; ROS: Reactive oxygen species; SHBG: Serum sex hormone-binding globulin; SOD: Ssuperoxide dismutase; SPF: Specific-pathogen-free; T: Testosterone; TT: Total testosterone; WHO: World Health Organization

Funding

This work was financed by the National "Twelfth Five-Year" Plan for Science and Technology Support (2012BAI32BC3 for purchasing most of the experimental reagents and materials, as well as the labor costs for the researchers and the fee for some antibodies).

Authors' contributions

YFJ and QF collected the data, performed the statistical analysis, interpreted the results, and drafted and revised the manuscript. YFJ and YQG conceived of and designed the study. ZYG, YG, FZ, KSZ, XWW, WHL, and XWL participated in data collection and performed the laboratory measurements. All authors read and approved the final manuscript.

Competing interest

The authors declare that they have no competing interests.

Author details

[1]Lanzhou University Second Hospital, Lanzhou 730020, People's Republic of China. [2]Xiyuan Hospital, China Academy of Traditional Chinese Medicine, Beijing 100091, People's Republic of China. [3]Graduate School of Peking Union Medical College, No. 9 Dongdansantiao, Dongcheng District, Beijing 100730, People's Republic of China. [4]National Health and Family Planning Key Laboratory of Male Reproductive Health, Department of Male Clinical Research, National Research Institute for Family Planning, Beijing 100081, People's Republic of China.

References

1. Matheus AS, Tannus LR, Cobas RA, Palma CC, Negrato CA, Gomes MB. Impact of diabetes on cardiovascular disease: an update. Int J Hypertens. 2013;2013:653789.
2. Finucane MM, Stevens GA, Cowan MJ, et al. National, regional, and global trends in body-mass index since 1980: systematic analysis of health examination surveys and epidemiological studies with 960 country-years and 9·1 million participants. Lancet. 2011;377:557–67.
3. Kahn BE, Brannigan RE. Obesity and Male infertility. Curr Opin Urol. 2017;27: 441–5.
4. Haslam DW, James WP. Obesity. Lancet. 2005;366:1197–209.
5. Poulain M, Doucet M, Major GC, et al. The effect of obesity on chronic respiratory diseases: pathophysiology and therapeutic strategies. CMAJ. 2006;174(9):1293.
6. Coviello AD, Legro RS, Dunaif A. Adolescent girls with polycystic ovary syndrome have an increased risk of the metabolic syndrome associated with increasing androgen levels independent of obesity and insulin resistance. J Clin Endocrinol Metab. 2006;91:492–7.
7. Landry D, Cloutier F, Martin LJ. Implications of leptin in neuroendocrine regulation of male reproduction. Reprod Biol. 2013;13:1–14.
8. Cabler S, Agarwal A, Flint M, du Plessis SS. Obesity: modern man's fertility nemesis. Asian J Androl. 2010;12:480–9.
9. McPherson NO, Lane M. Male obesity and subfertility, is it really about increased adiposity? Asian J Androl. 2015;17:450–8. https://doi.org/10.4103/1008-682X.148076. Pubmed:25652636.
10. MacDonald AA, Herbison GP, Showell M, Farquhar CM. The impact of body mass index on semen parameters and reproductive hormones in human males: a systematic review with meta-analysis. Hum Reprod Update. 2010; 16:293–311.
11. Tsao CW, Liu CY, Chou YC, Cha TL, Chen SC, Hsu CY. Exploration of the association between obesity and semen quality in a 7630 male population. Plos One. 2015;10(3):e0119458.
12. Dong X, Song W, Ge Z, et al. Effects of Jiangtang Xiaozhi tablets on expression of NFκB, CYP. Int J Clin Exp Med. 2016;9:18373–8.
13. Atilgan D, Parlaktas BS, Uluocak N, et al. Weight loss and melatonin reduce obesity-induced oxidative damage in rat testis. Ther Adv Urol. 2013;2013: 836121.
14. Johnsen SG. Testicular biopsy score count–a method for registration of spermatogenesis in human testes: normal values and results in 335 hypogonadal males. Horm Res Paediatr. 1970;1:2–25.
15. Zhu B, Zheng YF, Zhang YY, et al. Protective effect of L-carnitine in cyclophosphamide-induced germ cell apoptosis. J Zhejiang Univ Sci B. 2015;16:780–7.
16. Peskin AAV, Winterbourn CC. A microtiter plate assay for superoxide dismutase using a water-soluble tetrazolium salt (WST-1). Clin Chim Acta. 2000;293:157–66.
17. Draper HH, Hadley M. Malondialdehyde determination as index of lipid peroxidation. Methods Enzymol. 1990;186:421–31.
18. Hammoud AO, Meikle AW, Reis LO, Gibson M, Peterson CM, Carrell DT. Obesity and male infertility: a practical approach. Semin Reprod Med. 2012; 30:486–95.
19. Chavarro JE, Toth TL, Wright DL, Meeker JD, Hauser R. Body mass index in relation to semen quality, sperm DNA integrity, and serum reproductive hormone levels among men attending an infertility clinic. Fertil Steril. 2010; 93:2222–31.
20. Hammiche F, Laven JS, Boxmeer JC, Dohle GR, Steegers EA, Steegers-Theunissen RP. Sperm quality decline among men below 60 years of age undergoing IVF or ICSI treatment. J Androl. 2011;32:70–6.
21. Tunc O, Bakos HW, Tremellen K. Impact of body mass index on seminal oxidative stress. Andrologia. 2011;43:121–8.
22. Lee MO. Determination of the surface area of the white rat with its application to the expression of metabolic results. Am J Phys. 1929;89:24–33.
23. Levin BE. Arcuate npy neurons and energy homeostasis in diet-induced obese and resistant rats. Am J Physiol-Reg I. 1999;276:R382–7.
24. Chang S, Graham B, Yakubu F, Lin D, Peters JC, Hill JO. Metabolic differences between obesity-prone and obesity-resistant rats. Am J Phys. 1990;259: R1103–10.
25. Sermondade N, Faure C, Fezeu L, et al. BMI in relation to sperm count: an updated systematic review and collaborative meta-analysis. Hum Reprod Update. 2013;19:221–31.

26. Sermondade N, Faure C, Fezeu L, Lévy R, Czernichow S. Obesity-fertility collaborative group. Obesity and increased risk for oligozoospermia and azoospermia. Arch Intern Med. 2012;172:440–2.

27. Liu B, Ma D, Mao PF. Role of oxidative stress injury in male infertility. Natl J Androl. 2014;20:927–31.

28. Pasqualotto FF, Sharma RK, Pasqualotto EB, Agarwal A. Poor semen quality and Ros-TAC scores in patients with idiopathic infertility. Urol Int. 2008;81:263–70.

29. Garolla A, Torino M, Sartini B, et al. Seminal and molecular evidence that sauna exposure affects human spermatogenesis. Hum Reprod. 2013;28:877–85.

30. Mu Y, Yan WJ, Yin TL, Yang J. High-fat diet induces spermatogenesis dysfunction in male rats. J Med Res. 2015;44:88–91.

31. Xin W, Li X, Lu X, Niu K, Cai J. Involvement of endoplasmic reticulum stress-associated apoptosis in a heart failure model induced by chronic myocardial ischemia. Int J Mol Med. 2011;27:503–9.

32. Li CY, Dong ZQ, Lan XX, Zhang XJ, Li SP. Endoplasmic reticulum stress promotes the apoptosis of testicular germ cells in hyperlipidemic rats. Zhonghua Nan Ke Xue. 2015;21:402–7.

33. Rao PM, Kelly DM, Jones TH. Testosterone and insulin resistance in the metabolic syndrome and T2DM in men. Nat Rev Endocrinol. 2013;9:479–93.

34. Fui MNT, Dupuis P, Grossmann M. Lowered testosterone in male obesity: mechanisms, morbidity and management. Asian J Androl. 2014;16:223–31.

35. Camacho EM, Huhtaniemi IT, O'Neill TW, et al. Age-associated changes in hypothalamic–pituitary–testicular function in middle-aged and older men are modified by weight change and lifestyle factors. Eur J Endocrinol. 2013; 168:445–55.

36. Sharpe RM. Intratesticular factors controlling testicular function. Biol Reprod. 1984;30:29–49.

37. Liu TH, Yang RF, Kong XB, et al. Analysis of male serum total testosterone and serum free testosterone in different ages. Chin J Fam Plann Gynecotokol. 2014;6:16–8.

38. Blokhina O, Virolainen E, Fagerstedt KV. Antioxidants, oxidative damage and oxygen deprivation stress: a review. Ann Bot. 2003;91:179–94.

39. Vincent HK, Taylor AG. Biomarkers and potential mechanisms of obesity-induced oxidant stress in humans. Int J Obes. 2006;30:400–18.

40. Fang X, Xu QY, Jia C, Peng YF. metformin improves epididymal sperm quality and antioxidant function of the testis in diet-induced obesity rats. Zhonghua Nan Ke Xue. 2012;18:146–9.

22

Antihypertensive drugs use and the risk of prostate cancer

Liang Cao[1†], Sha Zhang[2†], Cheng-ming Jia[1], Wei He[2], Lei-tao Wu[1], Ying-qi Li[1], Wen Wang[1], Zhe Li[2*] and Jing Ma[1*]

Abstract

Background: Due to the lack of strong evidence to identify the relationship between antihypertensive drugs use and the risk of prostate cancer, it was needed to do a systematic review to go into the subject.

Methods: We systematically searched PubMed, Web of Science and Embase to identify studies published, through May 2015. Two evaluators independently reviewed and selected articles involving the subject. We used the Newcastle-Ottawa Scale (NOS) to assess the quality of the studies. All extracted results to evaluate the relationship between antihypertensive drugs usage and prostate cancer risk were pool-analysed using Stata 12.0 software.

Results: A total of 12 cohort and 9 case-control studies were ultimately included in our review. Most of the studies were evaluated to be of high quality. There was no significant relationship between angiotensin converting enzyme inhibitors (ACEI) usage and the risk of prostate cancer (RR 1.07, 95% CI 0.96–1.20), according to the total pool-analysed. Use of angiotensin receptor blocker (ARB) was not associated with the risk of prostate cancer (RR 1.09, 95% CI 0.97–1.21), while use of CCB may well increase prostate cancer risk based on the total pool-analysed (RR 1.08, 95% CI 1–1.16). Moreover, subgroup analysis suggested that use of CCB clearly increased prostate cancer risk (RR 1.10, 95% CI 1.04–1.16) in terms of case-control studies. There was also no significant relationship between use of diuretic (RR 1.09, 95% CI 0.95–1.25) or antiadrenergic agents (RR 1.22, 95% CI 0.76–1.96) and prostate cancer risk.

Conclusions: There is no significant relationship between the use of antihypertensive drugs (ACEI, ARB, beta-blockers and diuretics) and prostate cancer risk, but CCB may well increase prostate cancer risk, according to existing observational studies.

Keywords: Antihypertensive drugs, Prostate cancer, Meta-analysis

Background

The prevalence of hypertension is consistently high in older adults and regarded as a vital risk factor for cardiovascular diseases, congestive heart failure, and coronary heart disease [1, 2]. Antihypertensive drugs including angiotensin-converting enzyme inhibitors (ACEI), angiotensin II receptor blockers (ARB), calcium-channel blockers (CCB), alpha- and beta-blockers and diuretics, were mainly used for the control of blood pressure in patients with hypertension to prevent relevant cardiovascular diseases [3]. Beneficial therapeutic effects of these drugs, on blood pressure control, have been well established in previous literature [4].

However, antihypertensive drugs and cancer risk have long been raised as concerns [5]. It was first reported that Rauwolfia derivatives increased the risk of breast cancer [6]. After that, several classes of antihypertensive agents appeared to elevate cancer risk, but the relationship between antihypertensive drug usage and increased cancer risk could not be confirmed in numerous studies due to their short follow-up and the cancer risk from hypertension itself [7]. A retrospective cohort study

---
* Correspondence: lizhetcm@163.com; jingma@fmmu.edu.cn
†Equal contributors
2Shanxi University of Chinese Medicine, Xian yang 712046, People's Republic of China
1Department of Traditional Chinese Medicine, Xijing Hospital, Fourth Military Medical University, Xi'an 710032, People's Republic of China

showed that the use of ACE inhibitors has an association with a clearly decreased risk of overall cancer [8]. Meanwhile, a meta-analysis demonstrated that there was no association between the use of ACE inhibitors or angiotensin-receptor blockers and the overall risk of cancer [9]. A large-scale, population-based cohort study proposed that there was no substantial association between the use of calcium channel blockers (CCB) and the incidence rate of cancer or cancer mortality [10]. In a study by Hershel et al. study, there was small positive association between CCB usage and risk of cancer [11].

The incidence of prostate cancer is increasing, and it is the main cause of cancer death in males in the Western countries [12]. Studies on the association between antihypertensive drug usage and prostate cancer risk remain controversial. In vitro studies, CCB enhanced apoptosis of prostate cancer cells and might have a protective effect on prostate cancer [13]. Debes et al. found that CCB significantly decreased the risk of prostate cancer, and their results varied by family history of prostate cancer [14]. However, some case-control studies did not find the this relationship [15]. For instance, a study with 1,165,781 patients did not support the association between the long-term use of CCB and prostate cancer risk [16]. Some case-control studies showed significantly increased risk between ACE inhibitor usage and prostate cancer [15, 17], while a previous meta-analysis showed that ACE inhibitors or angiotensin-receptor blockers did not affect the occurrence of cancer [18]. In a study by Perron et al., beta-blockers were associated with a reduction in prostate cancer risk, while another study by Kemppainen et al. tended to show an increased risk of prostate cancer in patients treated by beta-blockers [15, 19]. One study reported the relationship between alpha- blockers or diuretic usage and prostate cancer risk and their results were also controversial [20].

Due to there being the long-term follow-up in the observational studies, we performed a systematic review of observational studies to confirm whether the use of antihypertensive drugs was able to result in the prostate cancer in the human body.

Methods

Our review was conducted in accordance with PRISMA (Preferred Reporting Items for Systematic Reviews and Meta-Analyses) and MOOSE (Meta-Analysis of Observational Studies in Epidemiology) guidelines.

Eligibility criteria

Studies were included if they met the following points: (1) Studies were cohort or case-control studies; and (2) the relationship between the use of one or more types of antihypertensive drugs and prostate cancer was reported in the study.

Search strategy

We systematically searched PubMed, Web of Science and Embase to identify studies published through May 2015. The search terms were composed of the following: "beta blockers", "angiotensin converting enzyme inhibitors", "angiotensin receptor blockers", "calcium channel blockers" "alpha blockers" "antihypertensive drugs" and "prostate cancer". The details of the search methods are summarized in the Additional file 1. We also screened the bibliographies of relevant articles to find additional articles that met the included standard. A language limitation was not set during the search process. We did not consider animal studies when we reviewed the records.

Study selection and data extraction

Two authors independently evaluated the studies retrieved from the databases to select the studies that met the inclusion criteria. Disagreements between the two reviewers were resolved by discussion or in consultation with an arbitrator. The following information was extracted from the included articles by the two authors independently: study design, geographic region, type of medication, sex, age range, follow-up time, adjusted factors in each study (Table1). The RR (relative risk), HR (hazard ratio), OR (odds ratio), SIR (standardized incidence ratio) along with their corresponding 95%CI (confidence interval), all of which indicated the relationship between antihypertensive drugs and prostate cancer were abstracted. If there was missing information in the article, we contacted the authors via e-mail or telephone. We used data from a 2×2 table to recalculate crude estimates when the outcome measures were unsuitable for meta-analysis and we failed to gain the data from the authors.

Methodological quality assessment

The quality of the observational studies was independently evaluated by two authors based on the Newcastle-Ottawa Assessment Scale(NOS) on the website (http://www.ohri.ca/programs/clinical_epidemiology/oxford.asp). The scale provided eight items consisting of three subscales: selection of subjects (four items), comparability of subjects (one item) and assessment of outcome/exposure (three items). The highest scores were nine for the eight items because there were two scores in the comparability of subjects. A study with greater than or equal to seven scores was considered to be of high methodological quality.

Data synthesis and analysis

Extracted RRs, HRs, ORs and SIRs and their 95% CIs that were adjusted for most confounders were pooled to compute the RR between antihypertensive drugs and prostate cancer risk [21]. The four measures of association above were expected to yield similar estimates of

RR, due to the incidence of prostate cancer being generally low [22]. For a single study that reported more than one type of cancer, only the data on the risk between prostate cancer and antihypertensive drugs were extracted and then pooled. If there were studies involving multi-drug treatment and we were not familiar with the data that reported which specific drug was associated with the incidence of prostate cancer in these studies, the data of the study would not be extracted to conduct a meta-analysis. In the included studies, the data that reported the risk between a single antihypertensive drugs and the occurrence of prostate cancer will be pooled for analysis based on the single drug category respectively. The meta-analysis was performed with Stata 12.0. Since the clinical and methodological heterogeneity were known, we used a random-effects model to calculate pooled RRs and their 95%CIs. Subgroup analyses were performed according to whether they corresponded to case-control or cohort studies. Between-study heterogeneity was assessed by using Cochran's Q statistic (significance level at $p < 0.1$) and by estimating I^2. If I^2 was more than 40%, there was significant heterogeneity among studies [23].

Results

Characteristic of included studies

Our search strategy yielded 729 records, A total of 193 and 491 records were excluded due to duplicated records and irrelevant subjects respectively. A total of 45 full-text articles were assessed and 21 studies that met our criteria were ultimately included (Fig. 1). These studies included 12 cohort studies [10, 20, 24–33], 4 nested case-control studies [11, 16, 34, 35] and 5 case-control studies [15, 17, 19, 36, 37]. The follow-up time in most cohort studies was more than 5 years. There were 11 studies that involved males only [10, 15, 19, 20, 24, 26, 28, 31, 35, 36, 38]. It was reported that the main outcomes of the included studies were adjusted for most of the confounding factors, and this information was missing in two studies (Tables 1 and 2) [10, 32].

Quality of included studies

The results of the quality assessment for the included studies are summarized in Tables 3 and 4. Quality scores for cohort studies ranged between 5 and 9, and those for case-control studies ranged between 7 and 9. Five

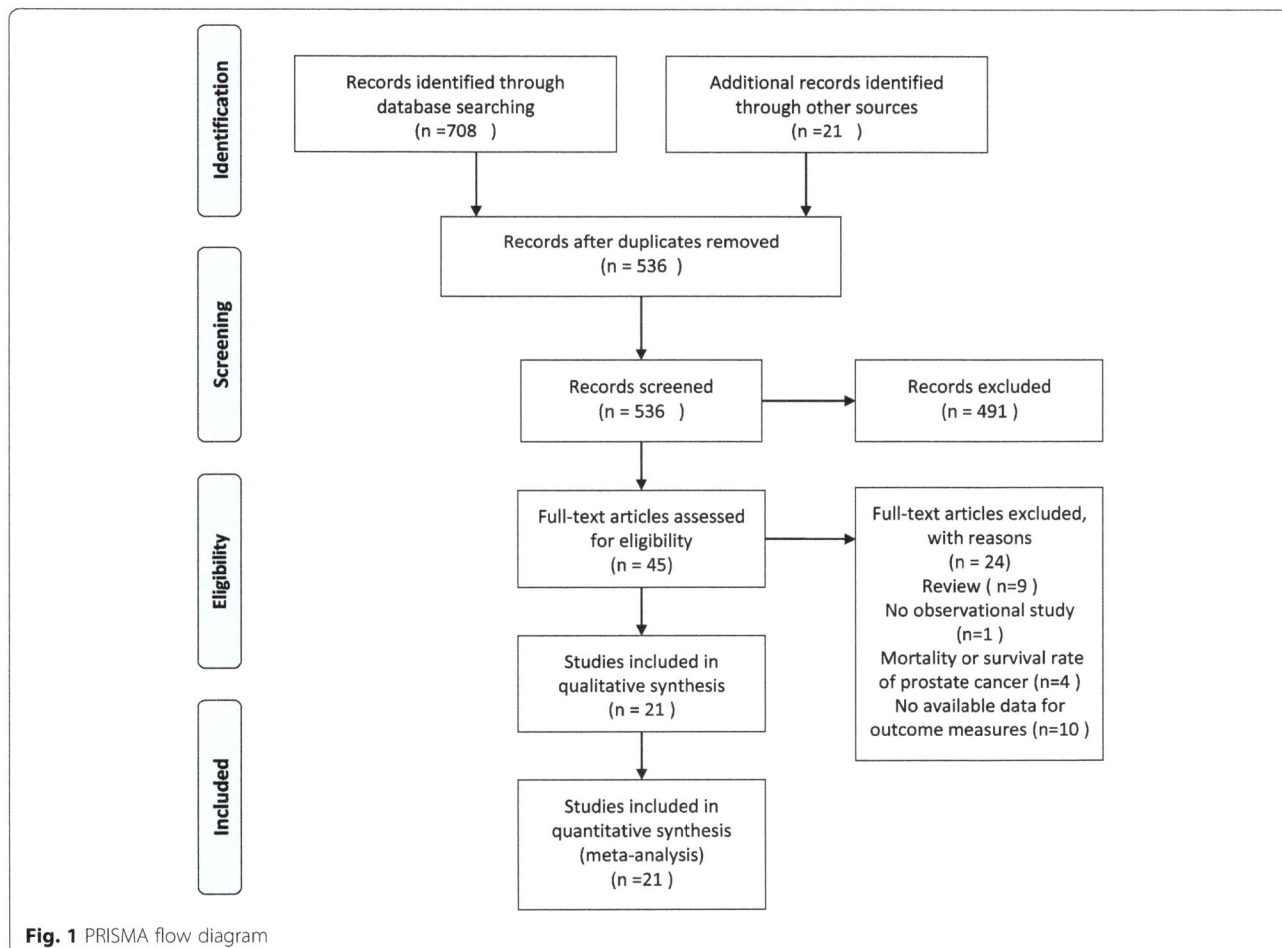

Fig. 1 PRISMA flow diagram

Table 1 Characteristics of cohort studies included in the meta-analysis

Studies	Types of studies	Population and selection of cases	NO. of participants	Type of medication (reference group)	Duration of follow-up,yr	Sex (%)	Mean age (range), yr	Adjustment
Pai, P.Y.et al. 2015 [20]	cohort study	Male patients with hypertension or without hypertension selected from CCHIA-NHI database	80,299	Diuretics, Alpha-blockersBeta-blockers, ARBsCCBs, ACEIOthers (no use of antihypertensive drugs)	9	Male (100)	69.28 VS 69.31(50-)	Age, urbanization level, income, comorbidities
Rao, G. A. et al. 2013 [24]	cohort study	Males patients receiving drug treatment from VA of U.S.A.	543,824	ARBs (no use of ARBs)	8	Male (100)	63.6 VS 63.6	All 54 variables that was used to compute propensity to receive treatment
Bhaskaran, K. et al. 2012 [25]	cohort study	Hypertensive patients receiving drug treatment from General Practice Research Database (GPRD) of U.K.	377,649	ARBs (no use of ARBs)	>5	M (52) F (48)	64 (18–103)	Age, sex, BMI, smoking, alcohol, diabetes (with or without metformin/insulin use), hypertension, heart failure, statin use, index of multiple deprivation score, calendar year.
Rodriguez, C. 2009 [26]	cohort study	Males patients receiving drug treatment from the CPS-II Nutrition Cohort of U.S.A	3031	CCBs, Beta-blockers, ACEIs, diuretics, and other anti-hypertensives (no use of anti-hypertensive drugs)	8	Males (100)	NA	Age at interview, race, education, BMI in 1997, family history of prostate cancer, history of diabetes, history of PSA screening,history of heart disease or bypass surgery, and use of cholesterol-lowering drugs
van der Knaap, R. et al. 2008 [27]	cohort study	Eligible individuals from the Rotterdam Study started with a baseline interview between July 1989 and July 1993.	7983	ACEI and/or angiotensin II type 1 receptor antagonist (no use of the drugs)	9.6	M (38.7) F (61.3)	70.4(50-)	Age, BMI, use of salicylates, diabetes mellitus, hypertension, and myocardial infarction.
Harris, A. M. et al. 2007 [28]	cohort study	Male patients receiving drug treatment seen at Lexington Veterans Affairs (VA) Hospital	27,138	a1-blockers (no use of a1-blockers)	>5	Male (100)	68 (50–89) VS 72 (46–99)	Unadjusted
Debes, J. D. et al. 2004 [29]	cohort study	Males from subgroup of Olmsted County Study of Urinary Symptoms and Health Status	2115	CCBs (no use of CCBs)	10	Male (100)	NA(40–79)	Age and family history of prostate cancer
Friis, S. et al. 2001 [30]	cohort study	Persons receiving drug treatment from Pharmacoepidemiological Prescription Research Database of North Jutland County, Denmark,	17,897	ACEI (no use of ACEI)	8	Male (50) Female (50)	62(NA)	Adjustment for age, gender, and duration of follow-up

Table 1 Characteristics of cohort studies included in the meta-analysis *(Continued)*

Studies	Types of studies	Population and slection of cases	NO. of participants	Type of medication (reference group)	Duration of follow-up,yr	Sex (%)	Mean age (range), yr	Adjustment
Fitzpatrick, A. L. 2001 [31]	cohort study	Individuals receiving drug treatment from chrot of the Cardiovascular Health Study (CHS) of USA	2442	CCBsACEIβ-blockersDiureticVasodilator (no use of antihypertensive drugs)	5.6	Male (100)	NA (65-)	Adjusted for age, race (black), and body mass index (BMI)
Sorensen, H. T. 2000 [10]	cohort study	Individuals taking CCBs from Pharmaco-Epidemiological Prescription Database of the County of North Jutland, Denmark	23, 167	CCBs (compared with the number expected, based on population rates from the Danish Cancer Registry)	3.2	Male (100)	63.4	NA
Olsen, J. H. 1997 [32]	cohort study	Individuals receiving treatment of CCBs from the County of North Jutland	17,911	CCBs (compared with the number expected, based on population rates from the Danish Cancer Registry)	1.8 years	Male (49), Female (51)	NA	NA
Pahor, M. 1996 [33]	cohort study	Individuals aged 65 years or older living in East Boston, Massachusetts, and in the counties of Iowa and Washington in the state of Iowa from epidemiologic studies of the elderly (EPESE) in U.S.	5052	CCBs (no use of CCBs)	3.6	Male (35.7), Female (64.3)	MA (65-)	Adjusted for age, sex, ethnic origin, heart failure, number of hospital admissions, cigarette smoking, and alcohol intake.

CCB calcium-channel blockers, *ACEI* angiotensin-converting enzyme inhibitors, *ARB* angiotensin II receptor blockers, *NA* not available

Table 2 Characteristics of case-control studies included in the meta-analysis

Studies	Types of studies	Case selection	NO. of participants	Collection of medication data (period)	Age of cases, yr., mean (range)	Sex of cases, %	Type of drugs (reference group)	Adjustment
Hallas, J. 2012 [17]	Case control	Review of data from the Danish Cancer Registry (DCR), the Danish National Registry of Patients (DNRP),the Prescription Database of the DanishMedicines Agency and the Danish Person Registry (2000–2005).	149, 417	Review of electronic medical records (1995 until cancer diagnosis)	69.4	Male (47.7), Female (52.3)	Use of ARBs or ACEI (never-use of the durgs)	(1)chronic obstructive pulmonary disease (COPD) as a crude marker of heavy smoking; (2) inflammatory bowel disease; (3) a modified Charlson Index that contains 19 categories of comorbidity and each category has an associated weight based on the adjusted risk of 1 year mortality; (4) non-steroidal antiinflammatory drugs (NSAIDs) or hig dose aspirin, oestrogen hormone therapy, oral contraceptives, finasteride or statins.
Azoulay, L. 2012 [39]	Nested case-control	Review of data from General Practice Research Database (GPRD)in U.K (1995–2010)	1,165,781	Review of computerized medical records (1995 until cancer diagnosis)	72.4	Male (52.7), Female (47.3)	use of ARBs or ACEIs or CCBs or alpha-blockers(use of Diuretics and/or beta-blockers)	Excessive alcohol use, body mass index, smoking, diabetes, previous cancer, and ever of aspirin, statins, and NSAIDs. In addition,cholecystectomy, inflammatory bowel disease and history of polyps for colorectal cancer; benign prostatic hyperplasia, 5-alpha reductase inhibitors, and number of PSA tests for prostate cancer; oophorectomy, use of hormone replacement therapy, and prior use of oral contraceptives for breast cancer.
Kemppainen, K. J. 2011 [15]	Case control	Review of data from the Finnish Cancer Registry (1995–2002)	25,029	Review of the prescription database of the Social Insurance Institution of Finland (1995 until cancer diagnosis)	NA	Males (100)	use of ARBs or ACEIs or CCBs or alpha-blockers or beta-blockers or diuretics (Nonusers of any antihypertensive medication)	Adjusted for age, place of residence, and use of cholesterol-lowering drugs, antidiabetic drugs, finasteride, or alpha-blockers.
Assimes, T. L. 2008 [34]	Nested case-control	Review of computerized database files of Saskatchewan Health (1980–2003)	11,697	Review of the linkable databases including the world's oldest electronic prescription database (1978 until cancer diagnosis)	71.8	Male (53.2) Female (46.8)	Use of β-blockers or CCBs or RAS inhibitors and never use of thiazide diuretics (use of thiazide diuretics and never use of β-blockers or CCBs or RAS inhibitors)	Adjusted for age, all measured comorbid conditions, and exposure to all other classes of antihypertensive not of interest except for potassium sparing diuretics.
Ronquist, G. 2004 [35]	Nested case-control	Review of the General Practice Research Database (GPRD) in U.K. (1995–1999)	243,331	Review of computerized medical records (1995 untilcancer diagnosis)	50–79	Males (100)	Use of diuretics, beta-blockers, ACE-inhibitors, CCBs, alpha-blockers and other antihypertensives (no use)	Adjusted for age, calendar year, prostatism and and other variables.

Table 2 Characteristics of case-control studies included in the meta-analysis *(Continued)*

Studies	Types of studies	Case selection	NO. of participants	Collection of medication data (period)	Age of cases, yr., mean (range)	Sex of cases, %	Type of drugs (reference group)	Adjustment
Perron, L. 2004 [19]	case-control	Review of the source population in Quebec cancer registry (1993–1995)	13,326	Review of computerized medical records (1981 untilcancer diagnosis)	75.7	Males(100)	Use of CCBs or ACEIs or beta-blockers or thiazidic diuretics and similars or others inlcusing vasodilatators and centrally acting adrenocep-tor antagonists. (no use)	Adjusted for age, recent medical contacts, and Aspirin use
Vezina, R. M. 1998 [36]	case-control	Monthly contact with the tumor registrar and review of Massachusetts Cancer Registry for males less than 70 years of age diagnosed with prostate cancers in Massachusetts (1992–1995)	2617	Telephone interview (lifetime until cancer diagnosis)	64	Males(100)	Use of CCBs or beta-blockers or ACEIs or Thiazides or others (no use)	Age; race; level of education; family history of prostate cancer; dietary fat intake; BMI; alcohol, tobacco, and coffee use; urologic symptoms; and physician visits 2 years previously.
Rosenberg, L. 1998 [37]	case-control	Interviewed patients aged 40 to 69 years in Boston, Mass, New York, NY, Philadelphia, Pa,and Baltimore, Md (1976–1996)	16,005	Interview with standard questionnaires by trained nurse (lifetime until cancer diagnosis)	56(40–69)	Males (41) Females (59)	Use of CCBs or beta-blockers or ACEIs (no use)	Age, BMI, interview year, annual visits to a physician 2 yr. before admission, smoking amount(pack year) for all cancers, and other additional risk factors for regressions for each cancer site)
Jick, H.1997 [11]	Nested case-control	Review of all hypertensive patients on the General Practice Research Database (GPRD) who were current users of beta-blockers only, ACEIs only, or CCBs only (with or without diuretics) and who had a first-time diagnosis of any cancer recorded in 1995.	2196	Review of computerized medical records (1987 until cancer diagnosis)	71.6 (NA)	Males (49.6) Females (50.4)	Use of CCBs (use of beta-blockers)	Smoking, BMI, change of medication, duration of hypertension, and diuretic use

CCB calcium-channel blockers, ACEI angiotensin-converting enzyme inhibitors, ARB angiotensin II receptor blockers, NA not available

Table 3 Assessment of the methodologic quality of the cohort studies included in meta-analysis

Studies	Slection				Comparability		Outcome			Total scores
	1	2	3	4	1	2	1	2	3	
Pai, P. Y.et al. 2015 [20]	+	+	+	+	+		+	+	+	8
Rao, G. A. et al. 2013 [24]	+	+	+	+	+	+	+	+	+	9
Bhaskaran, K. et al. 2012 [25]	+	+	+	+	+	+	+	+	+	9
Rodriguez, C. 2009 [26]	+	+	+	+	+	+		+	+	8
van der Knaap, R. et al. 2008 [27]	+	+	+	+	+	+	+	+	+	9
Harris, A. M. et al. 2007 [28]	+	+	+				+	+		5
Debes, J. D. et al. 2004 [29]	+	+	+	+	+		+	+	+	8
Friis, S. et al. 2001 [30]	+	+	+		+		+	+	+	7
Fitzpatrick, A. L. 2001 [31]	+	+	+	+	+	+	+	+	+	9
Sorensen, H. T. 2000 [10]	+	+	+				+		+	5
Olsen, J. H. 1997 [32]	+	+	+				+		+	5
Pahor, M. 1996 [33]	+	+	+	+	+	+	+	+	+	9

+: the article gain 1 score in the item

studies showed that their outcomes of interest were not present at the start of the study. Thirteen studies gained two scores in the section of comparability due to their well the control of confounding factors [15, 17, 24–27, 31, 33, 34–37, 39]. There was only one study whose ascertainment of exposure was deruved from self-report [26]. The duration of follow-up in two studies was less than 5 years [10, 32]. The non-response rate was low in the included cohort studies but the scores for this item were lacking in the case-control studies.

ACEI and prostate cancer risk

There were ten studies that reported the relationship between the use of ACE inhibitors and the risk of prostate cancer [15–17, 19, 26, 30, 31, 35–37]. We found no significant association between ACE inhibitor usage and the risk of prostate cancer in the meta-analysis of the ten studies (RR1.07, 95% CI0.96–1.20). However, obvious clear

heterogeneity existed among these studies ($I^2 = 86\%$). Subgroup analysis also showed no significant relationship between the use of ACE inhibitor and the risk of prostate cancer according to the poolanalysis of cohort studies (RR0.92, 95% CI0.77–1.11) and case-control studies (RR1.11, 95% CI0.98–1.26) (Fig. 2).

ARB and prostate cancer risk

Five studies reported the association between ARB usage and the risk of prostate cancer [15–17, 24, 25]. There was no significant relationship between ARB usage and the risk of prostate cancer according to the pool-analysis of all studies (RR1.09, 95% CI0.97–1.21). Subgroup analysis also suggested no significant connection between the use of ARB and the risk of prostate cancer according to the pooled-analysis of cohort studies (RR1.00, 95% CI0.83–1.20) and case-control studies (RR1.16, 95% CI0.98–1.38). However, heterogeneity among these studies was high ($I^2 = 83.7\%$) (Fig. 3).

Table 4 Assessment of the methodologic quality of the case-control studies included in meta-analysis

Studies	Slection				Comparability		Exposure			Total scores
	1	2	3	4	1	2	1	2	3	
Hallas, J. 2012 [17]	+	+	+	+	+	+	+	+	+	9
Azoulay, L. 2012 [39]	+	+	+	+	+	+	+	+		8
Kemppainen, K. J. 2011 [15]	+	+	+		+	+	+	+		7
Assimes, T. L. 2008 [34]	+	+	+	+	+	+	+	+		8
Ronquist, G. 2004 [35]	+	+	+	+	+	+	+	+		8
Perron, L. 2004 [19]	+	+	+	+	+			+	+	7
Vezina, R. M. 1998 [36]	+	+	+	+	+	+	+	+		8
Rosenberg, L. 1998 [37]	+	+	+	+	+	+	+	+	+	9
Jick, H. 1997 [11]	+	+	+	+	+			+	+	7

+: the article gain 1 score in the item

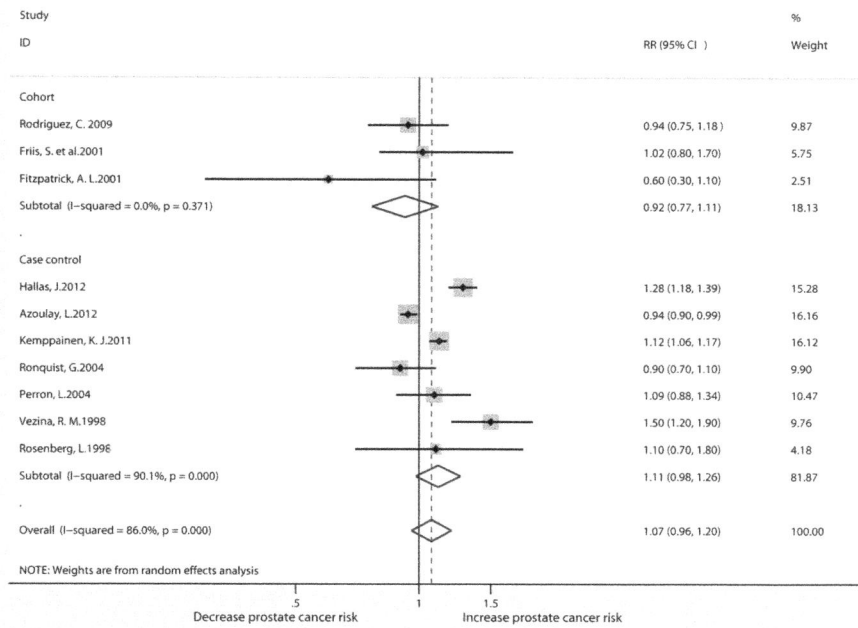

Fig. 2 Forest plot for ACEI use and prostate cancer risk (RR relative risk, CI confidence interval)

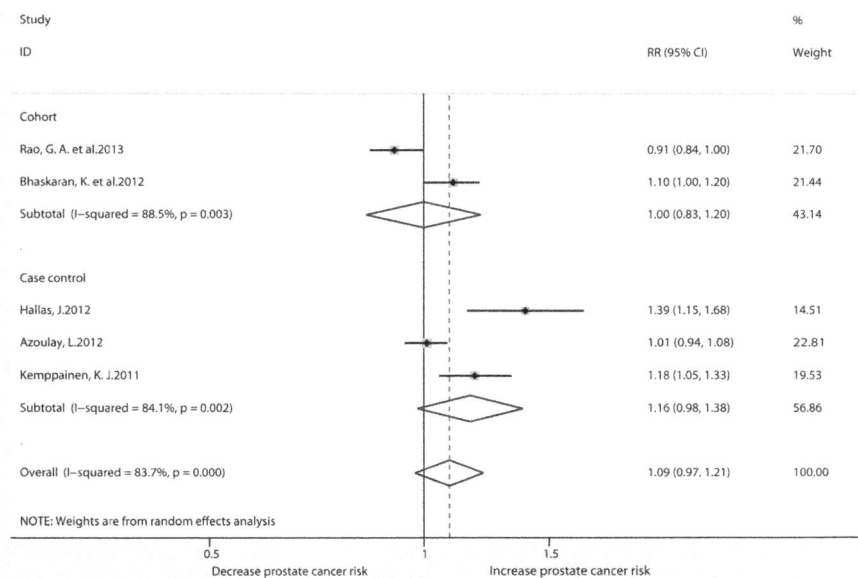

Fig. 3 Forest plot for ARB use and prostate cancer risk (RR relative risk, CI confidence interval)

CCB and prostate cancer risk

A total of 14 studies reported the connection between CCB usage and the risk of prostate cancer [10, 11, 15, 16, 19, 26, 31–35, 36–38]. There appeared to be a significant association between CCB usage and the risk of prostate cancer, according to the meta-analysis of all studies (RR1.08, 95% CI1.00–1.16). There was considerable heterogeneity existing among these studies ($I^2 = 57.4\%$). Subgroup analysis also indicated that without significant relationship between CCB usage and the risk of prostate cancer in terms of cohort studies (RR0.93, 95% CI0.71–1.21) but there was clear association between the use of CCB and the risk of prostate cancer according to the pool-analysis of case-control studies (RR1.10, 95% CI1.04–1.16) (Fig. 4).

Beta-blockers and prostate cancer risk

There were 8 studies involving the subject of the relationship between beta-blocker usage and the risk of prostate cancer [15, 19, 26, 31, 34–37]. The meta-analysis of all studies suggested that there was no significant association between beta-blocker usage and the risk of prostate cancer (RR0.91, 95% CI0.81–1.02). We also did not find a significant connection between beta-blocker usage and the risk of prostate cancer, according to the pooled analysis of cohort (RR0.85, 95% CI0.69–1.04) or case-control studies (RR0.92, 95% CI0.81–1.05). There

was significant heterogeneity existing among these studies ($I^2 = 70.1\%$) (Fig. 5).

Diuretics or antiadrenergic drugs and prostate risk

There were 5 and 4 studies involving the association between the use of diuretics [15, 31, 36, 35] and antiadrenergic drugs [15, 16, 28, 31, 35] and the risk of prostate cancer, respectively. We did not find significant association between the use of antiadrenergic drugs and the risk of prostate cancer (RR1.22, 95% CI0.76–1.96). The relationship between the use of diuretics and the risk of prostate cancer was demonstrated as not significant(RR1.09, 95% CI0.95–1.25). Significant associations between antiadrenergic drug usage and the risk of prostate cancer were found according to the cohort studies (RR0.71, 95% CI0.57–0.90) (Fig. 6).

Discussion

To the best of our knowledge, this is first meta-analysis to investigate the relationship between the use of antihypertensive drugs and the risk of prostate cancer. Our main findings suggested that there was no significant association between the use of ACE inhibitors, ARB, betablockers, diuretics or antiadrenergic drugs and the risk of prostate cancer. However, CCB usage appeared to be associated with the risk of prostate cancer. Moreover,

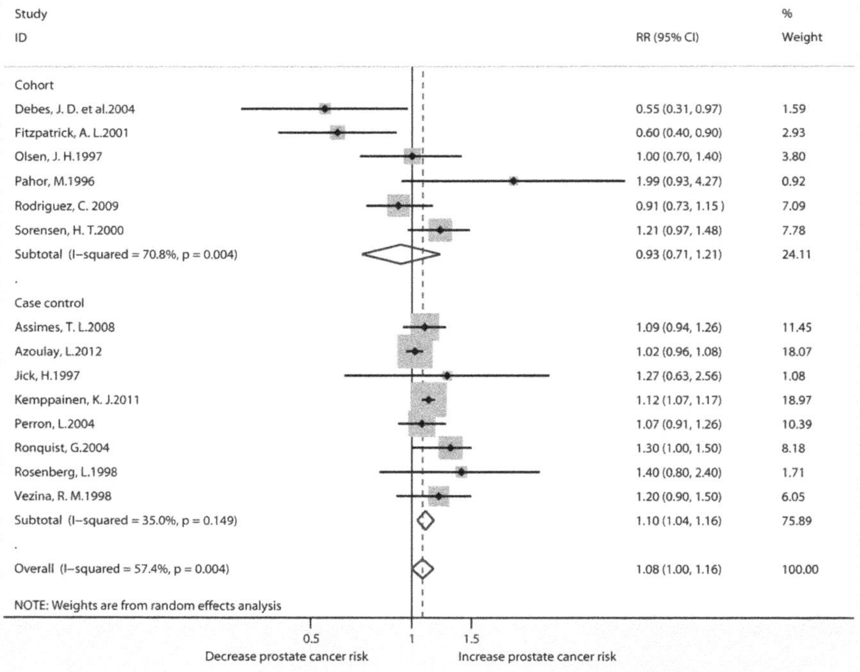

Fig. 4 Forest plot for CCB use and prostate cancer risk (RR relative risk, CI confidence interval)

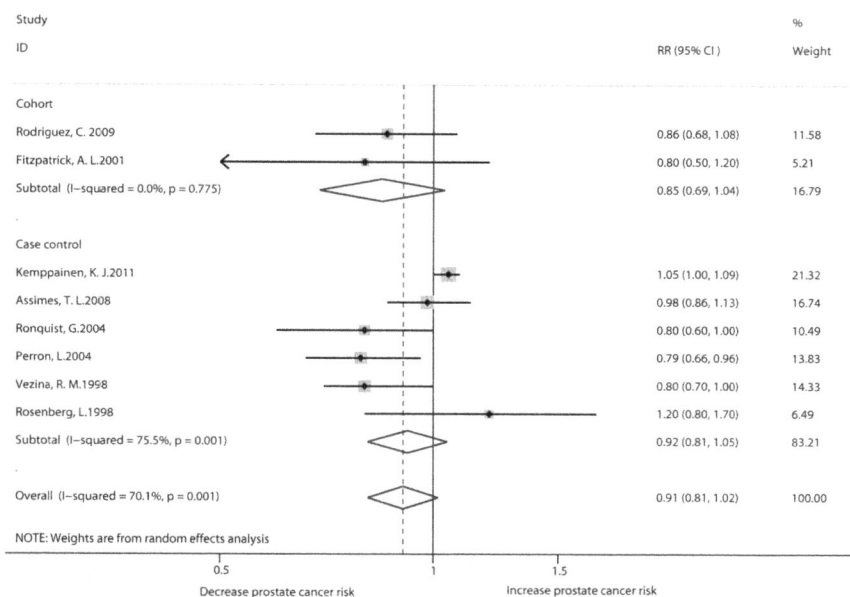

Fig. 5 Forest plot for beta-blockers use and prostate cancer risk (RR relative risk, CI confidence interval)

that considerable heterogeneity existed among the studies resulted in the reduction of evidence levels.

Prostate cancer is the most frequently diagnosed cancer diagnosed and the main causes of cancer death in older men in Western countries. Antihypertensive drugs such as ACE inhibitors and ARB are widely used for the management of hypertension and the prevention of cardiovascular disease events in high-risk persons [4, 40, 41]. Patients usually have long-term use of two or more different types of antihypertensive drugs to control their blood pressure [42]. The long-term ingestion of antihypertensive drugs can lead to adverse effects in patients, such as hypercholesterolemia, diabetes mellitus, chronic renal disease, and other cardiovascular diseases [43]. In addition, discussion of the connection between the use of antihypertensive drugs and the risk of cancer has consistently been a hot topic since the first relevant study was raised. We know that the older men are exposed to the condition of frequent use of antihypertensive drugs, and there is a high incidence of prostate cancer in this population [12, 44].

The topic of the relationship between the use of antihypertensive drugs and the risk of prostate cancer remain controversial, especially in the use of CCB and ACE inhibitors or ARB. The findings of a case-control study by Vezina, RM et al. suggested that there was no association between the use of CCB and the risk of prostate cancer in men younger than the age of 70 [36]. Debes, JD et al. found that there was an inverse

association between prostate cancer and the use of CCB, and the result varied according to a family history of prostate cancer [14]. Loughlin KR reviewed relevant literature and thought that CCB had a protective effect on the development of prostate cancer on a basic science level, although the association in clinical practice has been controversial [45].

ACEI and ARB have been successfully used as potent antihypertensive drugs for a long period of time, and some literatures have suggested that these drugs could serve as new anticancer drugs [46]. The increased expression of AngII type 1 receptor (AT1R) mRNA was found in prostate cancer tissues compared with expression levels in the normal human prostate [47]. According to the data from basic science, ACE inhibitors or ARB might have a protective role in cancer [48]. A meta-analysis of randomized controlled trials (RCT) suggested that ARB are associated with an increased risk of new cancer diagnoses, while another meta-analysis of observational studies did not find significant associations between the use of ACE inhibitors or ARB and the risk of cancer, noting that the previous meta-analysis of RCT had a short duration of follow-up [9, 18]. In a case-control study, Hallas J et al. found significantly elevated OR for prostate cancer (OR 1.28, 95% CI 1.18, 1.39) in the patients using ACE inhibitors [17]. A cohort study by Rodriguez, C et al. indicated that there was no significant relationship between the use of ACE inhibitors and the risk of prostate cancer [26].

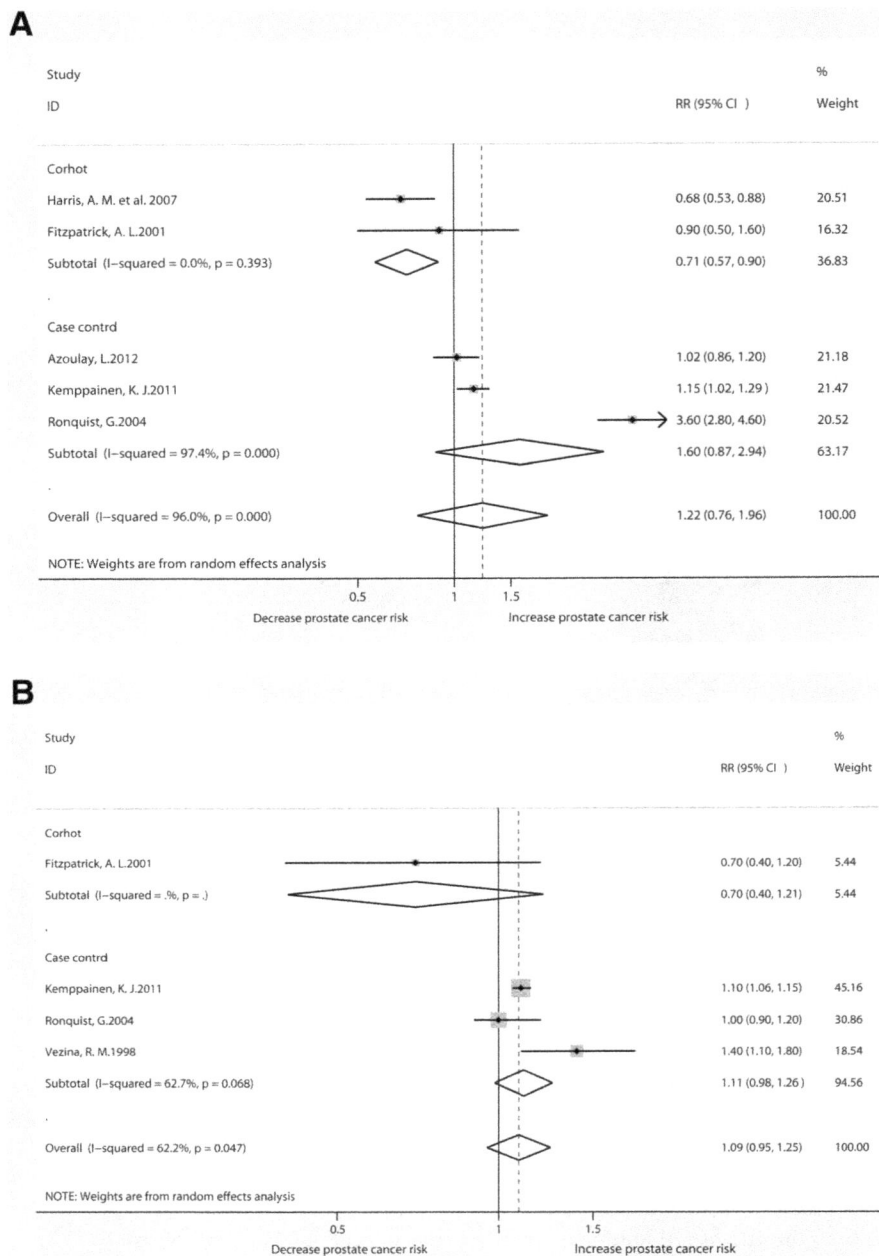

Fig. 6 Forest plot for use of antiadrenergic agents or diuretic and prostate cancer risk: **a** antiadrenergic agents and **b** diuretic. RR relative risk, CI confidence interval

A meta-analysis suggested that the use of BB was associated with reduced specific mortality among patients with prostate cancer [49]. However, the relationship between BB usage and the risk of prostate cancer lacks consistent evidence. Perron, L et al. found that the long-term use of BB might prevent prostate cancer (OR 0.79, 95% CI 0.66, 0.96) [19]. However, Kemppainen, KJ et al. found that beta-blockers were associated with a marginally elevated risk of prostate cancer (OR 1.05, 95% CI 1.00,1.09) [15].

Fewer studies have paid attention to the relationship between the use of diuretics or antiadrenergic drugs and prostate risk compared with other types of antihypertensive drugs and their use also had different results [15, 20].

The present systematic review and meta-analysis provided a summary analysis of previous relevant studies which could yield a conclusion characterized by compromise. According to the pooled analyses of cohort studies, we generally did not find significant associations between the use of antihypertensive drugs and the risk of prostate cancer. Nevertheless, CCB usage might contribute to the higher risk of prostate cancer, based on findings from the case-control studies. Moreover, antiadrenergic drugs had a protective effect on the development of prostate cancer, according to the meta-analysis of two cohort studies. As we know, there was longer duration of follow-up in observational studies and we only reviewed these studies to explore whether the long-term use of antihypertensive drugs affected the incidence of prostate cancer in natural population. In the present review, most of the studies had a follow-up time of at least five years, and we had a larger sample to analyse than any previous studies. The main confounding factors, such as age, BMI, and race were adjusted for in most of the studies. Although we included studies with samples containing females, the relative risk was calculated under an adjustment for sex. Moreover, most of the studies were assessed with a high quality of methodology. As a result, our pooled analyses provided a conclusion that was more closer to the truth.

Our studies also had some limitations. First, our evidence grade was compromised by the considerable heterogeneity, which might be caused by various factors, including study design, race, follow-up time, social background. Second, small sample were analysed on the association between diuretics or antiadrenergic drugs and prostate risk, and the results should be cautiously considered. Third, we did not detect the publication bias, although it might exist among these studies. Finally, we did not conduct a dose-response meta-analysis due to the lack of relevant data in the included studies.

Conclusions
We reviewed 21 observational studies and found that there was no significant association between use of antihypertensive drugs and the risk of prostate cancer. Nevertheless, CCB usage might contribute to the higher risk of prostate cancer based on findings from the case-control studies. Unfortunately, the high heterogeneity downgraded the evidence level and more well-designed studies with large samples are needed.

Abbreviations
ACEI: Angiotensin-converting enzyme inhibitors; ARB: Angiotensin II receptor blockers; CCB: Calcium-channel blockers; NOS: Newcastle-Ottawa Scale; RR: Relative risk; SMD: Standardized mean difference

Acknowledgments
Not applicable

Funding
The innovation program of Critical illness (Shaanxi administration of traditional Chinese medicine) no.2015-JDM.

Authors' contributions
LC: Project development, articles search, review, data extract, statistical analysis, and manuscript writing and revising; SZ: Project development, data extract, statistical analysis and articles search; CMJ: articles search, review, statistical analysis and manuscript writing; WH: review, data extract, statistical analysis, and manuscript writing and revising; LTW: data extract, statistical analysis, and manuscript writing and revising; YQL: data extract, and statistical analysis, and manuscript writing and revising; WW: articles search, review and pictures production; ZL: Project development and pictures production; JM: Project development, and manuscript writing and revising; All authors have read and approve of the final manuscript.

Competing interests
All authors declare that they have no conflict of interests.

References
1. Vokonas PS, Kannel WB, Cupples LA. Epidemiology and risk of hypertension in the elderly: the Framingham study. Journal Hypertens Suppl. 1988;6:S3–9.
2. Redmond N, Booth JN 3rd, Tanner RM, Diaz KM, Abdalla M, Sims M, et al. Prevalence of masked hypertension and its association with subclinical cardiovascular disease in African Americans: results from the Jackson heart study. J Am Heart Assoc. 2016;5:e002284.
3. Thomopoulos C, Parati G, Zanchetti A. Effects of blood pressure lowering on outcome incidence in hypertension: 4. Effects of various classes of antihypertensive drugs–overview and meta-analyses. J Hypertens. 2015;33:195–211.
4. Ettehad D, Emdin CA, Kiran A, Anderson SG, Callender T, Emberson J, et al. Blood pressure lowering for prevention of cardiovascular disease and death: a systematic review and meta-analysis. Lancet. 2016;387:957–67.
5. Aromaa A, Hakama M, Hakulinen T, Saxen E, Teppo L, Ida lan-Heikkila J. Breast cancer and use of rauwolfia and other antihypertensive agents in hypertensive patients: a nationwide case-control study in Finland. Int J Cancer. 1976;18:727–38.
6. Stanford JL, Martin EJ, Brinton LA, Hoover RN. Rauwolfia use and breast cancer: a case-control study. J Natl Cancer Inst. 1986;76:817–22.
7. Dyer AR, Stamler J, Berkson DM, Lindberg HA, Stevens E. High blood-pressure: a risk factor for cancer mortality? Lancet. 1975;1:1051–6.
8. Lever AF, Hole DJ, Gillis CR, McCallum IR, McInnes GT, MacKinnon PL, et al. Do inhibitors of angiotensin-I-converting enzyme protect against risk of cancer? Lancet. 1998;352:179–84.
9. Yoon C, Yang HS, Jeon I, Chang Y, Park SM. Use of angiotensin-converting-enzyme inhibitors or angiotensin-receptor blockers and cancer risk: a meta-analysis of observational studies. Can Med Assoc J. 2011;183:E1073–E84.
10. Sorensen HT, Olsen JH, Mellemkjaer L, Marie A, Steffensen FH, McLaughlin JK, et al. Cancer risk and mortality in users of calcium channel blockers. A cohort study. Cancer. 2000;89:165–70.
11. Jick H, Jick S, Derby LE, Vasilakis C, Myers MW, Meier CR. Calcium-channel blockers and risk of cancer. Lancet. 1997;349:525–8.
12. Dijkman GA, Debruyne FM. Epidemiology of prostate cancer. Eur Urol. 1996;30:281–95.
13. Jan CR, Lee KC, Chou KJ, Cheng JS, Wang JL, Lo YK, et al. Fendiline, an anti-anginal drug, increases intracellular Ca2+ in PC3 human prostate cancer cells. Cancer Chemother Pharmacol. 2001;48:37–41.
14. Debes JD, Roberts RO, Jacobson DJ, Girman CJ, Lieber MM, Tindall DJ, et al. Inverse association between prostate cancer and the use of calcium channel blockers. Cancer Epidem Biomar. 2004;13:255–9.
15. Kemppainen KJ, Tammela TL, Auvinen A, Murtola TJ. The associationbetween anti-hypertensive drug use and incidence of prostate cancer in Finland: a population-based case–control study. Cancer Causes Control. 2011;22:1445–52.
16. Azoulay L, Assimes TL, Yin H, Bartels DB, Schiffrin EL, Suissa S. Long-term use of angiotensin receptor blockers and the risk of cancer. PLoS One. 2012;7:e50893.
17. Hallas J, Christensen R, Andersen M, Friis S, Bjerrum L. Long term use of drugs affecting the renin-angiotensin system and the risk of cancer: a population-based case-control study. Br J Clin Pharmacol. 2012;74:180–8.
18. Sipahi I, Chou J, Mishra P, Debanne SM, Simon DI, Fang JC. Meta-analysis of randomized controlled trials on effect of Angiotensin-converting enzyme inhibitors on cancer risk. Am J Cardiol. 2011;108:294–301.
19. Perron L, Bairati I, Harel F, Meyer F. Antihypertensive drug use and the risk of prostate cancer (Canada). Cancer Causes Control. 2004;15:535–41.

20. Pai PY, Hsieh VC, Wang CB, Wu HC, Liang WM, Chang YJ, et al. Long term antihypertensive drug use and prostate cancer risk: a 9-year population-based cohort analysis. Int J Cardiol. 2015;193:1–7.

21. Greenland S. Quantitative methods in the review of epidemiologic literature. Epidemiol Rev. 1987;9:1–30.

22. Siristatidis C, Sergentanis TN, Kanavidis P, Trivella M, Sotiraki M, Mavromatis I, et al. Controlled ovarian hyperstimulation for IVF: impact on ovarian, endometrial and cervical cancer–a systematic review and meta-analysis. Hum Reprod Update. 2013;19:105–23.

23. Higgins JPT GS. Cochrane handbook for systematic reviews of interventions version 5.1.0 [updated march 2011]. The Cochrane collaboration. 2011; www.cochrane-handbook.org.

24. Rao GA, Mann JR, Bottai M, Uemura H, Burch JB, Bennett CL, et al. Angiotensin receptor blockers and risk of prostate cancer among United States veterans. J Clin Pharmacol. 2013;53:773–8.

25. Bhaskaran K, Douglas I, Evans S, van Staa T, Smeeth L. Angiotensin receptor blockers and risk of cancer: cohort study among people receiving antihypertensive drugs in UK general practice research database. BMJ. 2012;344:e2697.

26. Rodriguez C, Jacobs EJ, Deka A, Patel AV, Bain EB, Thun MJ, et al. Use of blood-pressure-lowering medication and risk of prostate cancer in the cancer prevention study II nutrition cohort. Cancer Causes Control. 2009;20:671–9.

27. van der Knaap R, Siemes C, Coebergh JW, van Duijn CM, Hofman A, Stricker BH. Renin-angiotensin system inhibitors, angiotensin I-converting enzyme gene insertion/deletion polymorphism, and cancer: the Rotterdam study. Cancer. 2008;112:748–57.

28. Harris AM, Warner BW, Wilson JM, Becker A, Rowland RG, Conner W, et al. Effect of alpha1-adrenoceptor antagonist exposure on prostate cancer incidence: an observational cohort study. J Urol. 2007;178:2176–80.

29. Debes JD, Roberts RO, Jacobson DJ, Girman CJ, Lieber MM, Tindall DJ, et al. Inverse association between prostate cancer and the use of calcium channel blockers. Cancer Epidemiol, Biomarkers Prev. 2004;13:255–9.

30. Friis S, Sorensen HT, Mellemkjaer L, McLaughlin JK, Nielsen GL, Blot WJ, et al. Angiotensin-converting enzyme inhibitors and the risk of cancer: a population-based cohort study in Denmark. Cancer. 2001;92:2462–70.

31. Fitzpatrick AL, Daling JR, Furberg CD, Kronmal RA, Weissfeld JL. Hypertension, heart rate, use of antihypertensives, and incident prostate cancer. Ann Epidemiol. 2001;11:534–42.

32. Olsen JH, Sorensen HT, Friis S, McLaughlin JK, Steffensen FH, Nielsen GL, et al. Cancer risk in users of calcium channel blockers. Hypertension. 1997;29:1091–4.

33. Pahor M, Guralnik JM, Ferrucci L, Corti MC, Salive ME, Cerhan JR, et al. Calcium-channel blockade and incidence of cancer in aged populations. Lancet. 1996;348:493–7.

34. Assimes TL, Elstein E, Langleben A, Suissa S. Long-term use of antihypertensive drugs and risk of cancer. Pharmacoepidemiol Drug Saf. 2008;17:1039–49.

35. Ronquist G, Garcia Rodriguez LA, Ruigomez A, Johansson S, Wallander MA, Frithz G, et al. Association between Captopril, other antihypertensive drugs and risk of prostate cancer. Prostate. 2004;58:50–6.

36. Vezina RM, Lesko SM, Rosenberg L, Shapiro S. Calcium channel blocker use and the risk of prostate cancer. Am J Hypertens. 1998;11:1420–5.

37. Rosenberg L, Rao RS, Palmer JR, Strom BL, Stolley PD, Zauber AG, et al. Calcium channel blockers and the risk of cancer. JAMA. 1998;279:1000–4.

38. Debes JD, Roberts RO, Jacobson DJ, Girman CJ, Lieber MM, Tindall DJ, et al. Inverse association between prostate cancer and the use of Calcium Channel blockers. Cancer Epidemio Biomark Prev. 2004;13:255–9.

39. Azoulay L, Assimes TL, Yin H, Bartels DB, Schiffrin EL, Suissa S. Long-term use of Angiotensin receptor blockers and the risk of cancer. PLoS One 2012;7:e50893.

40. Kario K, Saito I, Kushiro T, Teramukai S, Ishikawa Y, Mori Y, et al. Home blood pressure and cardiovascular outcomes in patients during antihypertensive therapy: primary results of HONEST, a large-scale prospective, real-world observational study. Hypertension. 2014;64:989–96.

41. Heerspink HJ, Gao P, de Zeeuw D, Clase C, Dagenais GR, Sleight P, et al. The effect of ramipril and telmisartan on serum potassium and its association with cardiovascular and renal events: results from the ONTARGET trial. Eur J Prev Cardiol. 2014;21:299–309.

42. Richards TR, Tobe SW. Combining other antihypertensive drugs with beta-blockers in hypertension: a focus on safety and tolerability. Can J Cardiol. 2014;30:S42–6.

43. Karagiannis A, Tziomalos K, Anagnostis P, Gossios TD, Florentin M, Athyros VG, et al. The effect of antihypertensive agents on insulin sensitivity, lipids and haemostasis. Curr Vasc Pharmacol. 2010;8:792–803.

44. Landahl S, Bengtsson C, Sigurdsson JA, Svanborg A, Svardsudd K. Age-related changes in blood pressure. Hypertension. 1986;8:1044–9.

45. Loughlin KR. Calcium channel blockers and prostate cancer. Urol Oncol. 2014;32:537–8.

46. Lindberg H, Nielsen D, Jensen BV, Eriksen J, Skovsgaard T. Angiotensin converting enzyme inhibitors for cancer treatment? Acta Oncol. 2004;43:142–52.

47. Uemura H, Ishiguro H, Nakaigawa N, Nagashima Y, Miyoshi Y, Fujinami K, et al. Angiotensin II receptor blocker shows antiproliferative activity in prostate cancer cells: a possibility of tyrosine kinase inhibitor of growth factor. Mol Cancer Ther. 2003;2:1139–47.

48. Deshayes F, Nahmias C. Angiotensin receptors: a new role in cancer? Trends Endocrin Met. 2005;16:293–9.

49. Lu H, Liu X, Guo F, Tan S, Wang G, Liu H, et al. Impact of beta-blockers on prostate cancer mortality: a meta-analysis of 16,825 patients. OncoTargets Ther. 2015;8:985–90.

23

Prognostic significance of epidermal growth factor receptor (EGFR) over expression in urothelial carcinoma of urinary bladder

Atif Ali hashmi[1], Zubaida Fida Hussain[1], Muhammad Irfan[1], Erum Yousuf Khan[1], Naveen Faridi[1], Hanna Naqvi, Amir Khan[3]* (iD) and Muhammad Muzzammil Edhi[2]

Abstract

Background: Epidermal growth factor receptor (EGFR) has been shown to have abnormal expression in many human cancers and is considered as a marker of poor prognosis. Frequency of over expression in bladder cancer has not been studied in our population; therefore we aimed to evaluate the frequency and prognostic significance of EGFR immunohistochemical expression in locoregional population.

Methods: We performed EGFR immunohistochemistry on 126 cases of bladder cancer and association of EGFR expression with tumor grade, lamina propria invasion, deep muscle invasion and recurrence of disease was evaluated.

Results: High EGFR expression was noted in 26.2% (33 cases), 15.1% (19 cases) and 58.7% (74 cases) revealed low and no EGFR expression respectively. Significant association of EGFR expression was noted with tumor grade, lamina propria invasion, deep muscle invasion and recurrence status while no significant association was seen with age, gender and overall survival. Kaplan- Meier curves revealed significant association of EGFR expression with recurrence while no significant association was seen with overall survival.

Conclusion: Significant association of EGFR overexpression with tumor grade, muscularis propria invasion and recurrence signifies its prognostic value; therefore EGFR can be used as a prognostic biomarker in Urothelial bladder carcinoma.

Keywords: Bladder cancer, Muscle invasion, Epidermal growth factor receptor, EGFR, Urothelial carcinoma

Background

Bladder cancer is the fifth commonest malignancy in males all over the world [1]. Most of the bladder tumors have transitional cell (urothelial) morphology and they have a natural propensity to progress from superficial non-invasive tumors to deep muscle invasive cancers [2] . Prognosis of bladder cancer depends upon grade and stage of the disease. The single most important factor for determining disease prognosis in bladder cancer is muscle invasion; the presence of which makes therapeutic approach more radical. The only therapeutic option for muscle invasive bladder cancer is radical cystectomy or radical radiotherapy; however 5 year survival remains poor [3, 4]. On the other hand, non-muscle invasive tumors can recur and progress with time to muscle invasive disease [5]. Therefore detection of abnormal expression of biological markers is under intense scrutiny in bladder cancer, which can serve as prognostic or predictive factors in bladder cancers. Epidermal growth factor receptor (EGFR) has been shown to have abnormal expression in many human cancers and is considered as a marker of poor prognosis [6]. Frequency of over expression in bladder cancer has not been studied in our population; therefore we aimed to evaluate the frequency and prognostic significance of EGFR immunohistochemical expression in locoregional population.

* Correspondence: dramirkhan04@gmail.com
[3]Kandahar University, Kandahar, Afghanistan
Full list of author information is available at the end of the article

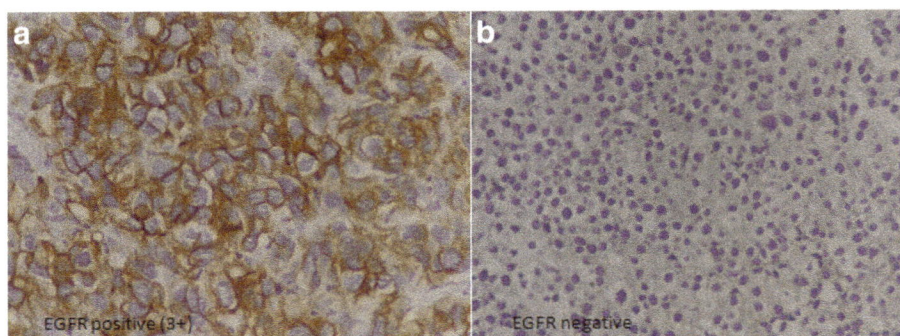

Fig. 1 Positive (Strong & diffuse) and negative EGFR expression in bladder cancer (400× magnification)

Methods
Selection of cases
Total 126 diagnosed cases of urothelial carcinoma specimens of urinary bladder were selected from records of pathology department. Cases of bladder cancer which were diagnosed other than urothelial carcinomas were excluded. All patients underwent surgeries at Liaquat National hospital, Karachi from January 2010 till December 2014 over a period of 5 years. The study was approved by research and ethical review committee of Liaquat National Hospital and informed written consent was taken from all patients at the time of surgery. Hematoxylin and eosin stained slides and paraffin blocks of all cases were retrieved and new sections were cut where necessary. Slides of all cases were reviewed by two senior histopathologists and pathologic characteristics like tumor grade, lamina propria invasion, muscularis propria invasion were evaluated. Deep muscle invasion was analyzed when thick muscle bundles of muscularis propria were present in transurethral resection specimen. Clinical records of 58 patients were available and are thus reviewed from institutional records to evaluate recurrence and survival status. Moreover, representative tissue blocks of each case were selected for EGFR immunohistochemistry.

Immunohistochemistry
EGFR immunohistochemistry was performed using using DAKO Monoclonal Mouse Anti-human Epidermal growth factor Receptor (EGFR), clone H11. 1:100 dilution was done using phosphate buffer saline (incubation time 30 mins at room temperature). To reduce background, incubation was done at room temperature for 20 min using proteinase K solution. Detection method was DAKO EnVision method, DAB was used as chromogen substrate (incubation time 1–3 min at room temperature) and counter stain was hematoxylin. Skin tissue was used as control. Both membranous and cytoplasmic staining for EGFR was both quantitatively and qualitatively evaluated. Intensity of staining was

categorized into no staining (0), weak (1+), intermediate (2+), strong (3+) while percentage of positively stained cells were measured as continuous variable. The following scoring approach in the assessment of EGFR immunostaining was used: score 0 = no staining, unspecific staining of tumor cells or less than 10% staining, score 1

Table 1 Demographic profile of patients involved in the study

	n (%)
Age (years)[a]	63.61 ± 14.49
Follow up (months)[a, b]	22.76 ± 13.66
EFGR (%)[a]	14.50 ± 22.41
Gender	
Male	91(72.2)
Female	35(27.8)
Specimen Type	
Transurethral resection	121(96)
Radical Cystectomy	5(4)
Tumor Grade	
Low Grade Papillary Urothelial Carcinoma	65(51.6)
High Grade Papillary Urothelial Carcinoma	61(48.4)
Lamina Propria Invasion	
Present	35(27.8)
Absent	91(72.2)
Deep Muscle Invasion	
Present	22(17.5)
Absent	59(46.8)
Can't Assessed	45(35.7)
Recurrence (n = 58)	
Yes	25(43.1)
No	33(56.9)
Survival Status (n = 58)	
Alive	49(84.5)
Expired	9(15.5)

[a]Mean ± SD
[b]58 cases

= membranous weak and incomplete staining of more than 10% of tumor cells, score 2 = moderate and complete membranous staining of more than 10% of tumor cells, score 3 = strong and complete membranous staining of more than 10% of tumor cells. Scored1+ tumors were classified as Low EGFR expression and those scored 2+ or 3+ were classified as High EGFR expression[18] (Fig. 1).

Follow-up and recurrence

Recurrence status and follow-up were evaluated by reviewing hospital medical records. Overall survival was taken as time from surgical excision till death or last follow-up and disease free survival was defined as time between surgical excision and local recurrence or distant metastasis, death or last follow-up.

Statistical analysis

Statistical package for social sciences (SPSS 21) was used for data compilation and analysis. Mean and standard deviation were calculated for quantitative variables. Frequency and percentage were calculated for qualitative variables. Chi-square was applied to determine association. Student t test or Mann witney test were applied to compare difference in means among groups. P-value ≤ 0.05 as significant. Survival curves were plotted using Kaplan- Meier method and the significance of difference between survival curves were determined using log-rank ratio. P-value ≤ 0.05 was taken as significant.

Results

Mean age of patients was 63.61 ± 14.49 years with male to female ratio of 2.6:1. 96% specimens were of transurethral resections. 48.4% (61 cases) were of high grade morphology,

Table 2 Association of EGFR Expression with clinicopathologic features of Urothelial carcinoma

	EFGR Expression n (%)				P-Value
	No Expression (n = 74)	Low EFGR Expression (n = 19)	High EFGR expression (n = 33)	Total (n = 126)	
Gender					
Male	54(73)	14(73.7)	23(69.7)	91(72.2)	0.930
Female	20(27)	5(26.3)	10(30.3)	35(27.8)	
Age Group[a]					
≤ 25 years	1(1.4)	0(0)	0(0)	0(0)	0.263
26–50 years	21(28.4)	2(10.5)	2(10.5)	5(15.2)	
> 50 years	52(70.3)	17(89.5)	17(89.5)	28(84.8)	
Specimen Type[a]					
Transurethral resection	72(97.3)	19(100)	30(90.9)	121(96)	0.209
Radical Cystectomy	2(2.7)	0(0)	3(9.1)	5(4)	
Tumor Grade					
Low Grade	48(64.9)	9(47.4)	8(24.2)	65(51.6)	0.000
High Grade	26(35.1)	10(52.6)	25(75.8)	61(48.4)	
Lamina Propria Invasion					
Present	15(20.3)	3(15.8)	17(51.5)	35(27.8)	0.002
Absent	59(79.7)	16(84.2)	16(48.5)	91(72.2)	
Deep Muscle Invasion[a]					
Present	9(12.2)	1(5.3)	12(36.4)	22(17.5)	0.012
Absent	38(51.4)	12(63.2)	9(27.3)	59(46.8)	
Can't Assessed	27(36.5)	6(31.6)	12(36.4)	45(35.7)	
Recurrence (n = 58)[a]					
Yes	15(40.5)	0(0)	10(66.7)	25(43.1)	0.017
No	22(59.5)	6(100)	5(33.3)	33(56.9)	
Survival Status (n = 58)[a]					
Alive	32(86.5)	6(100)	11(73.3)	49(84.5)	0.398
Expired	5(13.5)	0(0)	4(26.7)	9(15.5)	

Chi-Square test applied
[a]Fisher Exact test applied
P-Value≤0.05, considerd as significant

whereas 51.6% (65 cases) showed low grade histology. Lamina propria invasion was seen in 27.8% (35 cases), while muscularis propria invasion was noted in 17.5% (22 cases). Mean follow up of patients involved in the study was 22.76 ± 13.66 months and recurrence was seen in 43.1% (25 cases) as presented in Table 1. However, in 45 cases (35.7%) deep muscle was not present in the specimen and therefore deep muscle invasion couldn't be assessed.

According to scoring system used; high EGFR expression was noted in 26.2% (33 cases), 15.1% (19 cases) and 58.7% (74 cases) revealed low and no EGFR expression respectively.

Significant association of EGFR expression was noted with tumor grade, lamina propria invasion, deep muscle invasion and recurrence status while no significant association was seen with age, gender and overall survival (Table 2). Kaplan- Meier curves revealed significant association of EGFR expression with recurrence while no significant association was seen with overall survival (Figs. 2 and 3).

Discussion

In the current study, we evaluated EGFR expression in bladder cancers of locoregional population and found EGFR expression in 46% cases of bladder cancer. Moreover,

we found a significant association of EGFR expression with prognostic parameters like grade, lamina propria, deep muscle invasion and recurrence.

EGFR belongs to tyrosine kinase receptor family, all of which are encoded by c-erbB oncogenes. EGFR is the product of c-erbB1 proto-oncogene, which serves as a receptor for several growth factors like epidermal growth factor, transforming growth factor alpha, amphiregulin, heparin binding EGF like factor, betacellulin and epiregulin [7]. Activation of EGFR by one of its ligands leads to intracellular cascade of events resulting in transcriptional activation and cell proliferation [8, 9]. EGFR over expression occurs in many epithelial and solid malignancies like lung, breast and colon cancer. Several studies reported over expression of EGFR in bladder cancer. Results of most of the literature revealed that more than half of cases of bladder cancer overexpresses EGFR [10, 11]. Our data is in accordance with the reported literature; as we found significant association of EGFR expression with tumor grade, lamina propria and muscularis propria invasion; which are among most important prognostic factors in bladder cancer. Moreover, high frequency of recurrence was noted in patients with tumor showing intermediate and strong EGFR expression. Literature review revealed association of EGFR expression with high tumor grade, stage, tumor progression and poor clinical outcome

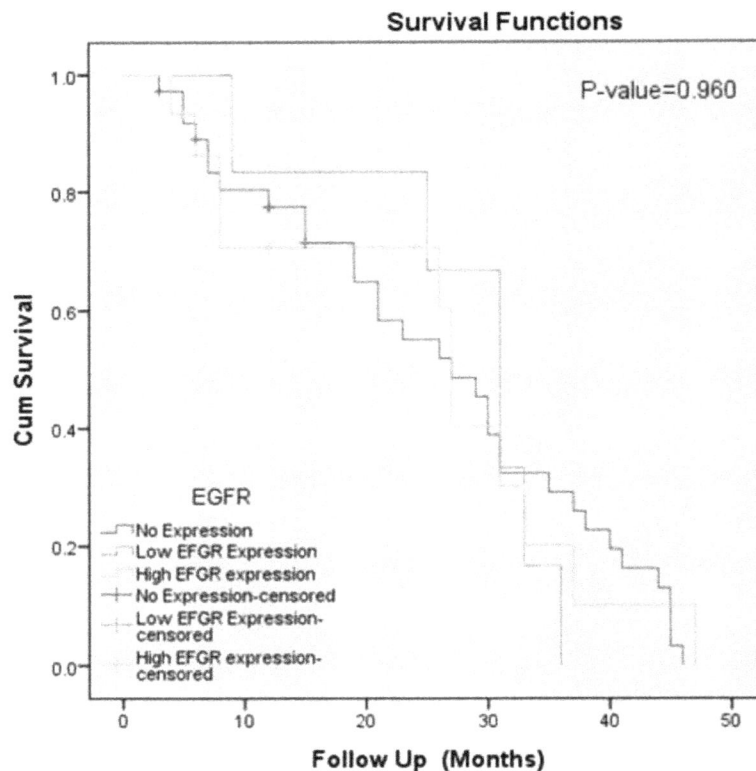

Fig. 2 Kalpien-Meier for EGFR overexpression (overall survival)

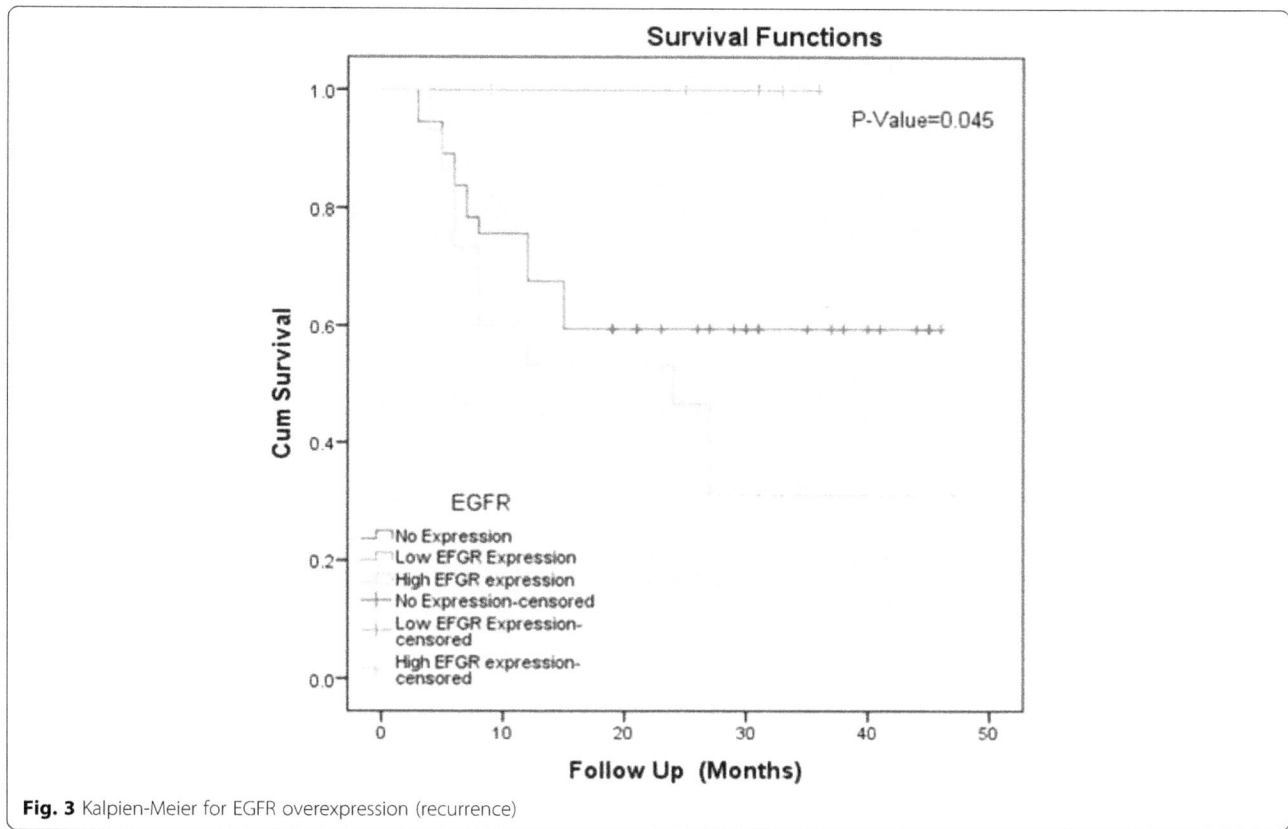

Fig. 3 Kalpien-Meier for EGFR overexpression (recurrence)

[6, 12, 13]. Carisson J et al., reported 71% EGFR expression in primary bladder tumors and co-expression of EGFR and Her2neu (c-erbB2) in more than half of patients [14]. Badaway AA et al., found EGFR expression in 86% cases of bladder cancer. They reported significant association of EGFR expression with grade and tumor stage [15]. Similarly, Arfaoni AT et al., reported statistically significant correlation of EGFR expression with tumor grade and stage [16].The mechanism of EGFR over expression resulting poor prognosis is still unclear. However, evidence suggests that activation of EGFR leads to activation of activator protein of transcription factor which results in induction of matrix metalloproteinases activity [17].

Conclusion

Significant association of EGFR overexpression with tumor grade, muscularis propria invasion and recurrence signifies its prognostic value; therefore EGFR can be used as a prognostic biomarker in Urothelial bladder carcinoma.

Abbreviation

EGFR: Epidermal growth factor receptor

Acknowledgments

We gratefully acknowledge all staff members of Pathology, Liaquat National Hospital, Karachi, Pakistan for their help and cooperation.

Authors' contributions

AAH and ZFH: main author of manuscript, have made substantial contributions to conception and design of study. MI, EYK and NF: been involved in drafting the manuscript, revising it critically for important intellectual content, and have been involved in requisition of data. HN, AK and MME have been involved in analysis of the data and revision of the manuscript. All authors read, revise and gave approval of the manuscript.

Competing interests

The authors declare that they have no competing interests.

Author details

[1]Liaquat National Hospital and Medical College, Karachi, Pakistan. [2]Brown University, Providence, RI, USA. [3]Kandahar University, Kandahar, Afghanistan.

References

1. Office of National Statistics. StatBase: cancer: incidence rates per 100,000 population 1998 by age and sex. London: ONS.
2. Lutzeyer W, Rubben H, Dahm H. Prognostic parameters in superficial bladder cancer: an analysis of 315 cases. J Urol. 1982;127:250–2.
3. Pearse HD, Reed RR, Hodges CV. Radical cystectomy for bladder cancer. J Urol. 1978;119:216–8.

4. Skinner DG, Lieskovsky G. Contemporary cystectomy with pelvic node dissection compared to preoperative radiation therapy plus cystectomy in the management of invasive bladder cancer. J Urol. 1984;131:1069–72.
5. Fitzpatrick JM, West AB, Butler MR, et al. Superficial bladder tumours (stages pTa, grade 1 and 2): the importance of recurrence pattern following initial resection. J Urol. 1986;135:920–2.
6. Neal DE, Sharples L, Smith K, et al. The epidermal growth factor receptor and the prognosis of bladder cancer. Cancer. 1990;65:1619–25.
7. Kondo I, Shimizu N. Mapping of the human gene for epidermal growth actor receptor (EGFR) on the p13 leads to q22 region of chromosome 7. Cytogenet Cell Genet. 1983;35:9–14.
8. Gullick WJ. Prevalence of aberrant expression of the epidermal growth factor receptor in human cancers. Br Med Bull. 1991;47:87–98.
9. Carpernter G, Cohen S. Epidermal growth factor receptor. J Biol Chem. 1990;265:7709–12.
10. Nicholson RI, Gee JMW, Harper MEEGFR. cancer prognosis. Eur J Cancer. 2001;37:S9–15.
11. Neal DE, Marsh C, Bennett MK, et al. Epidermal growth factor receptors in human bladder cancer: comparison of invasive and superficial tumours. Lancet 1985; i:366–368.
12. Nguyen PL, Swanson PE, Jaszcz W, et al. Expression of epidermal growth factor receptor in invasive transitional cell carcinoma of the urinary bladder: a multivariate survival analysis. Am J Clin Pathol. 1994;101:166–76.
13. Mellon JK, Wright C, Kelly P, et al. Long-term outcome related to EGFR status in bladder cancer. J Urol. 1995;153:919–25.
14. Carlsson J, Wester K, De La Torre M, Malmström PU, Gårdmark T. EGFR-expression in primary urinary bladder cancer and corresponding metastases and the relation to HER2-expression. On the possibility to target these receptors with radionuclides. Radiol Oncol. 2015 Mar 3;49(1):50–8.
15. Badawy AA, El-Hindawi A, Hammam O, Moussa M, Helal NS, Kamel A. Expression of epidermal growth factor receptor and transforming growth factor alpha in Cancer bladder: Schistosomal and non-Schistosomal. Curr Urol. 2017 Jan;9(4):192–201.
16. Arfaoui AT, Mejri S, Belhaj R, Karkni W, Chebil M, Rammeh S. Prognostic value of immunohistochemical expression profile of epidermal growth factor receptor in urothelial bladder cancer. J Immunoassay Immunochem. 2016;37(4):359–67.
17. Nutt JE, Mellon JK, Qureshi K, et al. Matrix metalloproteinase-1 is induced by epidermal growth factor in human bladder tumour cell lines and is detectable in the urine of patients with bladder tumours. Br J Cancer. 1998;78:215–20.

Efficacy analysis of self-help position therapy after holmium laser lithotripsy via flexible ureteroscopy

Jie Yang[1†], Rong-zhen Tao[1,3†], Pei Lu[1†], Meng-xing Chen[2], Xin-kun Huang[3], Ke-liang Chen[1], Ying-heng Huang[2], Xiao-rong He[2], Li-di Wan[2], Jing Wang[2], Xin Tang[2] and Wei Zhang[1*]

Abstract

Background: To observe the efficacy of self-help position therapy (SHPT) after holmium laser lithotripsy via flexible ureteroscopy (FURS).

Methods: From January 2010 to November 2015, 736 nephrolithiasis patients who had received FURS lithotripsy were analyzed retrospectively. In position group, 220 cases accepted SHPT after lithotripsies, and 428 cases as control, coming from another independent inpatient area in the same center. The stone-free status (SFS) between two groups were compared at the 2nd, 4th and 12th week ends by X-ray examinations.

Results: The preoperative incidence of hydronephrosis (25.9% vs. 18.0%, $p = 0.018$) or lower calyceal seeper (33.6% vs. 24.3%, $p = 0.012$) and the proportion of patients with > 2.0 cm stones (33.6% vs. 24.3%, $p = 0.003$) were all significantly higher in position group than in control group. There were no substantial difference between two groups in age, BMI, gender and medical histories. In postoperative followup, the incidence of hydronephrosis in position group was significantly lower than in control group (9.5% vs. 15.7%, $p = 0.032$) after removing double-J stents. In position group, the SFS of the 2nd week end (60.9% vs. 47.2%, $p = 0.001$), the 4th week end (74.1% vs. 62.8%, $p = 0.004$) and the 12th week end (86.9% vs. 79.4%, $p = 0.021$) were all significantly higher than those in control group.

Conclusions: SHPT after holmium laser lithotripsy via FURS may increase postoperative SFS, accelerate stone fragment clearance, and decrease the incidence of hydronephrosis after removal of double-J stents. The therapy does not require professional assistance and is economical, simple, and effective.

Keywords: Flexible ureteroscopy, Holmium laser lithotripsy, Self-help, Position therapy, Hydronephrosis

Background

Nephrolithiasis is one of the most frequently encountered diseases in urology practice. It varies in occurrence globally [1]. In 2011, the incidence was 1–5% in China and 2–19% in Western countries [2–4]. Minimally invasive procedures are being used more often for the treatment of nephrolithiasis. Flexible ureteroscopy (FURS) with holmium laser lithotripsy is the most popular and mature technology for small- and mid-size renal stones (≤2.5 cm). The documented advantages of FURS include minimal trauma, few complications, and rapid recuperation [5–7]. However, postoperative stone residue and fusion of drainable fragments (≤4 mm) are still intractable problems in clinical practice [8, 9]. Hyams et al. reported 120 cases undergoing FURS with holmium laser lithotripsy for renal stones 2–3 cm in size (mean 2.4 cm). During a 2-month follow-up, 56 (47%) patients were truly stone free, 20 (19%) had a residual burden of < 2 mm, and 24 (17%) had a residual burden of 2–4 mm [10]. Residual lower pole fragments < 2 mm in diameter can still be difficult to clear from the renal collecting system due to gravity and anatomy (the length and width

* Correspondence: trz1891597@126.com
†Equal contributors
[1]Department of Urology, First Affiliated Hospital of Nanjing Medical University, Nanjing 210029, Jiangsu, China
Full list of author information is available at the end of the article

of the lower caliceal infundibulum and the relative angle between the lower calyx and renal pelvis) [11–13].

To address this problem, the inversion-table treatment has been introduced for clinical use [14, 15]. It is a complicated operation requiring professional assistance and is expensive. These drawbacks have hindered its clinical application. The treatment is often unsuitable for patients with severe heart or brain vessel diseases.

Our long-term experience has indicated the value of self-help position therapy (SHPT) to increase the passive egress of stone fragments ≤4 mm in size. SHPT does not require professional assistance and appears to be safe, simple, effective, and suitable for most patients. To investigate its exact efficacy, data of 736 consecutive patients with nephrolithiasis who received holmium laser lithotripsy via FURS from January 2010 to November 2015 were retrospectively analyzed. The patients were divided into a position group and a control group to compare stone-expelling efficacy by postoperative stone free status (SFS) and stone expulsion time.

Methods
Patients
From January 2010 to November 2015, holmium laser lithotripsies via FURS were performed on a consecutive series of 736 adult patients with kidney stones by the same surgical team in our center. Applying strict inclusion criteria, 648 patients were ultimately included (Fig. 1). Outpatient and inpatient records for each enrollee were reviewed, which included admission and discharge records, laboratory examination reports, radiological images, operative records, and stone analysis reports. Information was collected in telephone or face-to-face interviews using a uniform questionnaire that consisted of general characteristics including population and practices between institutions, personal medical history including lithotripsy and double-J stent placement, lifestyle, occupational history, dietary habits, and family history. Consent for participation was obtained from all participants. This study was approved by the Ethic Committee of First Affiliated Hospital of Nanjing Medical University.

Perioperative and surgical procedure
All enrollees received a preoperative plain abdominal radiograph of the kidneys, ureters, and bladder (KUB) and unenhanced computed tomography (CT) to assess hydronephrosis and the size, location, and number of stones. The same imaging regimen was used for all

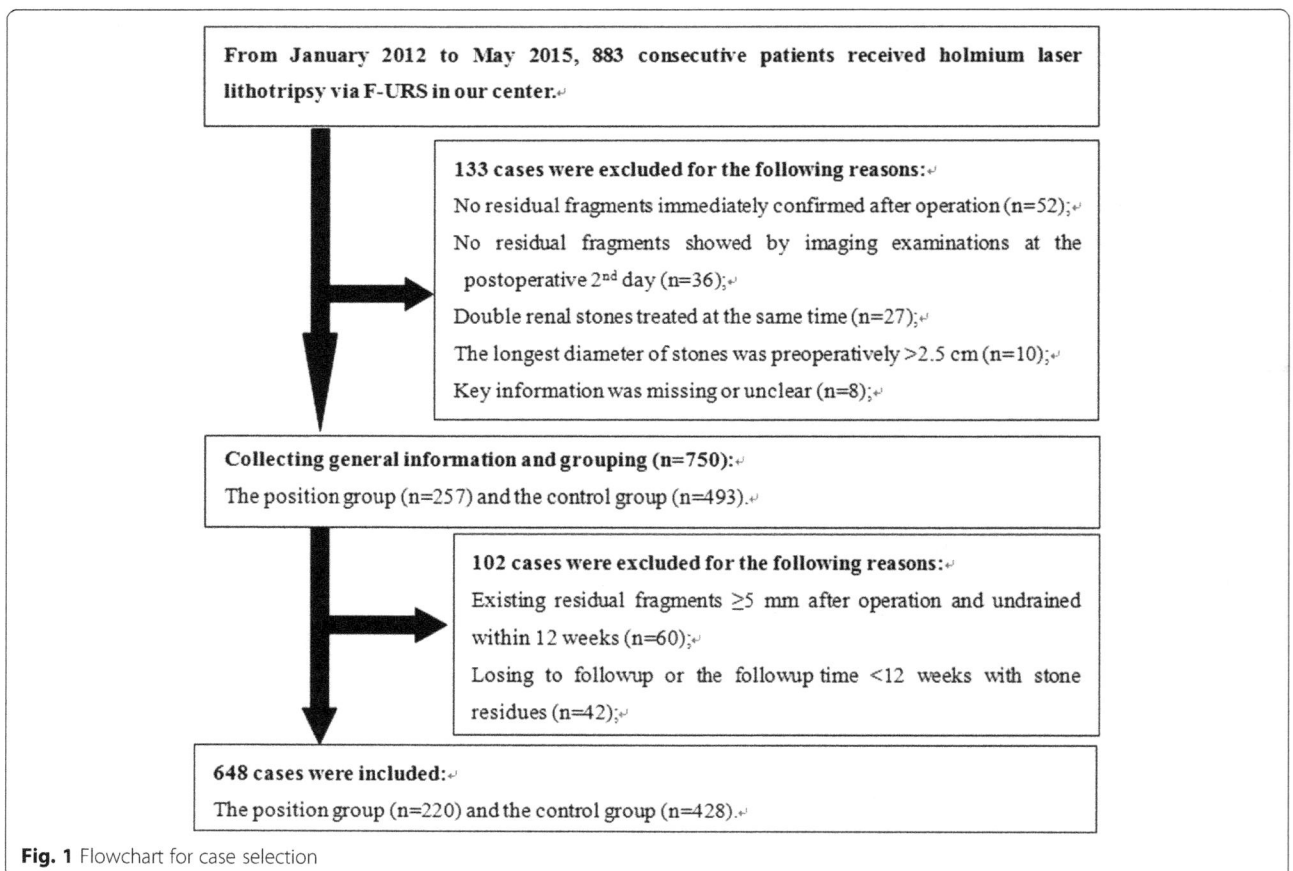

Fig. 1 Flowchart for case selection

patients. Stone size was determined by measuring the longest diameter on the preoperative radiologic images. In the case of multiple stones, the sum of the longest diameters of stones was used [16].

Patients were placed in a lithotomy position after general anesthesia, then a semirigid ureteroscope (8–9.8 F; Richard Wolf GmbH, Knittlingen, Germany) was retrogradely inserted into the upper urinary tract with the assistance of a Zebra guidewire (Cook Medical, Bloomington, IN, USA) to check the ureter and simplify the placement of a 12/14F ureteral access sheath (UAS; Cook Medical, Limerick, Ireland). A 7.5F fiberoptic FURS (P5; Olympus, Tokyo, Japan) was inserted into the renal pelvis via the UAS to search and fragment stones (≤2 mm). Fragmentation was done using a 200 um holmium laser fiber at an energy setting of 12–20 W based on the visually determined hardness of stones. Routinely, a 4.7F double-J stent (Bard Peripheral Vascular, Tempe, AZ, USA) was placed after lithotripsy. If the UAS could not be positioned due to ureter straitness, a 6F double-J stent (Bard Peripheral Vascular) was implanted for 2 weeks before lithotripsy.

A kidney, ureter, and bladder (KUB) examination was done on postoperative day 1. If residual fragments were found, patients in the position group were instructed to assume the SHPT, in which they adopted a contralateral head-down tilt position of at least 45° and maintained the position for 5 min (Fig. 2). The patients were instructed to perform the SHPT once a day during their hospitalization and for 12 weeks following discharge depending on the expelling efficacy of the stone. The control group comprised patients in another independent inpatient area of the same center. They were not given any information regarding position therapy for expelling of fragments. Both groups were suggested to receive medical expulsive therapy consisting of tamsulosin twice a day [17] and hydration with about 2 L of water each day. Implanted double-J stents were removed at postoperative 1–3 months on the basis of the stone-expelling efficacy.

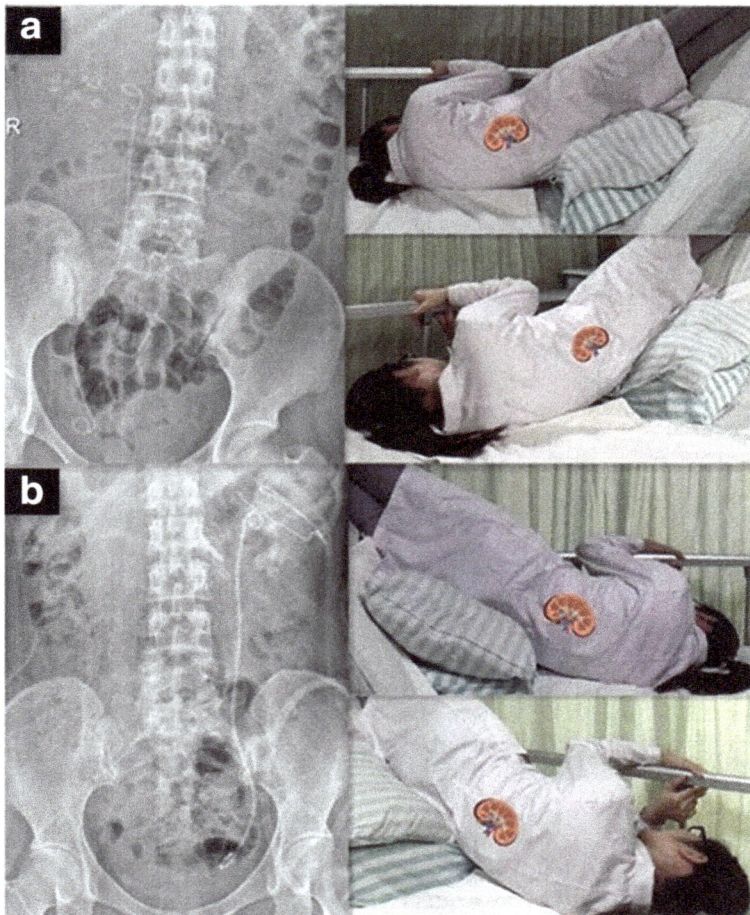

Fig. 2 The self-help position therapy (SHPT) after lithotripsies. **a** SHPT for right renal residual fragments; **b** SHPT for left renal residual fragments

Follow-up

Follow-up determinations included complete blood count, routine urinalysis, serum creatinine, and KUB examination. The determinations were done at postoperative week 2, 4, and 12 (Additional file 1: Figure S1). SFS was defined as no radiological evidence of stone or the presence of ≤2 mm asymptomatic fragments in the urinary tract [18–20].

Statistical analyses

SPSS v.16.0 for Windows (IBM Corp., Armonk, NY, USA) was used to perform statistical analyses. Continuous variables are presented as mean ± standard deviation. Patient demographics, follow-up time, and surgical outcomes between the two groups were compared using independent sample t test. The chi-squared test was used to compare other preoperative and postoperative clinical characteristics between the two groups. A p-value < 0.05 was considered significant.

Results

Demographics and preoperative clinical characteristics

The mean age at diagnosis in the position and control group was 46.4 and 44.1 years, respectively. The incidence of preoperative hydronephrosis (25.9% vs. 18.0%, p = 0.018) and lower calyceal seeper (33.6% vs. 24.3%, p = 0.012), and the proportion of patients with stones > 2.0 cm in size (33.6% vs. 24.3%, p = 0.003) were significantly higher in the position group than in the control group. The percentage of patients with stones that were exclusively located in the lower calyx was slightly and non-significantly higher in the position group than in the control group (47.3% vs. 37.6%, p = 0.164). There was no substantial difference between two groups in mean age, body mass index, gender, history of hypertension and diabetes, history of preoperative extracorporeal shock-wave lithotomy (ESWL), and nephrolithiasis surgery, preoperative renal function, and history of double-J stents placement (all p > 0.05) (Table 1).

Surgical outcomes and postoperative clinical characteristics

In postoperative follow-up, the incidence of hydronephrosis in the position group was significantly lower than in the control group (9.5% vs. 15.7%, p = 0.032). SFS in the position group was significantly higher than in the control group at week 2 (60.9% vs. 47.2%, p = 0.001), week 4 (74.1% vs. 62.8%, p = 0.004), and week 12 (86.9% vs. 79.4%, p = 0.021). However, there was no statistical significance between the groups concerning operative time, HGB decrease, hospital stay, postoperative anal aerofluxus time, stone composition, and postoperative renal function (all p > 0.05) (Table 2).

Table 1 Comparisons of patients' demographics and preoperative clinical characteristics between the two groups

Variables, mean ± SD or n (%)	Position group (n = 220)	Control group (n = 428)	P value
Age, year	46.4 ± 5.3	44.1 ± 3.7	0.782
BMI, kg/m2	22.1 ± 2.7	23.3 ± 1.5	0.635
Gender			
Male	123 (55.9)	222 (51.9)	–
Female	97 (44.1)	206 (48.1)	0.329
Hypertension history			
No	160 (72.7)	328 (76.6)	–
Yes	60 (27.3)	100 (23.4)	0.275
Diabetes history			
No	201 (91.4)	383 (89.5)	–
Yes	19 (8.6)	45 (10.5)	0.448
Stone size, cm			
< 1.0 cm	37 (16.8)	106 (24.8)	–
1.0–2.0 cm	109 (49.6)	218 (50.9)	0.108
2.0–2.5 cm	74 (33.6)	104 (24.3)	0.003**
Stone locations			
Pelvis or upper calyx	83 (37.7)	166 (38.8)	–
Middle calyx	33 (15.0)	101 (23.6)	0.077
Lower calyx	104 (47.3)	161 (37.6)	0.164
ESWL history			
No	115 (52.3)	245 (57.2)	–
Yes	105 (47.7)	183 (42.8)	0.228
Nephrolithiasis operation histories[a]			
No	164 (74.5)	297 (69.4)	–
Yes	56 (25.5)	131 (30.7)	0.170
Preoperative hydronephrosis			
No	163 (74.1)	351 (82.0)	–
Yes	57 (25.9)	77 (18.0)	0.018*
Preoperative lower calyceal seeper			
No	146 (66.4)	324 (75.7)	–
Yes	74 (33.6)	104 (24.3)	0.012*
Preoperative renal function			
Normal	199 (90.5)	394 (92.0)	–
Abnormal	21 (9.5)	34 (8.0)	0.488
Double-J stents placed histories			
No	140 (63.6)	288 (67.3)	–
Yes	80 (36.4)	140 (32.7)	0.352

BMI body mass index, *SD* standard deviation, *ESWL* extracorporeal shock wave lithotripsy
[a]Nephrolithiasis operation histories include flexible ureteroscope lithotripsy, percutaneous nephrolithotomy or nephrolithotomy
*p < 0.05, **p < 0.01

Table 2 Comparisons of surgical outcomes and postoperative clinical characteristics between two groups

Variables, mean ± SD or n (%)	Position group (n = 220)	Control group (n = 428)	P value
Follow-up, month	3.3 ± 0.4	3.6 ± 0.4	0.417
Surgical outcomes			
operative time, hour	1.7 ± 0.6	1.5 ± 0.5	0.243
HGB decrease (g/L)	4.9 ± 3.4	5.3 ± 3.7	0.915
Hospital stay, day	1.8 ± 0.4	1.9 ± 0.5	0.973
Postoperative anal aerofluxus time, day	1.2 ± 0.3	1.1 ± 0.4	0.853
Stone compositions			
Calcium oxalate	127 (57.7)	257 (60.0)	–
Struvite	51 (23.2)	84 (19.6)	0.322
Calcium phosphate	42 (19.1)	87 (20.4)	0.914
Postoperative renal function			
Normal	209 (95.1)	410 (95.8)	–
Abnormal	11 (4.9)	18 (4.2)	0.643
Postoperative hydronephrosis			
No	199 (90.5)	361 (84.3)	–
Yes	21 (9.5)	67 (15.7)	0.032*
SFS at the 2nd week end			
No	86 (39.1)	226 (52.8)	–
Yes	134 (60.9)	202 (47.2)	0.001**
SFS at the 4th week end			
No	57 (25.9)	159 (37.1)	
Yes	163 (74.1)	269 (62.9)	0.004**
SFS at the 12th week end			
No	29 (13.1)	88 (20.6)	
Yes	191 (86.9)	340 (79.4)	0.021*

SD standard deviation, HGB hemoglobin, SFS stone free status
*p < 0.05, **p < 0.01

Discussion

The clinical application of FURS was first reported in 1964 [21]. Since then, the equipment and optical imaging system have evolved quickly. FURS with holmium laser, which allows retrograde access to any calices of the renal collecting system, has increasingly become the first-line therapy for renal calculi, especially for patients with blood coagulation dysfunction, renal insufficiency, obesity, isolated kidney, or undergoing failed lithotripsies of ESWL or percutaneous nephrolithotomy (PCNL) [22–24].

The SFR is 70–90% after holmium laser lithotripsy using FURS at 3 months postoperatively [8, 9]. However, residual stone and gravel fusion remain troublesome problems. Residual calculi ≤2 mm in size in the absence of obstruction or infection are defined as clinically insignificant residual fragments [19, 20]. Although these fragments are usually clinically insignificant, they might

enlarge and lead to infection or obstruction of the urinary tract. In a study of 384 patients undergoing FURS, clinically insignificant residual fragments were present in 44 (11.5%) patients by abdominal CT from postoperative 3 weeks to 3 months [25]. Among them, 15 patients showed symptoms resulting from the enlargement or fusion of residual gravels. Therefore, promoting the discharge of clinically insignificant residual fragments from the urinary tract as soon as possible is prudent following lithotripsy.

Methods promoting the elimination of residual gravel and increasing postoperative SFR include drug-mediated dissolution of stones or stone discharge by movement or an inverted position. Position therapy has proven especially effective for lower pole residual gravel. Lower calices are the lowest parts of the renal collecting system, and are usually 2–3 cm distant from the calyceal bottom to the pelvic openings [26]. The distance will increase significantly with seeper in lower calices. Therefore, the lower pole residual stones are commonly difficult to expel with urine in the upright position due to the gravity and postoperative hydronephrosis, even if they have broken into small (< 2 mm) pieces. The effectiveness of inversion positioning prompted our center to initiate SHPT after holmium laser lithotripsy via FURS beginning in 2010 (Fig. 2), particularly for patients with preoperative hydronephrosis (Table 1).

Postoperative position therapy is also imperative for patients with large kidney stones (≤4 mm) after lithotripsy. If the stone pieces are not excreted during the first 3 months postoperatively, they will tend to fuse or growth, which can result in obstruction or infection in the urinary tract. Presently, although the preoperative rates of hydronephrosis and lower calyceal seeper were significantly higher in the position group than in the control group, the incidence of hydronephrosis was conspicuously lower in the position group after removal of double-J stents (Table 2). This highlights the importance of the timely expulsion of residual stones.

The discharge efficacy of residual stones with the assistance of inversion-table treatment has been confirmed. Pace et al. reported that a 60-degree tilt inversion combined with mechanical percussion effectively renders residual lower caliceal region stone-free, with a substantially higher SFR than that of the control group (40% vs. 3%, p < 0.01) 3 months after ESWL [14]. Another study also showed that inversion-table treatment group had higher SFR than control group in patients with lower calyceal stones undergoing FURS lithotripsy (97.4% vs. 81.8%, p < 0.05) [15]. However, the exact effect of an economic and easy-to-do SHPT has not been described. To provide clarity, the present retrospective study was undertaken to analyze the effect of SHPT in a consecutive cohort at our hospital. The

position group still had a significantly higher SFS than the control group, although the preoperative incidence of hydronephrosis or lower calyceal seeper and the proportion of patients with stones > 2.0 cm in size were both higher in position group. Especially, at postoperative week 2, the difference of SFS between the two groups was most significant (60.9% vs. 47.2%, $p = 0.001$). Thereafter the difference gradually lessening, but it remained statistically significant at week 12 (86.9% vs. 79.4%, $p = 0.021$) (Table 2). This indicates that inversion exceeding 45-degrees in a head-down position can speed up the expulsion of residual stones and compensate for the deficiency of gravel deposition in lower calices after renal stones are broken into < 2 mm pieces (the standard of CIRF) using FURS lithotripsy.

Our study chronicles the good curative effect of SHPT after holmium laser lithotripsy via FURS. However, therapeutic planning still needs to be individualized and optimized with respect to start time, frequency, duration, and inversion angles.

The study also has some limitations. It is a retrospective study, lacking the characteristics of random grouping and high homogeneity of patients between groups. Furthermore, we did not compare SHPT with inversion-table treatment in the effectiveness of expelling residual stones. Finally, the study is a single center study with relatively small sample size. There is the possibility of sampling error.

Conclusions

SHPT after holmium laser lithotripsy via FURS may increase postoperative SFS, accelerate stone fragment clearance, and decrease the incidence of hydronephrosis after removal of double-J stents. The therapy does not require professional assistance and is economical, simple, and effective. A prospective randomized controlled trial should be performed.

Abbreviations
CIRF: Clinically insignificant residual fragments; CT: Computed tomography; ESWL: Extracorporeal shock-wave lithotomy; FURS: Flexible ureteroscopy; KUB: Kidneys, ureters and bladder; PCNL: Percutaneous nephrolithotomy; SFR: Stone-free rate; SFS: Stone free status; SHPT: Self-help position therapy

Acknowledgements
JY and PL conceived and designed the study. JY and RZT drafted the manuscript. JY and RZT revised the manuscript. WZ provided technical help and writing assistance. All authors have read and approved the final version.

Funding
This study received no specific grant from any funding agency in the public, commercial or not-for-profit sectors.

Authors' contributions
JY and PL conceived and designed the study; YHH, XRH, LDW, XT and JW as corresponding researchers collected clinical information and interviewed patients in five medical teams; MXC and XKH organized and input the data; KLC checked and verified data input by MXC and XKH; RZT and WZ performed statistical analyses; JY and RZT drafted the manuscript; JY and RZT revised the manuscript. All authors have read and approved the final manuscript.

Competing interests
The authors declare that they have no competing interests.

Author details
[1]Department of Urology, First Affiliated Hospital of Nanjing Medical University, Nanjing 210029, Jiangsu, China. [2]First Clinical Medical College, Nanjing Medical University, Nanjing, Jiangsu, China. [3]Department of Urology, The Affiliated Jiangning Hospital with Nanjing Medical University, Nanjing, Jiangsu, China.

References
1. Trinchieri A. Epidemiology of urolithiasis. Arch Ital Urol Androl. 1996;68:203–49.
2. Zeng Q, He Y. Age-specific prevalence of kidney stones in Chinese urban inhabitants. Urolithiasis. 2013;41(1):91–3.
3. Turk C, Knoll T, Petrik A, et al. Guidelines on Urolithiasis. European Association of Urology: Arnhem; 2013.
4. Na YQ, Ye ZQ, Sun ZY, et al. The guideline of Chinese Association of Urology. Chinese Association of Urology: Beijing; 2011. p. 209.
5. Xu C, Song RJ, Jiang MJ, Qin C, Wang XL, Zhang W. Flexible ureteroscopy with holmium laser lithotripsy: a new choice for intrarenal stone patients. Urol Int. 2015;94(1):93–8.
6. Ding J, Xu D, Cao Q, et al. Comparing the efficacy of a multimodular flexible Ureteroscope with its conventional counterpart in the Management of Renal Stones. Urology. 2015;86(2):224–9.
7. Miernik A, Wilhelm K, Ardelt P, et al. Standardized flexible ureteroscopic technique to improve stone-free rates. Urology. 2012;80:1198–202.
8. Osman Y, Harraz AM, El-Nahas AR, et al. Clinically insignificant residual fragments: an acceptable term in the computed tomography era? Urology. 2013;81(4):723–6.
9. Delvecchio FC, Preminger GM. Management of residual stones. The Urol Clin North Am. 2000;27(2):347–54. 10778476
10. Hyams ES, Munver R, Bird VG, Uberoi J, Shah O. Flexible ureterorenoscopy and holmium laser lithotripsy for the management of renal stone burdens that measure 2 to 3 cm: a multi-institutional experience. J Endourol. 2010; 24(10):1583–8.
11. Burr J, Ishii H, Simmonds N, Somani BK. Is flexible ureterorenoscopy and laser lithotripsy the new gold standard for lower pole renal stones when compared to shock wave lithotripsy: comparative outcomes from a university hospital over similar time period. Cent European J Urol. 2015; 68(2):183–6.
12. Kosar A, Ozturk A, Serel TA, et al. Effect of vibration massage therapy after extracorporeal shockwave lithotripsy in patients with lower caliceal stones. J Endourol. 1999;13:705.
13. Sampaio FJ, Aragao AH. Limitations of extracorporeal shockwave lithotripsy for lower caliceal stones: anatomic insight. J Endourol. 1994;8:241.
14. Pace KT, Tariq N, Dyer SJ, Weir MJ, RJ DAH. Mechanical percussion, inversion and diuresis for residual lower pole fragments after shock wave lithotripsy: a prospective, single blind, randomized controlled trial. J Urol. 2001;166(6): 2065–71.
15. Chiong E, Hwee ST, Kay LM, Liang S, Kamaraj R, Esuvaranathan K. Randomized controlled study of mechanical percussion, diuresis, and inversion therapy to assist passage of lower pole renal calculi after shock wave lithotripsy. Urology. 2005;65(6):1070–4.
16. Tiselius H-G, Andersson A. Stone burden in an average Swedish population of stone formers requiring active stone removal: how can the stone size be estimated in the clinical routine? Eur Urol. 2003;43:275–81.
17. Yilmaz E, Batislam E, Basar MM. The comparison and efficacy of 3 different alpha1-adrenergic blockers for distal ureteral stones[J]. J Urol. 2005;173
18. Ghani KR, Wolf JS Jr. What is the stone-free rate following flexible ureteroscopy for kidney stones? Nat Rev Urol. 2015;12(7):363.

19. Dauw CA, Simeon L, Alruwaily AF, et al. Contemporary practice patterns of flexible Ureteroscopy for treating renal stones: results of a worldwide survey. J Endourol. 2015;29(11):1221–30.
20. Huang ZC, Fu FJ, Zhong ZH, et al. Flexible ureteroscopy and laser lithotripsy for bilateral multiple intrarenal stones: is this a valuable choice? Urology. 2012;80:800–4.
21. Marshall VF. Fiber optics in urology. J Urol. 1964;91:110–4.
22. Wen CC, Nakada SY. Treatment selection and outcomes: renal calculi. Urol Clin North Am. 2007;34(3):409–19.
23. Breda A, Ogunyemi O, Leppert JT, Lam JS, Schulam PG. Flexible ureteroscopy and laser lithotripsy for single intrarenal stones 2 cm or greater–is this the new frontier? J Urol. 2008;179(3):981–4.
24. Xu G, Wen J, Li Z, et al. A comparative study to analyze the efficacy and safety of flexible ureteroscopy combined with holmium laser lithotripsy for residual calculi after percutaneous nephrolithotripsy. Int J Clin Exp Med. 2015;8(3):4501–7.
25. Ozgor F, Simsek A, Binbay M, et al. Clinically insignificant residual fragments after flexible ureterorenoscopy: medium-term follow-up results. Urolithiasis. 2014;42(6):533–8.
26. Wolf JS Jr. Is lower pole caliceal anatomy predictive of extracorporeal shock wave lithotripsy success for primary lower pole kidney stones? Int Braz J Urol. 2002;28(6):572–3.

The effect of mirabegron, used for overactive bladder treatment, on female sexual function: a prospective controlled study

A. Zachariou[1,5]* (iD), C. Mamoulakis[2], M. Filiponi[3], F. Dimitriadis[1], J. Giannakis[1], S. Skouros[1], P. Tsounapi[4], A. Takenaka[4] and N. Sofikitis[1]

Abstract

Background: Aim of the study was to determine the effect of mirabegron, used for overactive bladder (OAB) treatment, on female sexual function.

Methods: Eighty five sexually active women suffering from overactive bladder were prospectively enrolled in this study. Females were divided into two groups. In Group A (control), 48 patients received no treatment and in Group B, 37 patients received mirabegron 50 mg/daily for 3 months. Patients were evaluated with FSFI-Gr at the beginning of the study and again after a period of 3 months.

Results: In Group B, there was a significant increase post-treatment compared to baseline ($p < 0.001$) in total FSFI (20.3 (3.8) to 26.6 (4.2)) and all domains (desire: 3.0 (1.2) to 4.8 (1.2)), arousal: 3.0 (0.8) to 4.8 (0.9), lubrication: 3.9 (1.1) to 4.8 (1.2), orgasm: 3.6 (0.8) to 4.8 (1.0), satisfaction: 3.2 (0.4) to 4.0 (0.8) and pain: 3.2 (0.8) to 4.4 (1.2)). In Group A, there were no statistically significant changes in pre- and post-observation values.

Conclusions: This study is one of the few demonstrating that management of OAB with mirabegron improves female sexual function.

Keywords: Female sexual dysfunction, Mirabegron, Overactive bladder

Background

Overactive bladder (OAB) is defined by the International Continence Society (ICS) as urinary urgency in the absence of any known infection or other obvious pathology. OAB is usually characterized by frequency and nocturia, but may or may not cause urinary incontinence [1]. It has been shown to affect up to 36% of adult women in Europe and US [2, 3].

Although not life threatening, OAB is a debilitating disease which can substantially impede the quality of life,

resulting in low self-esteem, anxiety, depression, impairment of work productivity and increase in the number of falls and fractures [4]. Women with OAB experience increased incidence of sexual problems, sometimes with consequent personal distress and sexual partner compatibility issues. [5]. The impact of OAB symptoms on sexual function in women has been evaluated in a few studies [6–9]. Patel et al. [6] reported that 25% of their female OAB population had some degree of sexual dysfunction, meaning that OAB has a greater effect on female sexual health than it does urinary incontinence.

Female sexual dysfunction (FSD) is traditionally classified into disorders of desire, arousal, lubrication, orgasm and pain. In the absence of detailed epidemiological data, current estimates have up to 43% of women complaining of at least one sexual issue [10]. Women are at

* Correspondence: zachariou@otenet.gr
Presented at the 19th Congress of the European Society of Sexual Medicine 2017 in Nice, France, February 1-3, 2017
[1]Department of Urology, School of Medicine, Ioannina University, Ioannina, Greece
[5]3 Spyridi Street, 38221 Volos, Greece
Full list of author information is available at the end of the article

risk of developing FSD due to physiologic, iatrogenic and psychological factors. Lower tract urinary tract infections are a further, independent FSD cause [10, 11]. To identify FSD, appropriate assessment guidelines should be applied. So as to ascertain sexual history and enable assessment, there are a number of self-reporting questionnaires available. The Female Sexual Function Index (FSFI) is a concise, multidimensional "gold standard" tool which is regarded in high-esteem [12].

Recently introduced as an oral treatment for OAB, mirabegron (a β3-adrenergic agonist compound) improves storage capacity of bladder without inducing anticholinergic adverse events [13]. In four, large–scale 12-week phase III studies [14–17], a pooled analysis [18] and 12-month study [19], mirabegron consistently demonstrated superiority over placebo with respect to reductions in incontinence episodes and micturition frequency, with a similar incidence of adverse effects as the placebo.

The objective of the current study is to evaluate the effect of the β3-adrenoceptor agonist, mirabegron, as used for OAB treatment on the sexual function of women (employing FSFI-Gr, a validated questionnaire translated into the Greek language).

Methods

Between January 2016 and December 2016, 85 sexually active women with confirmed OAB, had referred to the Urogynecology outpatient clinic and were prospectively enrolled in this study. OAB was determined using the International Continence Society definition [1]. The urination frequency of all women was 8 or more times a day, with urge symptoms independent of incontinence. OAB was present in all women for a minimum of 3 months and none of the women had undergone prior treatment for the condition. Other inclusion criteria were the willing of women to comply with the protocol and the capability to complete the voiding diaries and the questionnaires without assistance.

Subjects were excluded from inclusion if they had clinically significant stress urinary incontinence, neurogenic bladder and urinary retention or were at risk of these conditions. Women with a history of pelvic muscle training programs were excluded because it is accepted that pelvic floor muscle exercises improve female sexual function [20]. The protocol for the research project was approved by ELPIS HOSPITAL Ethics Committee and informed consent was taken from all the women.

The inclusion criteria also integrated women over the age of 18 being in a sexually active relationship. Women who stated that they were not sexually active were asked to indicate the reason and were excluded from further analysis. Women who considered that there was no need

for long-term treatment for OAB or were afraid of regimen's adverse effects were included in control group.

Patients were assessed using a comprehensive history, a detailed general and neurological physical examination, as well FSFI. According to the latest report of the International Consultation on Sexual Medicine, the FSFI remains the "gold standard" assessment tool, has a level of evidence 1 and recommendation grade A, for evaluating female sexual dysfunction [21]. Item selection and categories were based on the American Foundation for Urological Diseases classification system of female sexual dysfunction. Furthermore, FSFI has been translated and validated in the Greek language [22]. All women were asked to complete the Greek version of the FSFI, which evaluates the four phases of female sexual function and categorizes sexual dysfunction in the domains of (a) desire (b) arousal (c) lubrication (d) orgasm (e) satisfaction and (f) pain. The development of a scoring system, whereby higher scores indicate a healthier condition allowed the attainment of individual domain scores. Wiegel et al. [23] found that a total FSFI score of 26.5 is the optimal cut-off score for differentiating women with and without sexual dysfunction. We used the same cut-off scores in order to have comparable results with matching papers.

To determine the eligible women all females were asked to answer the question: "Do you have sexual distress associated with sexual dysfunction?" and only women who gave a negative answer were finally recruited for analysis, since sexual distress needs special questionnaires to be evaluated. Patients were divided into two groups. Group A, which is defined as a control group, consisted of 48 women. None of these females with OAB wished to receive any therapy. On the other hand, in Group B, 37 patients with OAB were treated with mirabegron 50 mg daily for 3 months.

Patients of Group A (without OAB therapy) completed a 3 day micturition diary prior to and after 3 month-observation-period. Patients of Group B completed a 3 day micturition diary prior to and immediately after the third month of mirabegron treatment. For each episode of urinary symptoms, the patient recorded the date and time, regardless of the presence of urgency and/or incontinence, the volume voided and the influence of the episode (of urinary symptoms) on the patient's sleep. All women within Group B attended monthly office visits to ensure patients' compliance with the treatment. In Group A, all women attended monthly office visits to ensure that they did not have any pharmacotherapy or behavioral therapy for OAB. Within Group A and Group B, voiding frequency, nocturia, urgency episodes, incontinent episodes, number of incontinence pads used, and voided volume were measured post-treatment using the 3 day micturition diary. All patients completed the FSFI questionnaire at the beginning and after the completion of the 3 month study.

All outcome variables were tested for normality using the Shapiro-Wilk W test. Concretely, the following continues/ordinal variables were tested per group: age, body weight, symptom duration, parity; pre- and post-observation/treatment FSFI domains (desire, arousal, lubrication, orgasm, satisfaction, pain), total score of sexual function and percentage (%) improvement in total score of sexual function; pre- and post-observation/treatment episodes of frequency, urgency, nocturia, incontinence; number of pads needed; and voided volumes. The potential presence of any correlation was investigated between the % of improvement in LUTS/incontinence and in sexual function (separately for each parameter) in order to evaluate the effect of OAB improvement on sexual function. Finally, % improvement in total score of sexual function was compared between groups and a multivariate linear regression analysis was performed in order to investigate the effect of several independent parameters on sexual function. The % improvement in total score of sexual function was used as dependent variable. The % improvements in frequency, urgency, nocturia, incontinence episodes, number of pads needed and voided volume were considered as independent variables. Data were analyzed using IBM Corp. Released 2016. IBM SPSS Statistics for Windows, Version 24.0. Armonk, NY: IBM Corp. Two-tailed $p < 0.050$ was considered significant.

Results

All tested variables showed significant departures from the normal distribution. The only exceptions were the pre- and post-observation/treatment total scores of sexual function and the voided volumes. Consequently, non-parametric tests (Mann Whitney U test and Wilcoxon signed-rank test, respectively) were performed for all comparisons (for uniformity purposes) between and within groups, respectively; all data are presented as medians (interquartile ranges; IQRs).

Among the 48 women who reported sexual activity in the last 4 weeks from Group A, 11 women reported during the monthly visits that they had decided to follow pharmacotherapy/behavioral therapy for OAB and were therefore excluded from the study. Furthermore, 2 women from Group A and 2 women from Group B refused to complete the FSFI questionnaire at the end of 3 month period and were also excluded. There were no adverse reactions from mirabegron administration during the study.

Demographic characteristics and baseline OAB/sexual scores did not differ significantly between groups (Table 1). Sixty-five percent of patients in Group B who were incontinent at baseline became continent by the study-endpoint. Furthermore, all urinary outcomes, all

Table 1 Demographic characteristics and baseline OAB/sexual scores of participants

Variable	Group A	Group B	P value
Age (yr)	43.5 (10.0)	43 (10)	0.838
Body weight (kg)	59.0 (14.0)	55.0 (14.0)	0.406
Symptom duration (yr)	4.2 (1.5)	4.2 (3.3)	0.821
Parity	2.0 (2.0)	2.0 (1.0)	0.738
Frequency	11.0 (1.0)	11.0 (2.0)	0.213
Urgency episodes	6.5 (1.0)	7.0 (2.0)	0.303
Nocturia episodes	2.0 (1.0)	2.0 (1.0)	0.227
Incontinence episodes	2.0 (1.0)	2.0 (1.0)	0.287
Incontinence pads	5.0 (2.0)	4.0 (2.0)	0.838
Voided volume (ml)	121.5 (31.0)	117.0 (33.0)	0.725
Desire	3.0 (0.6)	3.0 (1.2)	0.411
Arousal	3.6 (0.6)	3.0 (0.8)	0.281
Lubrication	3.6 (0.9)	3.9 (1.1)	0.214
Orgasm	3.6 (0.4)	3.6 (0.8)	0.253
Satisfaction	3.2 (0.4)	3.2 (0.8)	0.099
Pain	3.2 (0.4)	3.2 (0.8)	0.068
Total Score of Sexual Function	20.0 (2.5)	20.3 (3.8)	0.355

FSFI domain scores and the total score of sexual function improved significantly in Group B at 3 months, in contrast to Group A (Tables 2, 3 and 4). Spearman's rank-order correlation test yielded statistically significant (negative) correlations between % improvement in LUTS/incontinence and % improvement in sexual function were detected exclusively in Group B (frequency-lubrication, nocturia-arousal, incontinence-sexual satisfaction; Table 5).

Total score of sexual function improvement (%) differed significantly between groups (Group A vs. Group

Table 2 Urinary evaluation of the participants

Group A	Pre-observation	Post-observation	P value
Frequency	11.0 (1.0)	11.0 (1.0)	0.200
Urgency episodes	6.5 (1.0)	7.0 (1.0)	0.093
Nocturia episodes	2.0 (1.0)	1.0 (1.0)	0.231
Incontinence episodes	2.0 (1.0)	2.0 (2.0)	0.332
Incontinence pads	5.0 (2.0)	5.0 (2.0)	0.231
Voided volume (ml)	121.5 (31.0)	114.5 (27.0)	0.001
Group B	Pre-treatment	Post-treatment	P value
Frequency	11.0 (2.0)	9.0 (2.0)	< 0.001
Urgency episodes	7.0 (2.0)	4.0 (2.0)	< 0.001
Nocturia	2.0 (1.0)	1.0 (1.0)	< 0.001
Incontinence episodes	2.0 (1.0)	1.0 (1.0)	< 0.001
Incontinence pads	4.0 (2.0)	2.0 (2.0)	< 0.001
Voided volume (ml)	117.0 (33.0)	148.0 (26.0)	< 0.001

Table 3 Comparison of pre-observation and post-observation FSFI in Group A

	Pre-observation	Post-observation	P value
Desire	3.0 (0.6)	3.0 (0.6)	0.524
Arousal	3.6 (0.6)	3.6 (0.6)	0.628
Lubrication	3.6 (0.9)	3.9 (0.6)	0.713
Orgasm	3.6 (0.4)	3.6 (0.4)	0.505
Satisfaction	3.2 (0.4)	2.8 (0.4)	0.109
Pain	3.2 (0.4)	3.2 (0.8)	0.424
Total Score of Sexual Function	20.0 (2.5)	19.8 (2.0)	0.609

B: 1.0 (3.7) vs. 32.6 (7.9); $p < 0.001$. Multivariate linear regression analysis run to predict % improvement in total score of sexual function from group, as well as % improvements in frequency, urgency, nocturia, incontinence episodes, number of pads needed and voided volume revealed that Group and % improvements in frequency statistically significantly predicted % improvement in total score of sexual function, $F(7, 77) = 141.970$, $p < .001$, $R^2 = 0.928$. All seven variables added statistically significantly to the prediction, $p < 0.001$. The multivariate linear regression model is presented in Table 6.

Discussion

This study is one of the few, to our knowledge, to demonstrate the effect of mirabegron, the first β-3 adrenoceptor agonist, on sexual function of women suffering from OAB. Our data has indicated that after 3 months evaluation, females with OAB receiving mirabegron 50 mg revealed statistically significant changes in FSFI total score and all subscales.

OAB symptoms, urinary incontinence and sexual health in general are topics many find difficult to discuss. Not only may stigma make sufferers reluctant to approach a health professional, but it may also make health professionals embarrassed to confront patients. Self-reporting rather than interview-administered questionnaires greatly reduce this barrier. As FSFI allows a quantitative evaluation and can be used to study sexuality changes after therapeutic intervention, it has a distinct advantage over other assessment tools like diaries

or calendars [24]. This tool is a reliable self-reporting measure of FSD which only requires 15 min to complete. Although it excludes issues involving personal stress, it measures outcomes of therapeutic response by design.

Female sexual dysfunctions can interfere with intimacy, affect a marital relationship and ultimately erode well-being and overall health. Although sexual dysfunction is more likely in women than men, clinical FSD trials are rare compared to the available burgeoning data on men. Furthermore, the amount of data related to the effect of treatment agents used for OAB on the sexual function of women is insufficient in the literature while study comparisons should be made with caution because of differences in study designs and population.

The use of anticholinergics as a first-line treatment for OAB is well documented. However, many large trials exclude sexual function change assessment after their administration. Tolterodine and oxybutynin are two anticholinergic medications with high quality evidence supporting improvement in sexual function with use. According to Hajebrahimi et al. [7], tolterodine IR significantly improved all domains of sexual function of women with OAB. The FSD was evaluated with the Arizona Sexual Experience Scale (ASEX), a five-topic questionnaire. Rogers et al. [25] evaluated the effect of short term treatment with tolterodine ER on FSD using the Pelvic Organ Prolapse/Urinary Incontinence Sexual Function Questionnaire (PISQ) and Sexual Quality of Life – Female (SQOL-F). OAB symptoms improved with tolterodine ER, as did the scores of sexual health and

Table 4 Comparison of pre-treatment and post-treatment FSFI in Group B

	Pre-observation	Post-observation	P value
Desire	3.0 (1.2)	4.8 (1.2)	< 0.001
Arousal	3.0 (0.8)	4.8 (0.9)	< 0.001
Lubrication	3.9 (1.1)	4.8 (1.2)	< 0.001
Orgasm	3.6 (0.8)	4.8 (1.0)	< 0.001
Satisfaction	3.2 (0.8)	4.0 (0.8)	< 0.001
Pain	3.2 (0.8)	4.4 (1.2)	< 0.001
Total Score of Sexual Function	20.3 (3.8)	26.6 (4.2)	< 0.001

Table 5 Correlation between improvements (%) in lower urinary tract symptoms & female sexual function

	Desire		Arousal		Lubrication		Orgasm		Satisfaction		Pain		Total FSFI	
	r_s	P	r_s	P	r_s	P	r_s	P	r_s	P	r_s	P	r_s	P
Group A														
Frequency	−0.088	0.553	0.220	0.298	−0.201	0.171	−0.237	0.104	0.015	0.918	−0.105	0.479	−0.254	0.081
Urgency	0.168	0.253	0.041	0.781	−0.195	0.199	−0.240	0.135	0.035	0.815	0.013	0.928	−0.224	0.127
Nocturia	0.209	0.154	0.157	0.286	−0.188	0.201	0.062	0.674	0.240	0.101	−0.054	0.714	0.181	0.219
Incontinence	−0.007	0.960	0.158	0.283	0.134	0.364	−0.270	0.064	0.101	0.496	−0.076	0.610	−0.026	0.858
Pads	−0.114	0.442	−0.076	0.607	−0.076	0.609	−0.180	0.114	0.119	0.422	−0.128	0.384	−0.222	0.150
Voided Volume	0.041	0.782	−0.067	0.651	−0.114	0.441	−0.010	0.948	0.228	0.119	0.126	0.393	0.077	0.603
Group B														
Frequency	0.103	0.545	−0.284	0.089	−0.429	0.008	0.139	0.413	−0.037	0.826	−0.230	0.170	−0.267	0.110
Urgency	0.005	0.977	−0.002	0.991	0.163	0.335	−0.119	0.484	0.253	0.132	0.011	0.946	0.008	0.638
Nocturia	−0.041	0.808	−0.352	0.032	−0.145	0.391	−0.062	0.716	0.161	0.340	0.080	0.640	−0.056	0.743
Incontinence	0.178	0.292	−0.336	0.042	−0.009	0.957	−0.209	0.214	0.250	0.130	0.206	0.221	0.068	0.687
Pads	0.123	0.468	−0.253	0.131	0.068	0.689	0.125	0.461	0.298	0.073	0.202	0.230	0.156	0.357
Voided Volume	0.186	0.271	−0.170	0.314	−0.074	0.663	0.269	0.108	0.205	0.223	0.161	0.340	0.177	0.294

anxiety measures in sexually active women with OAB. Rogers et al. [26] revealed that in a population of racially diverse, sexually active women, long term tolterodine ER treatment for OAB resulted in a relief of symptoms as ascertained in bladder diaries. Their study also validated improved sexual health. Using three items from the King's Health Questionnaire and one item from the Beck Depression Inventory, Sand et al. [27] showed that transdermal oxybutynin treatment for OAB improved sexual function. Young et al. [28], in a prospective study using the FSFI questionnaire, demonstrated that OAB symptom management using solifenacin had a positive outcome on female sexual function, especially on the domains of arousal, desire and satisfaction. On the other hand, according to Jha [29] treatment of OAB symptoms with anticholinergics, in female patients evaluated with the PISQ questionnaire, does not guarantee improvement in sexual health. The small sample size and the uncontrolled design of the studies may not permit the

demonstration of a causal relationship between the regimen used for OAB treatment and FSD.

Other factors can have a greater effect on sexual life than urinary incontinence associated with intercourse. However, the enjoyment of intercourse can be adversely effected by urgency and frequency issues, along with the fear of leakage during stimulation and intercourse [30]. After 3 months of mirabegron treatment, results indicated statistically significant improvements in sexual function. These improvements may have played a critical role in overall women's sexual health wellness, as revealed by total FSFI scores and individual sexual domain scores, in Group B. Thus, the improvement of FSFI scores, in the current study, may at least partly be attributable to the established improvements in urgency and frequency.

Numerous studies have demonstrated that sexual function is negatively affected in women with bladder dysfunction [6, 30]. It is obvious that the improvement in lower urinary tract symptoms results in improvement of women's sexual life [7, 25–28]. These previous studies are consistent with our findings, demonstrating a positive influence of OAB symptom treatment with mirabegron on sexual health and quality of life. The fact that the number of incontinence pads used by patients was significantly reduced after treatment, might help women feel more desirable and willing to experience sexual relationships and may represent another mechanism to explain the improvement of FSFI demonstrated in the current study after mirabegron administration.

Extensive data exists on the β_3-adrenergic receptor subtype of the sympathetic nervous system [31, 32]. In a recent study, β_3-receptor stimulation caused rat aorta vasorelaxation via the activation of NO synthase and

Table 6 Multivariate linear regression analysis model

Variable	B	SE B	β	P value	95.0% CI	
Constant	1.162	0.752		0.126	−0.336	2.660
Group	24.193	3.688	0.741	< 0.001	16.849	31.538
Frequency	−0.155	0.079	−0.107	0.050	−0.312	− 0.001
Urgency	0.003	0.049	0.005	0.951	−0.095	0.101
Nocturia	−0.001	0.012	−0.003	0.931	−0.025	0.023
Incontinence	0.004	0.018	0.009	0.843	−0.032	0.039
Number of pads	−0.015	0.031	−0.036	0.629	−0.077	0.047
Voided volume	0.113	0.065	0.123	0.086	−0.016	0.243

the associated increase of tissue levels of cGMP [33]. Gur et al. [34] demonstrated that mirabegron markedly relaxed isolated human corpus cavernosum (HCC) and rat corpora cavernosa by activating β_3-adrenoceptors independently of the NO-cGMP pathway. Moreover, Cirino et al. [35] showed that the activation of the β_3-receptors present in human corpus cavernosum elicits a cGMP dependent but NO-independent vasorelaxation which involves the inhibition of the RhoA/Rho-kinase pathway and facilitates erectile function.

An up-regulation of Rho kinase-β protein in alloxan-induced diabetic rabbit corporal tissue [36] and in the human corpus cavernosum [37] has recently been shown to control corporal smooth muscle contraction induced by endothelin-1. This suggests that the RhoA/Rho kinase pathway plays a mediatory role in increased sensitivity and force generation of corporal smooth muscle. Additionally, β_3 receptor-mediated corporal smooth muscle relaxation involves the inhibition of RhoA/Rho-kinase [35]. Smooth muscle relaxation associated with phosphorylation and the resulting inhibition of RhoA is caused by the NO–cGMP signaling pathway mediated by the activation of the cGMP-dependent protein kinase [35, 38, 39]. As the cGMP-dependent protein kinase is found in human corpora cavernosa, this second mechanism is likely to occur in humans too. It seems, therefore,

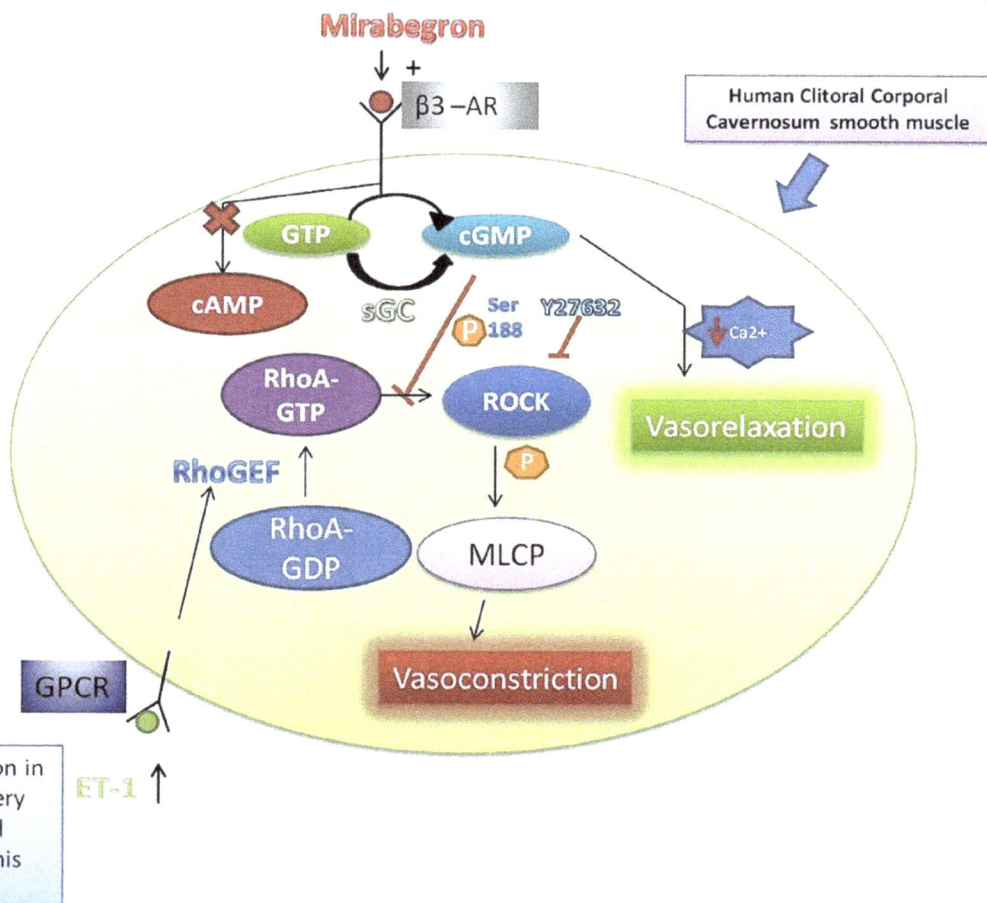

Fig. 1 Possible mechanism of mirabegron's effect, used for overactive bladder treatment, on female sexual function. β3- adrenergic receptor activation by mirabegron agonist is coupled to the generation of the second messenger cGMP, which causes human corporal cavernosum smooth muscle relaxation by lowering intracellular levels of free calcium. β3 receptor-mediated corporal smooth muscle relaxation involves inhibition of RhoA/Rho-kinase [34]. The Rho pathway is initiated by ET-1 agonist binding in the GPCR receptor, which activates RhoGEF, facilitating RhoA–GDP conversion to RhoA–GTP. RhoA–GTP binds to ROCK, facilitating autophosphorylation of ROCK that enhances its ability to phosphorylate and deactivate MLCP, promoting vasoconstriction. Relaxation is largely mediated by cGMP, which causes phosphorylation of RhoA, preventing interaction with ROCK and thereby inhibiting vasoconstriction. Endothelin-1-induced contraction of corporal smooth is mediated by an up-regulation of Rho kinase-β protein in alloxan-induced diabetic human corpus cavernosum [36]. Internal pudendal artery and clitoral artery are sensitive to the potent vasoconstrictor peptide, endothelin-1 (ET-1). The inhibition of Rho-kinase in the internal pudendal artery and clitoral artery reduces ET-1-mediated constriction [39].m. Abr. cGMP: cyclic GMP, GPCR: G-protein-coupled receptor, MLCP: myosin light chain phosphatase, RhoGEF: Rho guanine exchange factor, ROCK: Rho-associated protein kinase, sGC: soluble guanylyl cyclase, Y-27632: (R)-(+)-trans-N-(4-pyridyl)-4-(1-aminoethyl)-cyclohexanecarboxamide, ET-1: Endothelin-1

that the state of human corpus cavernosum tumescence may be regulated by the physiological function of these two pathways.

The clitoris is a complex structure that simulates the structure of penis, which is composed of two erectile bodies known as the corpora cavernosa. During sexual arousal, both the clitoris and the labia minora become engorged with blood. In addition, both vaginal and clitoral length and diameter increase. To date, the vascular contributions in FSD remain to be elucidated. The main blood supply to female genital tissue is via the internal pudendal artery (IPA) and clitoral artery (CA). A better understanding of female sexual arousal would be made possible if more was known about both these arteries. Allahdadi et al. [40] demonstrated that internal pudendal artery and clitoral artery are sensitive to the potent vasoconstrictor peptide, endothelin-1. Rho-kinase, however is a key component in endothelin-1 signaling. Furthermore, the inhibition of Rho-kinase in the internal pudendal artery and clitoral artery reduces ET-1-mediated constriction [40].

We may hypothesize that mirabegron, as a β_3-adrenoreceptor agonist, induces relaxation of the corpus cavernosum that may enhance blood flow in the female region-clitoris which might be accompanied by increased stimulation. This proposed mechanism of mirabegron explains our results, in which mirabegron treatment caused statistically significant improvements in arousal, desire, orgasm and satisfaction female sexual function domains, as well as in total FSFI score (Fig. 1).

However, the present study has some limitations. Our study had a control group with women not taking mirabegron treatment but there is no placebo group. Thus, there is no evaluation about the effect of placebo on sexual function. It was not possible to use a randomization method since the decision of female patients to receive mirabegron or not, was the reason for being in certain group. Someone could claim that it is a random process of selection although that can by chance lead to disparities. In spite of these limitations, significant results have been obtained, which are of value for clinicians working in this field.

Conclusions

Females with OAB should be assessed for their sexual function to provide better quality of life. According to the aforementioned data, OAB treatment with mirabegron improves female sexual function. The above documented improvement in female sexual function might be due to the improvement in the consequences of OAB pathophysiology. However an alternative mechanism may be raised attributing these beneficial effects in the women who received mirabegron treatment to mirabegron action per se. Our study is adherent to CONSORT guidelines.

Abbreviations

ASEX: Arizona Sexual Experience Scale; BDI: Beck depression inventory; CA: Clitoral artery; cGMP: Cyclic Guanosine Monophosphate; ET-1: Endothelin-1; FSD: Female sexual dysfunction; FSFI: Female sexual function index; FSFI-Gr: Female sexual function index –greek; HCC: Human corpus cavernosum; ICS: International Continence Society; IPA: Internal pudendal artery; KHQ: King's Health Questionnaire; NO: Nitric oxide; OAB: Overactive bladder; PISQ: Pelvic Organ Prolapse/Urinary Incontinence Sexual Function Questionnaire; SPSS: Statistical Package for the Social Sciences; SQOL-F: Sexual quality of life – female; Tolterodine ER: Tolterodine extended release; Tolterodine IR: Tolterodine immediate release

Acknowledgements

The authors would like to thank Mrs. D. Pantartzi, Scientific Secretary of the Clinical Trial Office, Department of Urology, University of Crete Medical School for the administrative and technical support.

Funding

ELPIS HOSPITAL.

Authors' contributions

ZA contributed to conception and design, collected data, contributed to the analysis and interpretation of data, drafted the manuscript and revised it critically for important intellectual content. CM led the analysis, made substantial contribution to the interpretation of data, has been involved in drafting the manuscript and revising it critically for important intellectual content. FM contributed to conception and design, collected data, contributed to the analysis and interpretation of data, drafted the manuscript and revised it critically for important intellectual content. DF, FJ, SS contributed to collection of data, contributed to the analysis and interpretation of data. TP, TA, SN contributed to conception and design, analysis and interpretation of data and helped revise the manuscript critically for important intellectual content. All authors read, approved and agree to be accountable for the final manuscript.

Competing interests

The authors declare that they have no competing interests.

Author details

[1]Department of Urology, School of Medicine, Ioannina University, Ioannina, Greece. [2]Department of Urology, University General Hospital of Heraklion, University of Crete, Medical School, Heraklion, Greece. [3]Department of Urology, ELPIS Hospital, Volos, Greece. [4]Department of Urology, School of Medicine, Tottori University, Yonago, Japan. [5]3 Spyridi Street, 38221 Volos, Greece.

References

1. Abrams P, Cardozo L, Fall M, Griffiths D, Rosier P, Ulmsten U, Van Kerrebroeck P, Victor A, Wein A, Standardisation sSub-Committee of the International Continence S. The standardisation of terminology in lower urinary tract function: report from the standardisation sub-committee of the International Continence Society. Urology. 2003;61(1):37_49.
2. Stewart WF, Van Rooyen JB, Cundiff GW, Abrams P, Herzog AR, Corey R, Hunt TL, Wein AJ. Prevalence and burden of overactive bladder in the United States. World J Urol. 2003;20(6):327–36.
3. Coyne KS, Sexton CC, Thompson CL, Milsom I, Irwin D, Kopp ZS, Chapple CR, Kaplan S, Tubaro A, Aiyer LP, et al. The prevalence of lower urinary tract symptoms (LUTS) in the USA, the UK and Sweden: results from the epidemiology of LUTS (EpiLUTS) study. BJU Int. 2009;104(3):352–60.
4. Coyne KS, Sexton CC, Irwin DE, Kopp ZS, Kelleher CJ, Milsom I. The impact of overactive bladder, incontinence and other lower urinary tract symptoms on quality of life, work productivity, sexuality and emotional well-being in men and women: results from the EPIC study. BJU Int. 2008;101(11):1388–95.
5. Cohen BL, Barboglio P, Gousse A. The impact of lower urinary tract symptoms and urinary incontinence on female sexual dysfunction using a validated instrument. J Sex Med. 2008;5(6):1418–23.

6. Patel AS, O'Leary ML, Stein RJ, Leng WW, Chancellor MB, Patel SG, Borello-France D. The relationship between overactive bladder and sexual activity in women. Int Braz J Urol. 2006;32(1):77–87.

7. Hajebrahimi S, Azaripour A, Sadeghi-Bazargani H. Tolterodine immediate release improves sexual function in women with overactive bladder. J Sex Med. 2008;5(12):2880–5.

8. Kim YH, Seo JT, Yoon H. The effect of overactive bladder syndrome on the sexual quality of life in Korean young and middle aged women. Int J Impot Res. 2005;17(2):158–63.

9. Zahariou A, Karamouti M, Tyligada E, Papaioannou P. Sexual function in women with overactive bladder. Female Pelvic Med Reconstr Surg. 2010; 16(1):31–6.

10. Laumann EO, Paik A, Rosen RC. Sexual dysfunction in the United States: prevalence and predictors. JAMA. 1999;281(6):537–44.

11. Hayes RD, Dennerstein L, Bennett CM, Fairley CK. What is the "true" prevalence of female sexual dysfunctions and does the way we assess these conditions have an impact? J Sex Med. 2008;5(4):777–87.

12. Rosen R, Brown C, Heiman J, Leiblum S, Meston C, Shabsigh R, Ferguson D, D'Agostino R Jr. The Female Sexual Function Index (FSFI): a multidimensional self-report instrument for the assessment of female sexual function. J Sex Marital Ther. 2000;26(2):191–208.

13. Yamaguchi O. Beta3-adrenoceptors in human detrusor muscle. Urology. 2002;59(5 Suppl 1):25–9.

14. Nitti VW, Auerbach S, Martin N, Calhoun A, Lee M, Herschorn S. Results of a randomized phase III trial of mirabegron in patients with overactive bladder. J Urol. 2013;189(4):1388–95.

15. Khullar V, Amarenco G, Angulo JC, Cambronero J, Hoye K, Milsom I, Radziszewski P, Rechberger T, Boerrigter P, Drogendijk T, et al. Efficacy and tolerability of mirabegron, a beta(3)-adrenoceptor agonist, in patients with overactive bladder: results from a randomised European-Australian phase 3 trial. Eur Urol. 2013;63(2):283–95.

16. Herschorn S, Barkin J, Castro-Diaz D, Frankel JM, Espuna-Pons M, Gousse AE, Stolzel M, Martin N, Gunther A, Van Kerrebroeck P. A phase III, randomized, double-blind, parallel-group, placebo-controlled, multicentre study to assess the efficacy and safety of the beta(3) adrenoceptor agonist, mirabegron, in patients with symptoms of overactive bladder. Urology. 2013;82(2):313–20.

17. Yamaguchi O, Marui E, Kakizaki H, Homma Y, Igawa Y, Takeda M, Nishizawa O, Gotoh M, Yoshida M, Yokoyama O, et al. Phase III, randomised, double-blind, placebo-controlled study of the beta3-adrenoceptor agonist mirabegron, 50 mg once daily, in Japanese patients with overactive bladder. BJU Int. 2014;113(6):951–60.

18. Nitti VW, Khullar V, van Kerrebroeck P, Herschorn S, Cambronero J, Angulo JC, Blauwet MB, Dorrepaal C, Siddiqui E, Martin NE. Mirabegron for the treatment of overactive bladder: a prespecified pooled efficacy analysis and pooled safety analysis of three randomised, double-blind, placebo-controlled, phase III studies. Int J Clin Pract. 2013;67(7):619–32.

19. Chapple CR, Kaplan SA, Mitcheson D, Klecka J, Cummings J, Drogendijk T, Dorrepaal C, Martin N. Randomized double-blind, active-controlled phase 3 study to assess 12-month safety and efficacy of mirabegron, a beta(3)-adrenoceptor agonist, in overactive bladder. Eur Urol. 2013;63(2):296–305.

20. Zahariou AG, Karamouti MV, Papaioannou PD. Pelvic floor muscle training improves sexual function of women with stress urinary incontinence. Int Urogynecol J Pelvic Floor Dysfunct. 2008;19(3):401–6.

21. Hatzichristou D, Kirana PS, Banner L, Althof SE, Lonnee-Hoffmann RA, Dennerstein L, Rosen RC. Diagnosing sexual dysfunction in men and women: sexual history taking and the role of symptom scales and questionnaires. J Sex Med. 2016;13(8):1166–82.

22. Zachariou A, Filiponi M, Kirana PS. Translation and validation of the Greek version of the female sexual function index questionnaire. Int J Impot Res. 2017;29(4):171–4.

23. Wiegel M, Meston C, Rosen R. The female sexual function index (FSFI): cross-validation and development of clinical cutoff scores. J Sex Marital Ther. 2005;31(1):1–20.

24. Chedraui P, Perez-Lopez FR, San Miguel G, Avila C. Assessment of sexuality among middle-aged women using the Female Sexual Function Index. Climacteric. 2009;12(3):213–21.

25. Rogers R, Bachmann G, Jumadilova Z, Sun F, Morrow JD, Guan Z, Bavendam T. Efficacy of tolterodine on overactive bladder symptoms and sexual and emotional quality of life in sexually active women. Int Urogynecol J Pelvic Floor Dysfunct. 2008;19(11):1551–7.

26. Rogers RG, Omotosho T, Bachmann G, Sun F, Morrow JD. Continued symptom improvement in sexually active women with overactive bladder and urgency urinary incontinence treated with tolterodine ER for 6 months. Int Urogynecol J Pelvic Floor Dysfunct. 2009;20(4):381–5.

27. Sand PK, Goldberg RP, Dmochowski RR, Mcllwain M, Dahl NV. The impact of the overactive bladder syndrome on sexual function: a preliminary report from the Multicenter Assessment of Transdermal Therapy in Overactive Bladder with Oxybutynin trial. Am J Obstet Gynecol. 2006;195(6):1730–5.

28. Young O, Hyo K, Won H, Jin B, Changhee Y, Goo L, Seon C. Clinical efficacy of solifenacin on female sexual dysfunction in patients with overactive bladder (SOS trial; Solifenacin on Overactive bladder and Sexual dysfunction). J Urol. 2013;189:e618–9.

29. Jha S. Impact of treatment of overactive bladder with anticholinergics on sexual function. Arch Gynecol Obstet. 2016;293(2):403–6.

30. Coyne KS, Margolis MK, Jumadilova Z, Bavendam T, Mueller E, Rogers R. Overactive bladder and women's sexual health: what is the impact? J Sex Med. 2007;4(3):656–66.

31. Strosberg AD. Structure and function of the beta 3-adrenergic receptor. Annu Rev Pharmacol Toxicol. 1997;37:421–50.

32. Guimaraes S, Moura D. Vascular adrenoceptors: an update. Pharmacol Rev. 2001;53(2):319–56.

33. Trochu JN, Leblais V, Rautureau Y, Beverelli F, Le Marec H, Berdeaux A, Gauthier C. Beta 3-adrenoceptor stimulation induces vasorelaxation mediated essentially by endothelium-derived nitric oxide in rat thoracic aorta. Br J Pharmacol. 1999;128(1):69–76.

34. Gur S, Peak T, Yafi FA, Kadowitz PJ, Sikka SC, Hellstrom WJ. Mirabegron causes relaxation of human and rat corpus cavernosum: could it be a potential therapy for erectile dysfunction? BJU Int. 2016;118(3):464–74.

35. Cirino G, Sorrentino R, di Villa Bianca R, Popolo A, Palmieri A, Imbimbo C, Fusco F, Longo N, Tajana G, Ignarro LJ, et al. Involvement of beta 3-adrenergic receptor activation via cyclic GMP- but not NO-dependent mechanisms in human corpus cavernosum function. Proc Natl Acad Sci U S A. 2003;100(9):5531–6.

36. Chang S, Hypolite JA, Changolkar A, Wein AJ, Chacko S, DiSanto ME. Increased contractility of diabetic rabbit corpora smooth muscle in response to endothelin is mediated via Rho-kinase beta. Int J Impot Res. 2003;15(1):53–62.

37. Wang H, Eto M, Steers WD, Somlyo AP, Somlyo AV. RhoA-mediated Ca2+ sensitization in erectile function. J Biol Chem. 2002;277(34):30614–21.

38. Sawada N, Itoh H, Yamashita J, Doi K, Inoue M, Masatsugu K, Fukunaga Y, Sakaguchi S, Sone M, Yamahara K, et al. cGMP-dependent protein kinase phosphorylates and inactivates RhoA. Biochem Biophys Res Commun. 2001;280(3):798–805.

39. Sauzeau V, Le Jeune H, Cario-Toumaniantz C, Smolenski A, Lohmann SM, Bertoglio J, Chardin P, Pacaud P, Loirand G. Cyclic GMP-dependent protein kinase signaling pathway inhibits RhoA-induced Ca2+ sensitization of contraction in vascular smooth muscle. J Biol Chem. 2000;275(28):21722–9.

40. Allahdadi KJ, Hannan JL, Tostes RC, Webb RC. Endothelin-1 induces contraction of female rat internal pudendal and clitoral arteries through ET(A) receptor and rho-kinase activation. J Sex Med. 2010;7(6):2096–103.

Surgical management of urolithiasis – a systematic analysis of available guidelines

Valentin Zumstein[1,2*†], Patrick Betschart[1†], Dominik Abt[1], Hans-Peter Schmid[1], Cedric Michael Panje[3] and Paul Martin Putora[3,4]

Abstract

Background: Several societies around the world issue guidelines incorporating the latest evidence. However, even the most commonly cited guidelines of the European Association of Urology (EAU) and the American Urological Association (AUA) leave the clinician with several treatment options and differ on specific points. We aimed to identify discrepancies and areas of consensus between guidelines to give novel insights into areas where low consensus between the guideline panels exists, and therefore where more evidence might increase consensus.

Methods: The webpages of the 61 members of the Societé Internationale d'Urologie were analysed to identify all listed or linked guidelines. Decision trees for the surgical management of urolithiasis were derived, and a comparative analysis was performed to determine consensus and discrepancies.

Results: Five national and one international guideline (EAU) on surgical stone treatment were available for analysis. While 7 national urological societies refer to the AUA guidelines and 11 to the EAU guidelines, 43 neither publish their own guidelines nor refer to others. Comparative analysis revealed a high degree of consensus for most renal and ureteral stone scenarios. Nevertheless, we also identified a variety of discrepancies between the different guidelines, the largest being the approach to the treatment of proximal ureteral calculi and larger renal calculi.

Conclusions: Six guidelines with recommendations for the surgical treatment of urolithiasis to support urologists in decision-making were available for inclusion in our analysis. While there is a high grade of consensus for most stone scenarios, we also detected some discrepancies between different guidelines. These are, however, controversial situations where adequate evidence to assist with decision-making has yet to be elicited by further research.

Keywords: Consensus, Guidelines, Urolithiasis, Management, Surgical, Decision tree

Background

A range of procedures is in use for the surgical treatment of urolithiasis. Treatment strategies are mainly based on stone location and size, and the patient's comorbidities and preferences. Guidelines have been developed to support clinicians in selecting the most appropriate treatment in controversial situations. Several institutions around the world have issued guidelines incorporating the latest evidence.

However, even the most commonly cited guidelines of the European Association of Urology (EAU) and the American Urological Association (AUA) leave the clinician with several treatment options and differ on specific points, such as cut-off values for stone size and recommendations for the treatment of choice [1–3]. Ambiguities and discrepancies between different guidelines may result from different interpretations of the evidence available and possible methodological differences in guideline creation. Therefore, careful analysis of the similarities and differences between different sources can provide additional insight [4].

We aimed to determine how many guidelines on the surgical management of urolithiasis actually exist and the urological associations that recommended them. We systematically analysed the criteria proposed for decision-making and the recommended surgical approaches in each guideline. In addition, we

---
* Correspondence: valentin.zumstein@gmail.com
†Equal contributors
[1]Department of Urology, Cantonal Hospital St. Gallen, St. Gallen, Switzerland
[2]Department of Urology, University Medical Center Hamburg-Eppendorf, Hamburg, Germany
Full list of author information is available at the end of the article

aimed to identify discrepancies and areas of consensus between guidelines, with particular attention to the two major guidelines, those of the EAU and AUA.

This work provides a systematic analysis of the recommended surgical management of urolithiasis worldwide, and gives novel insights into areas where low consensus between the guideline panels exists, and therefore where more evidence might increase consensus.

Methods

Guidelines were selected using the membership list of the Societé Internationale d'Urologie (SIU) (http://www.siu-urology.org/society/national-delegates). The webpages of all 61 members that are represented by delegates were analysed for mentions of and links to guidelines for the surgical management of renal and ureteral calculi.

Two authors (V.Z., P.B.) independently assessed all guidelines, and decision trees for the surgical management of urolithiasis were derived, followed by cross-checking and clarification of any differences by a third author (D.A.). The methodology of this approach has been recently described [5] and was successfully used in different fields including radiotherapy in prostate cancer [6], expert opinions of the systemic treatment of recurrent glioblastoma [7], renal cell carcinoma [8, 9] and sarcoma [10]. In cases where first-, second- and or even third-line recommendations were provided, all treatment options were included into the decision trees regardless of their hierarchical level. Although hierarchical levels were assessed, they were not incorporated into the decision trees. Decision trees were built based on the criteria used in the guidelines analysed. These were stone location, i.e. renal non-lower pole, renal lower pole, and proximal and distal ureter; and stone size, i.e. > 20 mm, 10–20 mm, < 10 mm for renal stones, and > 10 mm or < 10 mm for ureteral stones [1, 2]. All treatment modalities mentioned in the different guidelines were included in our analyses: shock wave lithotripsy (SWL), percutaneous nephrolithotomy (PNL/PCNL), ureterorenoscopy including flexible and semi-rigid URS, covering also the terms retrograde intrarenal surgery (RIRS) and cirurgia intrarenal retrograda (CIRR) as described in the EAU and Sociedad Argentina de Urologia (SAU) guidelines [2, 11, 12], and open surgery. Patient preference and contraindications were considered to be universal factors and were therefore omitted from the analysis. Moreover, recommendations on conservative treatment, special cases (e.g. stone management in pregnancy, staghorn stones, cysteine stones) and postoperative follow-up were not part of our systematic analysis.

All decision trees were analysed and compared to each other to determine consensus or discrepancies between each possible combination of parameters using web-based software (Diagnostic Nodes), as described previously [5–7, 13].

To evaluate discrepancies, a combined tree containing all recommendations was generated. A mode tree was also generated to identify the most common combination of recommendations for each possible situation.

Consensus was defined as complete overlap between the recommended treatments for any case. If all guidelines recommended only one therapy for a specific situation, agreement was 100%. However, if three of six guidelines recommended therapy A only, and the others therapy A or B, this resulted in only 50% agreement for therapy A.

In addition to comparing all guidelines, the two international and most frequently cited guidelines issued by the EAU and AUA were separately compared to highlight discrepancies or areas of consensus.

Results

Analysis of the websites of the 61 member associations represented by delegates of the SIU showed 6 national guidelines: AUA – American Urological Association [1, 3], SAU – Sociedad Argentina de Urologia [11, 12]; AFU – French Association of Urology [14]; DGU – German Society for Urology [15]; and SUA – Singapore Urological Association [16]; and the international guidelines from the EAU [2]. Some national guidelines (e.g. guideline of the Japanese Urology Association) were not included into the analysis due to linguistic difficulties caused by font systems or scripts. Eleven national urological societies refer website users to the EAU guidelines or the AUA guidelines (5 to both the EAU and AUA), 43 did not publish their own guidelines or refer readers to any others (Table 1).

Decision trees were able to be derived from all guidelines identified. The site of the stone is classified consistently, i.e. proximal or distal ureteral, and lower pole or non-lower pole renal calculi, in all guidelines, except the AFU guidelines, which do not explicitly classify lower pole renal stones as an entity in their own right.

While most guidelines distinguish between > 10 mm and < 10 mm for ureteral stones, stone size is not specifically mentioned for distal ureteral calculi in the DGU recommendations or for proximal ureteral calculi in the AFU guidelines.

With regard to renal stone size, thresholds of < 10 mm, 10–20 mm and > 20 mm are used in the EAU, DGU and SAU guidelines, whilst the AUA guidelines differentiate between lower pole calculi > 10 mm and ≤ 10 mm, and non-lower pole stones > 20 mm and ≤ 20 mm. The SUA guidelines provide recommendations for lower pole calculi

Table 1 Recommendations of the SIU members represented by delegates regarding surgical stone treatment

SIU Member	Own guideline	Reference to other guideline	Language / latest version
Albania	No	No	
Argentina	Yes		Spanish / 2014
Australia	No	EAU	
Austria	No	EAU / AUA	
Brazil	No	No	
Canada	No[a]	No	
China	No	No	
Colombia	No[b]	No	
Costa Rica	No	No	
Cuba	No	No	
Cyprus	No	No	
Czech Rep.	No	EAU	
Egypt	No	EAU / AUA	
Finland	No	No	
France	Yes		French / 2004
Germany	Yes		German / 2016
Ghana	No	No	
Greece	No	No	
Guyana	No	No	
Haiti	No	No	
Hungary	No	No	
India	No	No	
Indonesia	No	No	
Iran	No	No	
Israel	No	No	
Italy	No	No	
Jamaica	No	No	
Japan	Yes		Japanese
Jordan	No	EAU / AUA	
Kenya	No	No	
Latvia	No	No	
Liberia	No	No	
Libya	No	No	
Lithuania	No	No	
Malaysia	No	EAU	
Mauritius	No	No	
Morocco	No	No	
Myanmar	No	No	
Netherlands	No	EAU	
Nigeria	No	No	
Norway	No	No	
Pakistan	No	No	

Table 1 Recommendations of the SIU members represented by delegates regarding surgical stone treatment *(Continued)*

SIU Member	Own guideline	Reference to other guideline	Language / latest version
Palestine	No	No	
Peru	No	No	
Portugal	No	EAU	
Puerto Rico	No	AUA	
Romania	No	No	
Russia	No	No	
Serbia	No	No	
Singapore	Yes		English / 2001
Slovakia	No	No	
South Africa	No	EAU/AUA	
South Korea	No	No	
Sudan	No	No	
Sweden	No	No	
Switzerland	No	EAU / AUA	
Turkey	No	No	
Ukraine	No	No	
United Kingdom	No[c]	EAU	
United States	Yes	AUA	
Zimbabwe	No	No	

[a]No guidelines for surgical management of renal calculi
[b]No guidelines for surgical management of ureteral calculi
[c]Guidelines for renal and ureteric stones in development (anticipated publication Feburary 2019)

regardless of size, and the AFU guidelines differentiate between > 20 mm and < 20 mm for all renal stones.

Figure 1 shows the consensus decision tree resulting from semi-automatic comparison of all decision trees. SWL and URS were the most commonly recommended procedures for all stone sizes and locations. Moreover, PNL is mentioned as a treatment option for all renal calculi by all guidelines except for the AUA and SUA guidelines, which do not recommend it for the treatment of smaller non-lower pole renal calculi.

Comparative analysis assessing the most often recommended combination of procedures revealed an agreement ranging from 50 to 83% for different stone sizes and locations (Fig. 2). A high degree of consensus was found in particular for lower pole renal stones below 20 mm (83% of the guidelines recommend 'SWL or URS or PNL') and distal ureteral stones (83% of the guidelines recommend 'SWL or URS').

In contrast, we saw a low level of agreement for the treatment of proximal ureteral stones. The EAU, AUA and DGU guidelines recommend SWL or URS, whereas the other 3 guidelines additionally list PNL and open

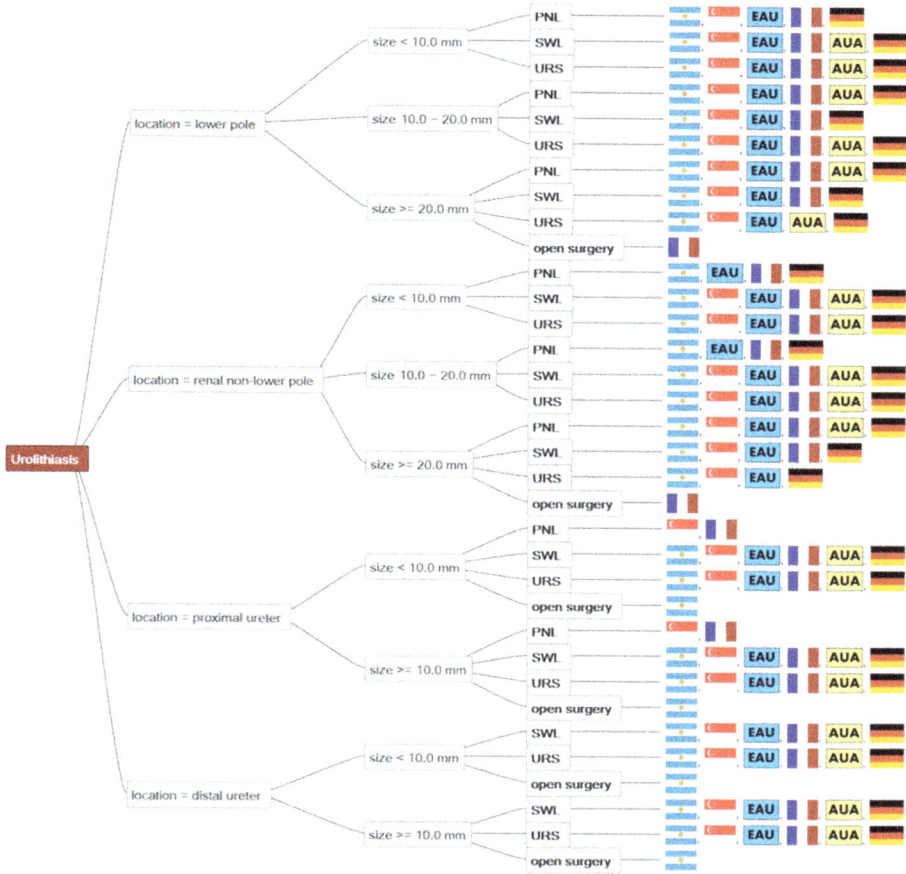

Fig. 1 Consensus tree listing decision criteria and recommended treatments of all guidelines. (Note that URS for proximal ureteral calculi > 10 mm involves ante- and retrograde approach in the EAU-Guidelines)

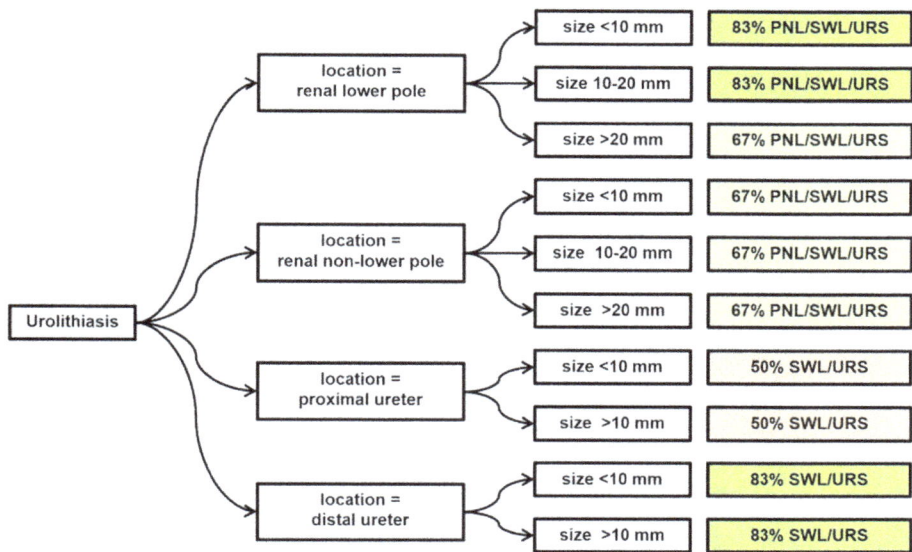

Fig. 2 Mode tree listing the degree of agreement for the most often recommended therapeutic options. (Note that URS for proximal ureteral calculi > 10 mm involves ante- and retrograde approach in the EAU-Guidelines)

surgery, resulting in a 50% consensus for 'SWL or URS' as the most common recommendation.

An intermediate level of agreement was found for the remaining situations (67% consensus for renal non-lower pole calculi and lower pole calculi > 20 mm).

A separate comparison of the EAU and AUA guidelines including all recommended treatment options regardless of hierarchical level showed complete consensus for the treatment of ureteral calculi (Fig. 3). However, the EAU guidelines provide wider scope for decision-making regarding the treatment of renal stones, especially for larger non-lower pole calculi, and the use of PNL.

All guidelines provide a hierarchical listing of the recommended therapies for each situation (Table 2). The best agreement between the hierarchical recommendations in the six guidelines was found for distal ureteral calculi.

SWL is recommended as first line therapy in all guidelines for smaller non-lower pole renal stones (< 20 mm), whilst only the AFU guidelines recommend SWL as first choice for > 20 mm calculi. The situation for PNL in non-lower pole and lower pole calculi is different: for small calculi < 10 mm, PNL is first choice in only the SUA guidelines, whereas for larger renal calculi > 20 mm, PNL is listed in all guidelines as first-line therapy.

Regarding proximal ureteral calculi < 10 mm, SWL is first-line therapy in all guidelines except those of the AUA, where URS is recommended as first line and SWL as second line. PNL is not recommended in this situation except for by the AFU and SUA guidelines.

URS is recommended as first line for all distal ureteral calculi, regardless of size.

Discussion

If surgical treatment of ureteral or renal stones is indicated, clinicians face the challenge of choosing the most appropriate treatment for each patient. In ambiguous situations, evidence-based guidelines can help the urologist with decision-making.

Our systematic search covering all members of the SIU showed that the EAU and AUA guidelines are the most frequently referenced guidelines worldwide for the treatment of urolithiasis. Treatment recommendations are based on stone size and location in all available guidelines. Remarkably, the websites of most national urological associations neither refer to a reference guideline nor provide their own guidelines. However, efforts are made to improve this situation such as those by the British Association of Urological Surgeons (BAUS) in collaboration with the National Institute for Health and Care Excellence (NICE). Besides a linked guideline on laparoscopic stone removal, new guidelines covering the management of renal and ureteric calculi are supposed to be published by February 2019 (https://www.nice.org.uk/guidance/conditions-and-diseases/kidney-conditions/renal-stones). We suggest that urological associations without own guidelines should refer to one of the cited guidelines to provide a reliable source their members can refer to.

Regarding location – except for the AFU guidelines [14] – all guidelines consider calculi in the lower renal pole separately because of a reduced possibility of

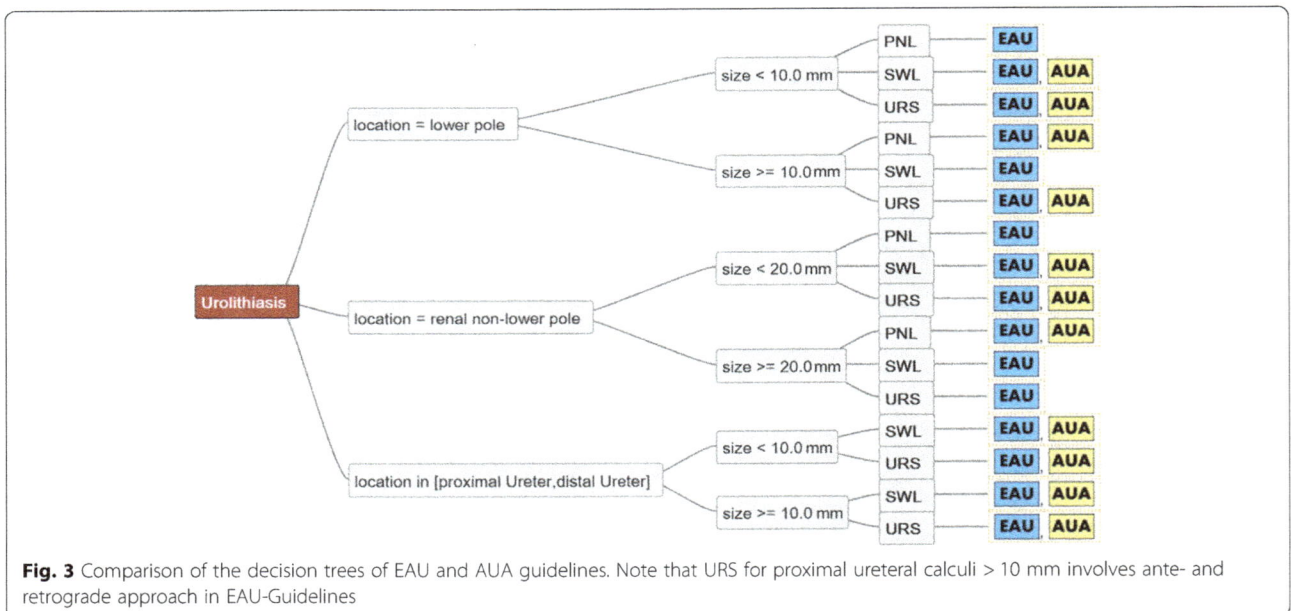

Fig. 3 Comparison of the decision trees of EAU and AUA guidelines. Note that URS for proximal ureteral calculi > 10 mm involves ante- and retrograde approach in EAU-Guidelines

Table 2 Hierarchical levels of the most commonly recommended therapies (SWL, URS, PNL) in different guidelines

renal

	non lower pole			lower pole		
	< 10 mm	10-20 mm	> 20 mm	< 10 mm	10 - 20 mm	> 20 mm
	S U P E	S U P E	S U P E	S U P E	S U P E	S U P E
EAU	GR B	GR B	GR B	GR B	GR B	GR B
AUA	LE B	LE B	LE C	LE B	LE B	LE C
DGU	100%	100%	100%	100%	100%	100%
AFU	-	-	-	-	-	-
SAU	-	-	-	-	-	-
SUA	-	-	-	-	-	-

ureteral

	proximal		distal		
	< 10 mm	> 10 mm	< 10 mm	> 10 mm	
	S U P E	S U P E	S U P E	S U P E	
EAU	GR A	GR A	GR A	GR A	■ first choice
AUA	LE B	LE B	LE B	LE B	second choice
DGU	96%	96%	96%	96%	third choice
AFU	-	-	-	-	no option
SAU	-	-	-	-	
SUA	-	-	-	-	

S SWL, *U* URS, *P* PNL, *E* Evidence declaration with GR Grade of recommendation in EAU, *LE* Level of evidence in AUA, Degree of Panel consensus in DGU

passage of fragments [15, 17–20]. Most guidelines categorize stone size into < 10 mm, 10–20 mm, and > 20 mm. However, the AUA guidelines for renal calculi only differentiate between ≤10 mm and > 10 mm for lower-pole stones and between ≤20 mm and > 20 mm for non-lower pole stones [1, 3]. There is also some deviation from the most common classifications in the AFU guidelines [14], SAU guidelines [11, 12], and SUA guidelines [16].

Surgical treatment of ureteral calculi depends on stone location and size. The AUA guidelines state that earlier classifications split the ureter into thirds and that this was because of the surgical approaches available. Nowadays, the ureter is divided into two sections marked by the crossing of the iliac vessels. All guidelines use a cut-off level of 10 mm to define the surgical approach.

Concerning hierarchical recommendations, all guidelines give treatment options in multiple scenarios, listed as equal or, in some cases, as first-, second- or third-line surgical treatment. To prevent the loss of recommended second- or third-line surgical therapies in our comparative analysis, we included all surgical procedures proposed as "standard procedures", regardless of their hierarchical position in the guideline text.

Our consensus tree showed a high degree of consensus for most recommended procedures in nearly all ureteral and renal stone scenarios. We did, however, detect some

significant differences, mainly concerned with the rating of SWL, where little consensus between guidelines for larger renal, distal ureteral and small proximal ureteral calculi was found. One reason for that might be geographical discrepancies in the technical performance of interventions, such as the strict use of X-ray-localisation systems for SWL in the United States compared to the widely available ultrasound guidance in Europe. Considering the rapid technological improvements of URS and PNL, further evidence seems to be required here.

While the mode tree showed a high degree of agreement for lower pole renal stones of < 10 mm and 10–20 mm and distal ureteral stones, a low level of agreement was found for proximal ureteral stones. This can be explained by the AFU and SUA guidelines also recommending PNL for proximal ureteral stones, and the SAU guidelines also recommending open surgery. However, the reason for this might be rather missing updates of some guidelines in the recent past, than a real lack of evidence for these scenarios. Thus, the last revisions of the SUA [16] and AFU guidelines [14] were issued in 2001 and 2004 and do not, therefore, reflect the latest developments.

All other guidelines clearly focus on SWL and URS in such cases. However, at this point it must be mentioned, that EAU guidelines consider a percutaneous approach for proximal ureteral calculi under the term "antegrade URS" and state that percutaneous antegrade removal of ureteral stones should be considered in selected cases [2].

The comparison of the EAU and AUA guidelines as the most commonly cited guidelines worldwide revealed several discrepancies. In general, the EAU guidelines give more therapeutic options for specific situations, delegating the choice of the appropriate treatment to the urologist and patient's preference.

Since several approaches may be appropriate in specific situations, guidelines also rate procedures hierarchically in such cases. Our analysis of these hierarchical listings revealed a number of discrepancies between guidelines, showing that for the choice between SWL and URS, available data might have been interpreted differently. While the AUA guidelines refer to an unpublished systematic review conducted by the guidelines-panel [1], the EAU guidelines recommendation is based on a meta-analysis [18] and a work carried out by Hong et al. [19].

Moreover, PNL is mentioned as a treatment option for all renal calculi by all guidelines, except for the AUA and SUA guidelines, which do not recommend it for the treatment of smaller non-lower pole renal calculi. Although recent developments in minimal invasive PNL techniques are mentioned in the EAU and AUA guidelines, these procedures are not yet listed separately in the recommendations. The comparison of recent advances in PNL is particularly difficult because different approaches are associated with substantially different degrees of invasiveness and technical complexity.

SWL still plays an important role in all guidelines. This is remarkable because several recent studies have shown that technical advances with URS achieved higher stone-free rates and had fewer complications than previously [21, 22]. However, lower morbidity and economic aspects [2, 23, 24] support the use of SWL, and this explains its continuing prominence in all guidelines. A further explanation is that, based on the published decision tree and consensus tree, the EAU guidelines state that more than 90% of renal and ureteral calculi might be suitable for SWL according to the recent literature [25–27].

One limitation of our study was disregarding hierarchical recommendations when comparing recommended approaches. Since comparing decision trees with multiple weighted recommendations would have resulted in an exuberant consensus tree, we decided to include all recommended therapies for each specific situation and weight them equally to avoid distortion of the comparative analysis through oversimplification. To compensate for this, hierarchical recommendations of different treatment options were analysed separately in our comparative analysis (Table 2). Guideline language is usually restricted to the nation's main language. Due to linguistic difficulties caused by different font systems or scripts, some national guidelines could not be included in our analysis (e.g. the guidelines of the Japanese Urology Association) or might have remained unnoticed. Moreover, our systematic analysis excluded stone composition, postoperative management, follow-up and specific situations such as staghorn calculi, urolithiasis in pregnancy or in children. Techniques such as laparoscopic and open surgery are part of many guidelines (e.g. SAU, AFU, EAU and AUA). While these approaches are part of the standard treatment recommendations in SAU and AFU guidelines, EAU and AUA guidelines mention the use of these approaches in limited special scenarios only, which is why we did not include the latter in our comparative analysis. Of course, these aspects must be additionally considered in decision-making.

Conclusion

Six guidelines with recommendations for the surgical treatment of urolithiasis to support urologists in decision-making were available for inclusion in our analysis. While there is generally a high grade of consensus for most stone scenarios, we also detected some relevant discrepancies between different guidelines. In particular, lower consensus was found for the treatment of proximal ureteral stones and hierarchical levels of recommended treatments for specific situations. These are, however, controversial situations where adequate evidence to assist with decision-making has yet to be elicited by further research.

Acknowledgements
Not applicable

Funding
None

Authors' contributions
VZ contributed in project development, data collection, data analysis and manuscript writing. PB contributed in project development, data collection, data analysis and manuscript writing. DA contributed in project development, data analysis and manuscript writing. HPS contributed in project development, data collection and data analysis and manuscript writing. CP contributed in project development, data collection, data analysis and manuscript writing. PMP contributed in project development, data collection, data analysis and manuscript writing. All authors read and approved the final manuscript.

Competing interests
The authors declare that they have no competing interests.

Author details
[1]Department of Urology, Cantonal Hospital St. Gallen, St. Gallen, Switzerland. [2]Department of Urology, University Medical Center Hamburg-Eppendorf, Hamburg, Germany. [3]Department of Radiation Oncology, Cantonal Hospital St. Gallen, St. Gallen, Switzerland. [4]Department of Radiation Oncology, Inselspital, Bern University Hospital, Bern, Switzerland.

References

1. Assimos D, Krambeck A, Miller NL, Monga M, Murad MH, Nelson CP, Pace KT, Pais VM Jr, Pearle MS, Preminger GM, et al. Surgical Management of Stones: American urological association/Endourological society guideline, PART I. J Urol. 2016;196(4):1153–60.
2. Turk C, Petrik A, Sarica K, Seitz C, Skolarikos A, Straub M, Knoll T. EAU guidelines on interventional treatment for urolithiasis. Eur Urol. 2016; 69(3):475–82.
3. Assimos D, Krambeck A, Miller NL, Monga M, Murad MH, Nelson CP, Pace KT, Pais VM Jr, Pearle MS, Preminger GM, et al. Surgical Management of Stones: American urological association/Endourological society guideline, part II. J Urol. 2016;196(4):1161–69.
4. Putora PM, Oldenburg J. Swarm-based medicine. J Med Internet Res. 2013; 15(9):e207.
5. Panje CM, Glatzer M, von Rappard J, Rothermundt C, Hundsberger T, Zumstein V, Plasswilm L, Putora PM. Applied swarm-based medicine: collecting decision trees for patterns of algorithms analysis. BMC Med Res Methodol. 2017;17(1):123.
6. Panje CM, Dal Pra A, Zilli T, Zwahlen DR, Papachristofilou A, Herrera FG, Matzinger O, Plasswilm L, Putora PM. Consensus and differences in primary radiotherapy for localized and locally advanced prostate cancer in Switzerland: a survey on patterns of practice. Strahlenther Onkol. 2015; 191(10):778–86.
7. Hundsberger T, Hottinger AF, Roelcke U, Roth P, Migliorini D, Dietrich PY, Conen K, Pesce G, Hermann E, Pica A, et al. Patterns of care in recurrent glioblastoma in Switzerland: a multicentre national approach based on diagnostic nodes. J Neuro-Oncol. 2016;126(1):175–83.
8. Rothermundt C, Bailey A, Cerbone L, Eisen T, Escudier B, Gillessen S, Grunwald V, Larkin J, McDermott D, Oldenburg J, et al. Algorithms in the first-line treatment of metastatic clear cell renal cell carcinoma–analysis using diagnostic nodes. Oncologist. 2015;20(9):1028–35.
9. Rothermundt C, von Rappard J, Eisen T, Escudier B, Grunwald V, Larkin J, McDermott D, Oldenburg J, Porta C, Rini B, et al. Second-line treatment for metastatic clear cell renal cell cancer: experts' consensus algorithms. World J Urol. 2017;35(4):641–8.
10. Rothermundt C, Fischer GF, Bauer S, Blay JY, Grunwald V, Italiano A, Kasper B, Kollar A, Lindner LH, Miah A, et al. Pre- and postoperative chemotherapy in localized extremity soft tissue sarcoma: a European Organization for Research and Treatment of Cancer expert survey. Oncologist. 2017; https://doi.org/10.1634/theoncologist.2017-0391.
11. SAU-Sociedad-Argentina-de-Urologia: GUIAS EN TRATAMIENTO DE LITIASIS RENAL. 2014.
12. SAU-Sociedad-Argentina-de-Urologia: GUIAS EN TRATAMIENTO DE LITIASIS URETERAL. 2014.
13. Putora PM, Panje CM, Papachristofilou A, Dal Pra A, Hundsberger T, Plasswilm L. Objective consensus from decision trees. Radiat Oncol. 2014;9:270.
14. Conort P, Dore B, Saussine C, Comite Lithiase de l'Association Francaise dU. Guidelines for the urological management of renal and ureteric stones in adults. Prog Urol. 2004;14(6):1095–102.
15. Knoll T, Bach T, Humke U, Neisius A, Stein R, Schonthaler M, Wendt-Nordahl G. S2k guidelines on diagnostics, therapy and metaphylaxis of urolithiasis (AWMF 043/025) : compendium. Urologe A. 2016;55(7):904–22.
16. SUA-Singapore-Urological-Association: The Management of Urolithiasis. 2001.
17. Danuser H, Muller R, Descoeudres B, Dobry E, Studer UE. Extracorporeal shock wave lithotripsy of lower calyx calculi: how much is treatment

outcome influenced by the anatomy of the collecting system? Eur Urol. 2007;52(2):539–46.
18. Pearle MS, Lingeman JE, Leveillee R, Kuo R, Preminger GM, Nadler RB, Macaluso J, Monga M, Kumar U, Dushinski J, et al. Prospective, randomized trial comparing shock wave lithotripsy and ureteroscopy for lower pole caliceal calculi 1 cm or less. J Urol. 2005;173(6):2005–9.
19. Sahinkanat T, Ekerbicer H, Onal B, Tansu N, Resim S, Citgez S, Oner A. Evaluation of the effects of relationships between main spatial lower pole calyceal anatomic factors on the success of shock-wave lithotripsy in patients with lower pole kidney stones. Urology. 2008;71(5):801–5.
20. Srisubat A, Potisat S, Lojanapiwat B, Setthawong V, Laopaiboon M. Extracorporeal shock wave lithotripsy (ESWL) versus percutaneous nephrolithotomy (PCNL) or retrograde intrarenal surgery (RIRS) for kidney stones. Cochrane Database Syst Rev. 2009;4:CD007044.
21. Mi Y, Ren K, Pan H, Zhu L, Wu S, You X, Shao H, Dai F, Peng T, Qin F, et al. Flexible ureterorenoscopy (F-URS) with holmium laser versus extracorporeal shock wave lithotripsy (ESWL) for treatment of renal stone <2 cm: a meta-analysis. Urolithiasis. 2016;44(4):353–65.
22. Dell'Atti L, Papa S. Ten-year experience in the management of distal ureteral stones greater than 10 mm in size. G Chir. 2016;37(1):27–30.
23. Knoll T, Fritsche HM, Rassweiler J. Medical and economic aspects of extracorporeal shock wave lithotripsy. Aktuelle Urol. 2011;42(6):363–7.
24. Tiselius HG, Chaussy CG. Arguments for choosing extracorporeal shockwave lithotripsy for removal of urinary tract stones. Urolithiasis. 2015;43(5):387–96.
25. Wen CC, Nakada SY. Treatment selection and outcomes: renal calculi. Urol Clin North Am. 2007;34(3):409–19.
26. Miller NL, Lingeman JE. Management of kidney stones. BMJ. 2007;334(7591): 468–72.
27. Galvin DJ, Pearle MS. The contemporary management of renal and ureteric calculi. BJU Int. 2006;98(6):1283–8.

Scrotal hemorrhage after testicular sperm aspiration may be associated with phosphodiesterase-5 inhibitor administration

Yong-tong Zhu[1†], Rui Hua[1†], Song Quan[1], Wan-long Tan[3], Qing-jun Chu[1*] and Chun-yan Wang[2*]

Abstract

Background: Scrotal hemorrhage after testicular sperm aspiration (TESA) is uncommon in clinical operation. Phosphodiesterase-5 inhibitors (PDE5i) are commonly given to men who have difficulty providing a sperm sample for assisted reproductive technique such as in vitro fertilization. In this study, we examine the incidence of scrotal hemorrhage after TESA in men who received a PDE5i.

Methods: In this retrospective study, 504 men with TESA operation in Center for Reproductive Medicine, Nanfang Hospital, Southern Medical University were collected. Men in the drug group had taken orally PDE5i before TESA. Men in the control group only operated TESA. The testis volume, coagulation function were measured. Sonographic examination with Doppler imaging was performed when scrotal hemorrhage appeared.

Results: A total of 504 men with a mean age of 28.63 ± 4.22 years were included in the analysis. Of these, 428 did not receive a PDE5i prior to TESA and 76 received a PDE5i prior to TESA. Measures of coagulation function were not different between the groups. The incidence of hemorrhage was 0.0% in the control group and the drug group was 5.3%. The incidence of hemorrhage between two groups was different significantly ($P = 0.000$).

Conclusion: In summary, the results of this study suggest that a PDE5i administration increases the risk of scrotal hemorrhage in men undergoing TESA, although the study design does not allow drawing a conclusion of cause and effect. Given the potential risk of scrotal hemorrhage after the ingestion of PDE5i, it may be wise not to administer it to men in whom a TESA may be performed.

Keywords: Scrotal hemorrhage, Testicular sperm aspiration, Phosphodiesterase-5 inhibitor

Background

Over the past several decades, in vitro fertilization and intracytoplasmic sperm injection (ICSI) have come into routine practice. On the day of oocyte retrieval, the male partner is typically asked to provide sperm by masturbation. However, a small number of males are able to provide sperm by masturbation due to psychologic stress and anxiety. These individuals are generally provided psychological guidance and administered a phosphodiesterase-5 inhibitor (PDE5i). When these measures are not successful, testicular sperm aspiration (TESA) is performed. Unfortunately, several males experienced scrotal hemorrhage after TESA.

As the worsening of the doctor-patient relationship in China, the violence in hospitals in China was growing and Chinese doctors were under tremendous stress [1]. It is necessary to look for the possible reason of scrotal hemorrhage after TESA and avoid such events. Surprisingly, none of azoospermia patients appeared scrotal hemorrhage after biopsy with the same TESA operation. It is assumed that scrotal hemorrhage after TESA may

* Correspondence: 13763339658@163.com; zhuyongtong@sina.com
†Equal contributors
[1]Reproductive Medicine Center, Department of Obstetrics and Gynecology, Nanfang Hospital/ The First School of Clinical Medicine, Southern Medical University, Guangzhou, China
[2]Department of Neurology, Integrated Hospital of Traditional Chinese Medicine, Southern Medical University, Guangzhou, China
Full list of author information is available at the end of the article

be associated with PDE5i administration. To our knowledge, reports about such cases are scarce. Therefore, this retrospective study was designed to summarize the data and answer this question.

Methods

Study design

We retrospectively reviewed the records of 504 men who underwent TESA at the Center for Reproductive Medicine, Nanfang Hospital, Guangzhou, China From 2012 to 2015. This study was approved by the Clinical Medical Local Ethical Review Committee of the Southern Medical University. Informed written consent was provided by all men in the study.

The men were classified into 2 groups; those who received a PDE5i before TESA and those who did not receive a PDE5i. Briefly, if men were unable to provide a sperm sample by masturbation due to stress/anxiety, and met the criteria described below, they were given tadalafil 20 mg and attempted to provide a sample by masturbation again. If a sample could not be provided TESA was performed. The time from tadalafil administration to TESA was approximately 3 h. The criteria of men in whom TESA was performed directly (not given the option of masturbation, control group) are described below.

Five hundred four men in this study were all infertility more than 1 year. Inclusion criteria for the drug group were: (1) had ejaculation by masturbation successfully more than twice, (2) were not able to ejaculation on the day of oocyte retrieval, (3) sperm were identified on semen analyses. Inclusion criteria for the control group were: (1) previously identified azoospermia, which contained obstruction azoospermia and non- obstruction azoospermia, or cryptozoospermia [2], (2) testis volumes were more than 8 mL. Patients in the drug group were all sperm retrieval performed by TESA successfully. In order to compare consistently, patients with prior epididymal sperm aspiration (PESA), testicular sperm extraction (TESE) or micro-TESE were excluded from this study.

TESA procedure

The testis was anesthetized using 1% lidocaine. A 23 gauge needle was passed through the scrotal skin into the testicular tissue. Suction was applied with a 5 mL syringe, and the backpressure was maintained by hand. The needle was pushed in different directions into the testicular tissue to obtain a sample. Once an adequate sample was obtained, the needle was slowly removed from the testis while the negative pressure was maintained (Fig. 1). The sample was placed on a sterile plate, and the small tubules recovered were picked up by an assistant using 2 pairs of fine tweezers. Sperm in

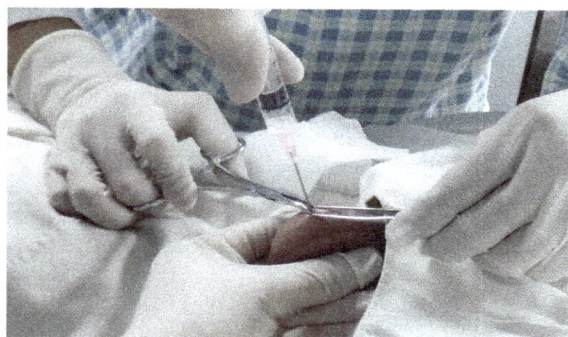

Fig. 1 The testicular sperm aspiration procedure

aspirated tissue was retrieved for ICSI or biopsy. All procedures were performed by Dr. Chu and Dr. Zhu.

Follow-up

Patients were given wound care instructions, and instructed to keep the puncture site dry and clean for 3 days. They were asked about light level of activity following the procedures, and abstained from strenuous exercise for 1 month. Patients were seen for follow-up at 3 day, 1 week, and 1 month after TESA. At the follow-up visits, examination of the scrotum was performed for identification of hematoma formation. Patients were also asked the following 2 questions at each visit: (1) Did you avoid the strenuous exercise? (2) Did you feel uncomfortable in your scrotum?

Sonographic examination with Doppler imaging was performed if physical examination was consistent with a scrotal hemorrhage. If a hemorrhage did not self-absorb during 4- week period, an evacuation procedure was performed to remove the remaining blood products and clots.

Statistical analysis

Calculations were analyzed by using SPSS 19.0 software (SPSS Inc., Chicago, Illinois, USA). All numeric data were presented as the mean value ± standard deviation. Frequencies were expressed as percentages. Students t-test was used for comparisons between 2 groups, and Fischer's exact test was used for comparison of proportions. Values of $P < 0.05$ were considered to indicate statistically significant differences.

Results

A total of 504 men who received TESA from 2012 to 2015 were included in the analysis. Mean age of the men was 28.63 ± 4.22 years. The testis size, character and the presence of testicular mass, or asymmetry was assessed via manual palpation and orchidometer. Mean testis volume was 11.8 ± 2.6 ml (Table 1). Coagulation function, which contained Thrombin time, Activated partial

Table 1 Characteristics of patients

	Control group	Drug group	Overall	P value
Number	428	76	504	
Age (years)	28.40 ± 3.86	29.07 ± 4.11	28.63 ± 4.22	P > 0.05
Testis volume (mL)	12.0 ± 4.3	11.5 ± 2.9	11.8 ± 3.6	P > 0.05
Coagulation function				
Thrombin time (sec)	15.24 ± 2.11	14.98 ± 2.03	15.11 ± 2.14	P > 0.05
Activated partial thromboplastin time (sec)	25.71 ± 3.23	26.01 ± 3.17	25.89 ± 3.26	P > 0.05
International normalized ratio	0.89 ± 0.23	0.91 ± 0.22	0.90 ± 0.22	P > 0.05
Prothrombin time (sec)	11.65 ± 1.09	12.02 ± 1.16	11.87 ± 1.18	P > 0.05
Fibrinogen (g/L)	2.55 ± 1.03	2.64 ± 1.06	2.62 ± 1.07	P > 0.05
Incidence of hemorrhage (%)	0(0.0)	4(5.3)	4(0.8)	P = 0.000

thromboplastin time, International normalized ratio, Prothrombin time and Fibrinogen were not different between the 2 groups. There were 428 men in the control group (no PDE5i) and 76 men in the drug group. The overall incidence of scrotal hemorrhage in the 504 men was 0.8%. However, the incidence in the control group was 0.0%, and in the PDE5i group was 5.3% (4 men) (P = 0.000). All 4 patients required an evacuation procedure. No other post-operative complications were noted.

Discussion
TESA, which was developed in 1992, is a method for retrieving sperm for use in assisted reproductive technology [3]. The procedure is also used to perform biopsy of the testis. Compared to TESE, TESA is a simpler procedure with minimal physiological consequences [4]. The majority of patients in the control group were obstructive patients. While azoospermic patients who had smaller testicular volume (< 8 mL), especially in the setting of testicular hypofunction, TESE or micro-TESE would be more appropriate in these patients.

It has been reported that intra-testicular hematoma formation occurs in 29% of diagnostic testicular biopsies [5]. However, scrotal hemorrhage was a relatively rare clinical event after TESA. In the current study of 504 TESA procedures, the incidence was only 0.8%. The difference in rates may be due to the increased use of sonographic examination. Most patients do not feel uncomfortable after TESA, and routine sonographic examination is not performed, and thus small areas of hemorrhage maybe overlooked.

At our institution, during the period from 2013 to 2015, 76 men successfully ejaculated by masturbation more than 2 times, but they were not able to ejaculation on the day of oocyte retrieval. Patients on intracavernosal injection treatment had high withdrawal rates. The most common reason for withdrawal was poor response to the therapy, followed by the inconvenience of use [6].

So they did not receive such therapy in our centre. These men passed through a procedure of relaxation, given pornographic material, mood adjusting and PDE5i drug taking, selected TESA operation finally to retrieve sperm. Although the proportion of these men who developed a scrotal hemorrhage was only 2.6%, no scrotal hemorrhage occured after same operation in the other 428 patients who did not receive a PDE5i. The results suggest that the scrotal hemorrhage in these 4 patients was related to the use of a PDE5i.

PDE5i, such as sildenafil (Viagra), vardenafil (Levitra) and tadalafil (Cialis), are used to treat erectile dysfunction. PDE5i increases nitrous oxide (NO) and cyclic guanosine monophosphate (cGMP) in the smooth muscles of the corpus cavernosum. For a PDE5i to be effective, sufficient sexual stimulation is essential [7]. The men who received a PDE5i still could not relax enough to achieve sexual arousal and could not successfully ejaculate. PDE5i are generally safe and well tolerated [8], have not been reported in association with scrotal hemorrhage events. As men were not able to ask to stop PDE5i before any surgical procedure, the rationale for excess bleeding in men taking PDE5i may not exist. Although our results showed a correlation between taking a PDE5i and scrotal hemorrhage, a cause-effect relationship could not be determined from the study design. However, the mechanism by which a PDE5i increases the risk of a scrotal hemorrhage may be as follows. First, a PDE5i results in vasodilation, and redistribution of arterial blood flow that is associated with rupture of vessels. Second, the NO and cGMP pathway might be responsible for inhibition of platelet aggregation and activation. Finally, PDE5i are considered as an antithrombotic agent [9].

The limitations of this study include its retrospective design. A prospective study should be done to validate our results. Although a large number of patients participated in this study, it appears as there were only 4 events (hematoma) in the 504 patients, which may be not enough to draw the conclusion and the results maybe only anecdotal. As ultrasound was only performed after the physician suspected a hematoma on physical exam post procedure. This may introduce significant bias and lack of certainty if there actually were many other patients that did not develop hematomas that were not detected by the clinician performing a 3 days post procedure exam. So it would be better to perform ultrasound exam at 3 days after TESA.

Although there were no sufficient evidences which could support that scrotal hemorrhage after TESA was caused by the administration of a PDE5i. Given the potential risk of scrotal hemorrhage after the ingestion of a PDE5i, it should be cautious to prescribe this medicine when the patient is likely to perform TESA. Patients were on anti-coagulants, anti-platelets, taking NSAIDs and ice scrotum may be beneficial after TESA. Although it is difficult to predict ahead who have difficulty producing a semen sample of the day of assisted reproductive technique, as all patients in the drug group had been able to produce ejaculated sperm twice prior to the procedure date. We should gain information by detailed inquiry. It would be better to prepare frozen sperm before the day of the retrieval once patient were categorized as masturbation difficulty males.

Conclusion

In summary, the results of this study suggest that a PDE5i administration increases the risk of scrotal hemorrhage in men undergoing TESA, although the study design does not allow drawing a conclusion of cause and effect. Given the potential risk of scrotal hemorrhage after the ingestion of PDE5i, it may be wise not to administer it to men in whom a TESA may be performed.

Abbreviations
cGMP: Cyclic guanosine monophosphate; ICSI: Intracytoplasmic sperm injection; NO: nitrous oxide; PDE5i: Phosphodiesterase type5 inhibitor; PESA: Epididymal sperm aspiration; TESA: Testicular sperm aspiration; TESE: Testicular sperm extraction

Acknowledgments
This research was supported by The Chinese Medical Association of Clinical Medicine Research Special Fund (No. 16020530669, 16020170633), Natural Science Foundation of Guangdong Province (No. 2016A030310403, 2015A030310367), Medical Scientific Research Foundation of Guangdong Province (No. A2016092), and Merck Serono China Research Fund.

Authors' contributions
YZ and RH contributed equally to this work. YZ, CW, RH, WT and QC conceived and designed the study; YZ and CW collected data; YZ, CW, RH, WT and QC performed data analysis; YZ, CW, RH, SQ, WT and QC prepared the manuscript; All authors read and approved the final manuscript.

Competing interests
The authors declare that they have no competing interests.

Author details
[1]Reproductive Medicine Center, Department of Obstetrics and Gynecology, Nanfang Hospital/ The First School of Clinical Medicine, Southern Medical University, Guangzhou, China. [2]Department of Neurology, Integrated Hospital of Traditional Chinese Medicine, Southern Medical University, Guangzhou, China. [3]Department of Urology, Nanfang Hospital, Southern Medical University, Guangzhou, China.

References
1. Yang T, Zhang H, Shen F, Li JW, Wu MC. Appeal from Chinese doctors to end violence. Lancet. 2013;382(9906):1703–4.
2. Zhu YT, Luo C, Li Y, Li H, Quan S, Deng YJ, Yang Y, Hu YH, Tan WL, Chu QJ. Differences and similarities between extremely severe oligozoospermia and cryptozoospermia in intracytoplasmic sperm injection. Asian J Androl. 2016; 18(6):904–7.
3. Nowroozi MR, Ahmadi H, Ayati M, Jamshidian H, Sirous A. Testicular fine-needle aspiration versus testicular open biopsy: comparable sperm retrieval rate in selected patients. Indian J Urol. 2012;28(1):37–42.
4. Westlander G, Ekerhovd E, Granberg S, Lycke N, Nilsson L, Werner C, Bergh C. Serial ultrasonography, hormonal profile and antisperm antibody response after testicular sperm aspiration. Hum Reprod. 2001;16(12):2621–7.
5. Harrington TG, Schauer D, Gilbert BR. Percutaneous testis biopsy: an alternative to open testicular biopsy in the evaluation of the subfertile man. J Urol. 1996;156(5):1647–51.
6. Sung HH, Ahn JS, Kim JJ, Choo SH, Han DH, Lee SW. The role of intracavernosal injection therapy and the reasons of withdrawal from therapy in patients with erectile dysfunction in the era of PDE5 inhibitors. Andrology. 2014;2(1):45–50.
7. Sharma R. Novel phosphodiesterase-5 inhibitors: current indications and future directions. Indian J Med Sci. 2007;61(12):667–79.
8. Yuan J, Zhang R, Yang Z, Lee J, Liu Y, Tian J, Qin X, Ren Z, Ding H, Chen Q, Mao C, Tang J. Comparative effectiveness and safety of oral phosphodiesterase type 5 inhibitors for erectile dysfunction: a systematic review and network meta-analysis. Eur Urol. 2013;63(5):902–12.
9. Stefanovic-Budimkic M, Jovanovic DR, Beslac-Bumbasirevic L, Ercegovac MD. Recurrent ischemic stroke associated with sildenafil and tadalafil use in a young adult. Clin Neurol Neurosurg. 2012;114(4):405–7.

28

Fibroblast growth factor receptor 3 (FGFR3) aberrations in muscle-invasive urothelial carcinoma

Young Saing Kim[1], Kyung Kim[2], Ghee-Young Kwon[3], Su Jin Lee[2] and Se Hoon Park[2]* (iD)

Abstract

Background: Recent studies suggest that *FGFR3* is a potential therapeutic target in urothelial carcinoma (UC). The purpose of this study was to evaluate the rates and types of *FGFR3* aberrations in patients with muscle-invasive UC who received radical resection.

Methods: We analyzed surgical tumor samples from 74 UC patients who had received radical cystectomy ($n = 40$) or ureteronephrectomy ($n = 34$). Ion AmpliSeq Cancer Hotspot Panel v2 and nCounter Copy Number Variation Assay were used to detect *FGFR3* aberrations.

Results: Fifty-four patients (73%) had high-grade tumors, and 62% had lymph node involvement. Sixteen patients (22%) harbored *FGFR3* alterations, the most common of which was *FGFR3* mutations ($n = 13$): Y373C ($n = 3$), N532D ($n = 3$), R248C ($n = 2$), S249C ($n = 1$), G370C ($n = 1$), S657S ($n = 1$), A797P ($n = 1$), and 746_747insG ($n = 1$). Three additional patients had a *FGFR3-TACC3* rearrangement. The frequency of *FGFR3* aberrations was higher in bladder UC (25%) than in UC of the renal pelvis and ureter (18%) but the difference was not statistically significant ($P = 0.444$). Genes that were co-aberrant with *FGFR3* included *APC* (88%), *PDGFRA* (81%), *RET* (69%), and *TP53* (69%).

Conclusions: We report the frequency and types of FGFR3 aberrations in Korean patients with UC. Patients with *FGFR3* mutations or *FGFR3-TACC3* fusion may constitute potential candidates for a novel FGFR-targeted therapy in the perioperative setting.

Keywords: Urothelial carcinoma, FGFR, Mutation, Fusion

Background

Urothelial carcinoma (UC), a cancer involving the transitional epithelium of the urinary tract, is the seventh most common malignancy in Korea [1]. The majority of cases arises in the bladder, whereas only about 5 to 10% occurs in the upper urinary tract including the renal pelvis and ureter [2]. Because of the relative rarity of upper tract urothelial carcinoma (UTUC), clinical decision making for patients with UTUC depends on data available for urinary bladder urothelial carcinoma (UBUC) [3].

For metastatic or advanced UC, platinum-based chemotherapy is considered standard treatment. There is a need to develop new therapeutic options focused on the molecular aberrations driving UC, as patients who fail to respond or have progressed after platinum-based chemotherapy have a grim prognosis. Recently, molecular analysis has identified subsets of UC expressing distinct molecular signatures. Genomic alterations in the fibroblast growth factor receptor 3 (*FGFR3*) are well described in UC and have led to extensive clinical investigations evaluating FGFR3 inhibitors [4]. FGFR3, which belongs to the family of tyrosine kinase, is responsible for the FGF signal transduction. FGFR3 signaling is involved in development, differentiation, cell survival, migration, angiogenesis, and carcinogenesis [5]. The most common types of *FGFR3* aberrations in UC are activating mutations, followed by gene rearrangements and amplification [6, 7]. *FGFR3* mutations are predominantly found in genetically stable UC [8], and have been

---
* Correspondence: hematoma@skku.edu
[2]Division of Hematology-Oncology, Department of Medicine, Sungkyunkwan University Samsung Medical Center, Sungkyunkwan University School of Medicine, 81 Irwon-ro, Gangnam-gu, Seoul 06351, South Korea
Full list of author information is available at the end of the article

associated with oncogenic progression in UC [9]. *FGFR3* gene rearrangements generate constitutively activated and oncogenic FGFR3 kinase protein products, and cellular dependence on these drivers confers sensitivity to selective FGFR inhibition [10, 11]. Furthermore, studies indicate that *FGFR3* mutation status could be used to guide anti-FGFR3 therapy [12]. However, previous molecular studies were performed mainly in patients with UBUC. Data on FGFR3 aberrations in the UTUC, particularly in the muscle invasive type, are not yet sufficient. Based on these considerations, this retrospective study aimed to evaluate the frequency and types of *FGFR3* gene aberrations in radically resected UC. We also compared the frequency of *FGFR3* alterations between UBUC and UTUC.

Methods

Patients

This study is a part of the Samsung Medical Center (SMC) Oncology Biomarker study (ClinicalTrials.gov identifier: NCT01831609). Tumor samples were collected from 74 consecutive patients with UC who underwent radical cystectomy or nephroureterectomy between 2012 and 2014, and had adequate specimen for molecular analysis. All patients provided written informed consent for the use of tumor tissues as well as their clinical data. This study was performed in accordance with the Declaration of Helsinki and approved by the Institutional Review Board of SMC (Seoul, Korea).

Genomic DNA extraction

Our dedicated genitourinary pathologist (G.Y.K.) reviewed all pathology specimens to ensure the samples contained > 80% tumor cells with < 20% necrosis. Genomic DNA was extracted from the primary tumor tissues using a QIAamp DNA Mini Kit (Qiagen, Valencia, CA, USA). After extraction, we measured concentration as well as 260/280 and 260/230 nm ratio by spectrophotometer (ND1000, Nanodrop Technologies, Thermo-Fisher Scientific, MA, USA). Each sample was then quantified with the Qubit fluorometer (Life technologies, Carlsbad, CA, USA). Genomic DNA with > 10 ng measured by Qubit fluorometer was subjected to library preparation.

DNA sequencing and copy number variations

We used the Ion Torrent Ampliseq™ cancer panel v2 to detect frequent somatic mutations that were selected based on a literature review. This panel examines 2855 mutations in 50 commonly mutated oncogenes and tumor suppressor genes (Additional file 1: Table S1). We constructed libraries using 10 ng of genomic DNA with

the Ion AmpliSeq Library Kit and Ion Xpress Barcodes (Life Technologies). For barcoded library preparations, barcoded adapters from the Ion Xpress Barcode Adapters 1–96 Kit were substituted for the non-barcoded adapter mix in the Ion AmpliSeq Library Kit. Next, the multiplexed barcoded libraries were enriched by clonal amplification using emulsion polymerase chain reaction (PCR) on Ion Sphere Particles (Ion PGMTemplate 200 Kit) and loaded on an Ion 316 Chip. Massively parallel sequencing was carried out on an Ion PGM using the Ion PGM Sequencing 200 Kit v2. The primary filtering process was performed using Torrent Suite v3.6.0 and Ion Torrent Variant Caller v3.6 software. The pipeline included signaling processing, base calling, quality score assignment, adapter trimming, read alignment to 19 human genome references, mapping quality control, coverage analysis, and variant calling. For detection of copy number variations (CNV), nCounter Copy Number Variation CodeSets (NanoString Technologies, Seattle, WA, USA) were used with 300 ng of purified genomic DNA extracted from 2 to 3 sections of 4-µm-thick, formalin-fixed, paraffin-embedded (FFPE) representative tumor blocks using a QIAamp DNA FFPE Tissue Kit (Qiagen, Hilden, Germany). DNA was fragmented via AluI digestion and denatured at 95uC. Fragmented DNA was hybridized with the codeset of 257 genes (Additional file 2: Table S2) in the nCounter Cancer CN Assay Kit (Nanostring Technologies) for 18 h at 65uC and processed according to the manufacturer's instructions. The nCounter Digital Analyzer counted and tabulated the signals of reporter probes.

Bioinformatics and statistical analyses

We used cutoff values of greater than 6% variant frequency and more than 100X coverage to detect true mutational changes in accordance with previous reports and our own experience. Variant calls were further analyzed using the ANNOVAR, which included variant filtering and annotation using the Catalogue of Somatic Mutations in Cancer (COSMIC, http://cancer.sanger.ac.uk/cancergenome/projects/cosmic) database, dbSNP build 137, and amino acid change information. Variant calls from Ion AmpliSeq were further evaluated to reduce potential false-positives. Coverage (> 100X) and quality score (> 30) were considered as filtering criteria. For gene expression data from the NanoString nCounter assay, filtering of samples using quality control criteria was performed according to the manufacturer's recommendations. All statistical analyses were performed by the Biostatistics and Clinical Epidemiology Center at our institute. The R for Windows v2.11.1 software (R Core Team, Vienna, Austria; http://www.r-project.org) was used for

Table 1 Patient characteristics

	All patients (n = 74)	UTUC (n = 34)	UBUC (n = 40)
Age, years			
Median	64	65	64
Range	37 to 83	50 to 79	37 to 83
Gender			
Male	64 (86%)	25 (74%)	37 (93%)
Female	10 (14%)	9 (26%)	3 (8%)
pT			
1	3 (4%)	1 (3%)	2 (5%)
2	14 (19%)	5 (15%)	9 (23%)
3	55 (74%)	27 (79%)	28 (70%)
4	2 (3%)	1 (3%)	1 (3%)
pN			
0	11 (15%)	7 (21%)	4 (10%)
1	19 (26%)	4 (12%)	15 (38%)
2	23 (31%)	6 (18%)	17 (43%)
3	4 (5%)	1 (3%)	3 (8%)
Not evaluated	17 (23%)	16 (47%)	1 (3%)
Grade			
2	20 (27%)	11 (32%)	9 (23%)
3	54 (73%)	23 (68%)	31 (78%)
Lymphovascular invasion			
No	34 (46%)	15 (44%)	19 (48%)
Present	40 (54%)	19 (56%)	21 (53%)
Type of surgery			
Open	41 (55%)	15 (44%)	26 (65%)
Laparoscopic/robot-assisted	33 (45%)	19 (56%)	14 (35%)
Perioperative chemotherapy			
None	21 (28%)	10 (29%)	11 (28%)
Neoadjuvant	27 (36%)	1 (3%)	26 (65%)
Adjuvant	26 (35%)	23 (68%)	3 (8%)

UTUC Upper tract urothelial carcinoma, *UBUC* Urinary bladder urothelial carcinoma; *pT* pathological T stage, *pN* pathological N stage

analysis of all data. We implemented the method found in the R "compound.Cox" package.

Results

A total of 74 patients with primary tumor samples available were included: 34 patients for UTUC and 40 patients for UBUC (Table 1). Median age at the time of surgery of all patients was 64 years (range, 37 to 83). UC patients were predominantly male (86%), but the proportion of female patients was a bit higher in UTUC than in UBUC (26% vs. 8%, respectively). All but one UBUC had undergone lymph node dissection whereas it was performed in 53% of UTUC patients. In UBUC cohort, more than half of patients (65%) received neoadjuvant chemotherapy prior to radical

cystectomy. In all patients, perioperative chemotherapy was a combination of gemcitabine plus either cisplatin or carboplatin, based on the patients' renal function. There was no significant difference in other clinicopathological features including histology, tumor grade, pathological T (pT) stage, pathological N (pN) and lymphovascular invasion between UBUC and UTUC. Since all tumor samples were obtained at the time of radical surgery, the cohorts lacked early stage, superficial UC.

Among 74 tumor samples tested, we found 16 (22%) actionable *FGFR3* gene aberrations. Table 2 presents the clinical and pathological characteristics of the 16 patients with *FGFR3* aberrations. In addition to 13 patients with *FGFR3* mutations, we identified three patients with

Table 2 Clinical and pathological characteristics of patients with *FGFR3* gene aberrations detected in surgical specimens

Patient	Age	Gender	Primary site	Pathologic stage	Grade	LVI	FGFR3
TCC_03	64	M	Bladder	pT3N0	3	No	FGFR3-TACC3 fusion
TCC_07	58	M	Bladder	pT2N0	2	No	Y373C
TCC_13	47	M	Bladder	pT2N2	2	Yes	R248C
TCC_14	61	M	Bladder	pT3N0	2	No	G370C
TCC_19	66	M	Bladder	pT3N0	2	No	746_747insG (NM_000142)
TCC_41	55	M	Renal pelvis	pT3Nx	2	No	FGFR3-TACC3 fusion
TCC_44	71	M	Renal pelvis	pT3Nx	3	Yes	N532D
TCC_48	50	M	Bladder	pT4N3	3	No	S249C
TCC_49	63	M	Bladder	pT1N2	2	Yes	A797P
TCC_50	59	F	Ureter	pT3N1	2	No	N532D
TCC_55	73	M	Bladder	pT2N0	2	No	S675S
TCC_56	54	F	Renal pelvis	pT3Nx	2	No	Y373C
TCC_61	78	M	Ureter	pT3Nx	3	No	Y373C
TCC_63	55	M	Ureter	pT3N2	3	Yes	R248C
TCC_70	66	M	Bladder	pT4N0	2	No	N532D
TCC_71	80	M	Bladder	pT2N0	2	No	FGFR3-TACC3 fusion

FGFR3 Fibroblast growth factor receptor 3, *LVI* Lymphovascular invasion

translocation involving *FGFR3-TACC3* (Chr4) which was already considered a promising therapeutic target [13]. There was no significant difference in the frequency of *FGFR3* aberrations between UTUC (18%) and UBUC (25%) cohorts ($P = 0.444$). 31% of tumors with *FGFR3* aberrations were of grade 3 (i.e., poorly-differentiated, according to the WHO 1973 classification). Grade 3 and lymphovascular invasion were associated with a lower frequency of *FGFR3* aberrations (Table 3).

We next investigated other genetic alterations in 16 patients with *FGFR3* gene aberrations (Fig. 1). As

Table 3 Rates of *FGFR3* gene aberrations according to patient characteristics

Characteristics	Total No.	FGFR3 aberration No.	P value
Primary site			0.444[a]
UBUC	40	10 (25%)	
UTUC	34	6 (18%)	
Gender			1.000[b]
Male	64	14 (22%)	
Female	10	2 (20%)	
Grade			< 0.001[b]
2	20	11(55%)	
3	54	5 (9%)	
Lymphovascular invasion			0.008[a]
No	34	12 (35%)	
Yes	40	4 (10%)	

[a]Chi-squared test
[b]Fisher's exact test

expected, we found no relevant differences in the incidence of both inactivating and activating mutations between UTUC and UBUC. The most frequently observed genetic mutation was *APC*, followed by *PDGFRA*, *KDR*, *FLT3*, and *STK11*. *HRAS* mutations were found in 7 patients. Interestingly, three of these *HRAS* mutations were found to be activating, actionable mutations (G12S, G13R and Q61R), unlike the previous study suggesting a mutual exclusion of *RAS* and *FGFR3* [14].

Discussion

Radical cystectomy is the treatment of choice for muscle invasive UBUC [15], and radical nephroureterectomy is considered the standard treatment for UTUC [16]. However, the high rate of recurrence in these tumors necessitates novel approaches to systemic therapy. FGFR3 is considered a potential therapeutic target in UC, because recent studies show that FGFR3 activation is an important contributor to tumor development and angiogenesis in UC [17, 18]. Molecular tumor analysis and rational selection of patients are necessary in order to perform clinical trials involving FGFR-targeted agents. The present study demonstrated that *FGFR3* abnormalities are present in 22% of patients with UC who underwent radical resection. The majority of aberrations were *FGFR3* point mutations.

Although UTUC and UBUC have a similar histologic feature, there are epidemiologic and clinicopathologic differences between them [19]. Recently, several studies have reported molecular profiles of UTUC and UBUC [20–22], but controversy remains regarding whether

Gene	UTUC TCC_61	TCC_44	TCC_50	TCC_56	TCC_63	TCC_41	UBUC TCC_71	TCC_13	TCC_03	TCC_48	TCC_07	TCC_19	TCC_14	TCC_49	TCC_70	TCC_55	Freq(%)
FGFR3																	100
APC																	88
PDGFRA																	81
KDR																	81
FLT3																	75
STK11																	75
CSF1R																	69
RET																	69
TP53																	69
ERBB4																	63
EGFR																	50
HRAS																	44
SMO																	44
ALK																	38
KIT																	38
ABL1																	38
ATM																	38
SMAD4																	38
FBXW7																	38
RB1																	31
ERBB2																	31
GNAQ																	25
PTPN11																	25
PIK3CA																	25
NOTCH1																	25
GNA11																	19
PTEN																	19
FGFR1																	19
VHL																	19
FGFR2																	13
MLH1																	13
MET																	13
IDH2																	13
KRAS																	6
HNF1A																	6
CDH1																	6
IDH1																	6
SMARCB1																	6

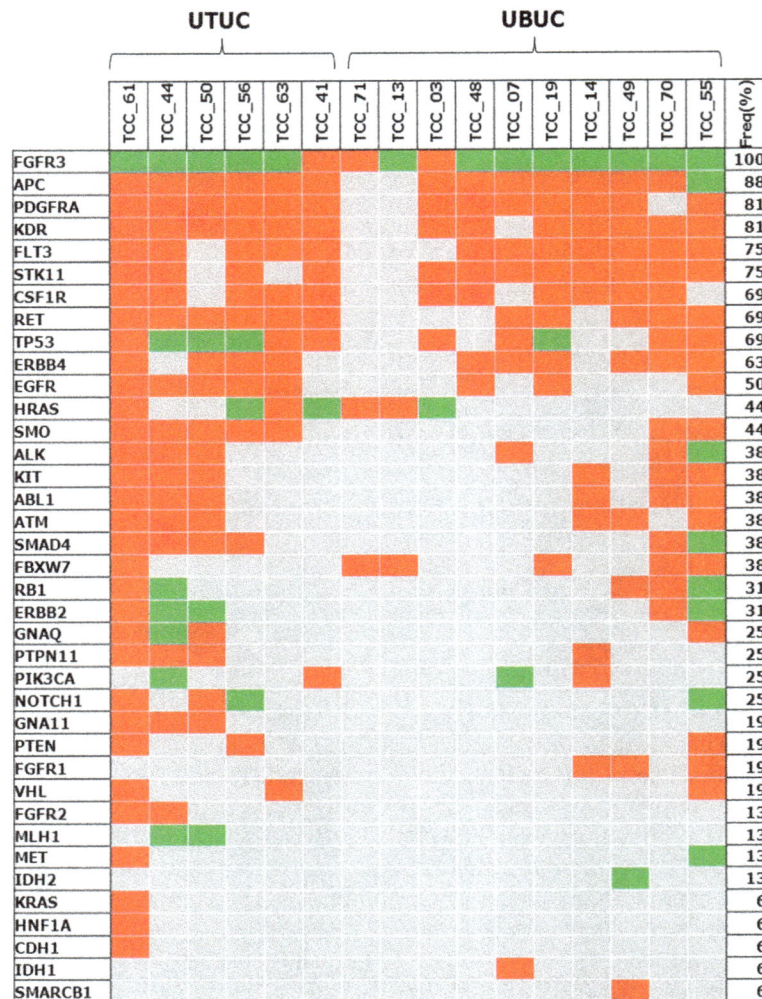

Fig. 1 Distribution of additional mutations identified by Ampliseq (*n* = 16). Red squares indicate inactivating mutation. Green squares indicate activating mutation. *UTUC* Upper tract urothelial carcinoma, *UBUC* Urinary bladder urothelial carcinoma

UTUC is biologically distinct from UBUC. This is because, in part, of the relative rarity of UTUC hindering large-scale molecular studies. Our study focused on *FGFR3* aberrations in muscle-invasive UC and compared UTUC with UBUC. Compared to previous studies, relatively many cases of UTUB (*n* = 34) were included in the analysis and the results showed no significant difference in the frequency of *FGFR3* aberrations between UBUC (25%) and UTUC (18%). On the other hand, in a study comparing high-grade UTUC (*n* = 59) with UBUC (*n* = 102), overall landscape of genetic alterations was similar in both groups, although *FGFR3* were more frequently altered in UTUC than in UBUC (36% vs. 22%, respectively) [22]. In a comprehensive study of the genetics of UTUC, whole exome sequencing was performed in samples from 27 patients; *FGFR3* alteration was detected in 60% (9 of 15) of high-grade tumors and in 37.5% (3 of 8) of > pT2 tumors [21].

FGFR3 mutations are common in low grade and early stage UCs, while they are less common in muscle-invasive tumors. In a previous meta-analysis for *FGFR3* mutations in UBUC, the frequency of *FGFR3* mutations decreased with increasing stage and grade: 65% in pTa, 30.2% in pT1, 11.5% in pT2–4 and 69.8% in G1, 68% in G2 and 18.6% in G3 [23]. The frequency of *FGFR3* mutations in the present study was infrequent with 18%; it is explained by that in our study, 96 and 73% had pT2–4 and G3 disease, respectively. We identified eight different mutations, including R248C, S249C, and Y373C, which consist more than 95% of mutations from radical cystectomy specimens in a previous study [12]. Preclinical models and early clinical trials suggest that these mutations have sensitivity to FGFR3 inhibitors [18, 24, 25]. Furthermore, we found four additional mutations (N532D, S676S, A797P, and 746_747insG) which have not been reported previously in the COSMIC database (accessed December 2017). Further studies are needed in order to evaluate if these mutations are pathogenic and represent valid targets for anti-FGFR3 therapy.

FGFR3 fusion proteins are additional type of mutational events in a subset of UCs with up-regulated FGFR3 expression. FGFR3 fusions with TACC3 and BAIAP2L1 have been reported in UC cell lines and tissues [10, 18]. The clinical relevance of FGFR3-TACC3 fusion in UC has been highlighted by results from preclinical and early clinical studies reporting promising responses to the treatment with FGFR inhibitors. In a phase I trial with FGFR inhibitor JNJ-42756493 (n = 65), five responses were observed; two of them harbored FGFR3-TACC3 translocation [26]. It has been reported that the prevalence of FGFR3-TACC3 fusion in UC ranged 2 to 6% [6, 22, 27]. As the majorities of studies analyzed samples from muscle-invasive cancer, the association between FGFR3 fusion and tumor grade or stage is still uncertain. In our study, FGFR3-TACC3 translocation was observed in three patients (4%): one patient with high-grade tumor and two patients with low-grade tumor. On the other hand, Sfakianos et al. reported that all five FGFR3-TACC3 translocations were detected only in high-grade UTUCs (n = 59) but in no low-grade tumors (0 of 23) [22].

Recent studies have reported encouraging data of FGFR3-targeted therapies in patients with advanced UC harboring FGFR3 alterations. In a phase I expansion cohort study [28], 67 patients with FGFR3-altered UC were enrolled and treated with BGJ398, a selective FGFR1–3 inhibitor; 70.1% had received two or more systemic therapies. BGJ398 monotherapy was well tolerated and had response rate of 25.4% with a disease control rate of 64.2%. In a Phase II trial of erdafitinib [29], a pan-FGFR inhibitor, the 99 patients enrolled had a verified mutation in FGFR3 (74.7%) or fusion in FGFR2/FGFR3 (25.3%); 88.1% had received ≥1 line of prior systemic treatment. Erdafitinib showed a response rate of 40.4% and a disease control rate of 79.8%. Responses occurred in patients without prior exposure to chemotherapy (41.7%) as well as those previously treated with chemotherapy (40.2%). These results suggest that FGFR3-targeted therapies may represent a viable strategy for the treatment of FGFR3-altered UC in metastatic as well as perioperative settings.

Several limitations of our study warrant consideration. First, the results should be interpreted with caution given the limited number of patients and retrospective nature. Second, analysis using matched normal tissues was not performed. Third, the imbalance in the administration of neoadjuvant chemotherapy between UBUC and UTUC may affect the results, because it is known that neoadjuvant chemotherapy can induce mutational shift [30, 31]. Similarly, it should be noted that previous

intravesical therapy may influence the results of mutational analysis in UBUC, although our study included only three patients who had received intravesical therapy.

Conclusions
We report that FGFR3 gene aberrations were detected in 22% of curatively-resected UC. The frequency was similar between UTUC and UBUC. Patients with FGFR3 mutations or FGFR3-TACC3 fusion may constitute potential candidates for a novel FGFR-targeted therapy in the perioperative setting. Further studies are warranted to reveal the functional significance of the FGFR3 aberrations and better define subset of patients that benefit from anti-FGFR therapy.

Abbreviations
CNV: Copy number variation; COSMIC: Catalogue of somatic mutations in cancer; FFPE: Formalin-fixed, paraffin-embedded; FGFR3: Fibroblast growth factor receptor 3; PCR: Polymerase chain reaction; pN: Pathological N; pT: Pathological T; SMC: Samsung Medical Center; UBUC: Urinary bladder urothelial carcinoma; UC: Urothelial carcinoma; UTUC: Upper tract urothelial carcinoma

Funding
No funding source

Authors' contributions
YSK contributed to study design and drafted the manuscripts. KK and SJL participated in data collection and analysis. GYK carried out pathologic review of tissue samples and participated in genetic studies. SHP contributed to study design, data interpretation, and editing the manuscript. All authors read and approved the final manuscript.

Competing interests
The authors declare that they have no competing interests.

Author details
[1]Division of Medical Oncology, Department of Internal Medicine, Gil Medical Center, Gachon University College of Medicine, Incheon, South Korea. [2]Division of Hematology-Oncology, Department of Medicine, Sungkyunkwan University Samsung Medical Center, Sungkyunkwan University School of Medicine, 81 Irwon-ro, Gangnam-gu, Seoul 06351, South Korea. [3]Department of Pathology and Translational Genomics, Sungkyunkwan University Samsung Medical Center, Seoul, South Korea.

References
1. Jung KW, Park S, Kong HJ, Won YJ, Lee JY, Park EC, Lee JS. Cancer statistics in Korea: incidence, mortality, survival, and prevalence in 2008. Cancer Res Treat. 2011;43(1):1–11.
2. Munoz JJ, Ellison LM. Upper tract urothelial neoplasms: incidence and survival during the last 2 decades. J Urol. 2000;164(5):1523–5.
3. Roupret M, Zigeuner R, Palou J, Boehle A, Kaasinen E, Sylvester R, Babjuk M, Oosterlinck W. European guidelines for the diagnosis and management of upper urinary tract urothelial cell carcinomas: 2011 update. Eur Urol. 2011; 59(4):584–94.

4.   Sethakorn N, O'Donnell PH. Spectrum of genomic alterations in FGFR3: current appraisal of the potential role of FGFR3 in advanced urothelial carcinoma. BJU Int. 2016;118(5):681–91.

5.   Turner N, Grose R. Fibroblast growth factor signalling: from development to cancer. Nat Rev Cancer. 2010;10(2):116–29.

6.   Cancer Gemone Atlas Network. Comprehensive molecular characterization of urothelial bladder carcinoma. Nature. 2014;507(7492):315–22.

7.   Helsten T, Elkin S, Arthur E, Tomson BN, Carter J, Kurzrock R. The FGFR landscape in Cancer: analysis of 4,853 tumors by next-generation sequencing. Clin Cancer Res. 2016;22(1):259–67.

8.   van Rhijn BW, Vis AN, van der Kwast TH, Kirkels WJ, Radvanyi F, Ooms EC, Chopin DK, Boeve ER, Jobsis AC, Zwarthoff EC. Molecular grading of urothelial cell carcinoma with fibroblast growth factor receptor 3 and MIB-1 is superior to pathologic grade for the prediction of clinical outcome. J Clin Oncol. 2003;21(10):1912–21.

9.   Parker BC, Engels M, Annala M, Zhang W. Emergence of FGFR family gene fusions as therapeutic targets in a wide spectrum of solid tumours. J Pathol. 2014;232(1):4–15.

10. Williams SV, Hurst CD, Knowles MA. Oncogenic FGFR3 gene fusions in bladder cancer. Hum Mol Genet. 2013;22(4):795–803.

11. Wu YM, Su F, Kalyana-Sundaram S, Khazanov N, Ateeq B, Cao X, Lonigro RJ, Vats P, Wang R, Lin SF, et al. Identification of targetable FGFR gene fusions in diverse cancers. Cancer Discov. 2013;3(6):636–47.

12. Pouessel D, Neuzillet Y, Mertens LS, van der Heijden MS, de Jong J, Sanders J, Peters D, Leroy K, Manceau A, Maille P, et al. Tumor heterogeneity of fibroblast growth factor receptor 3 (FGFR3) mutations in invasive bladder cancer: implications for perioperative anti-FGFR3 treatment. Ann Oncol. 2016;27(7):1311–6.

13. Daly C, Castanaro C, Zhang W, Zhang Q, Wei Y, Ni M, Young TM, Zhang L, Burova E, Thurston G. FGFR3-TACC3 fusion proteins act as naturally occurring drivers of tumor resistance by functionally substituting for EGFR/ERK signaling. Oncogene. 2017;36(4):471–81.

14. Jebar AH, Hurst CD, Tomlinson DC, Johnston C, Taylor CF, Knowles MA. FGFR3 and Ras gene mutations are mutually exclusive genetic events in urothelial cell carcinoma. Oncogene. 2005;24(33):5218–25.

15. Bellmunt J, Orsola A, Leow JJ, Wiegel T, De Santis M, Horwich A. Bladder cancer: ESMO Practice Guidelines for diagnosis, treatment and follow-up. Ann Oncol. 2014;25(Suppl 3):iii40–8.

16. Roupret M, Babjuk M, Comperat E, Zigeuner R, Sylvester RJ, Burger M, Cowan NC, Bohle A, Van Rhijn BW, Kaasinen E, et al. European Association of Urology guidelines on upper urinary tract urothelial cell carcinoma: 2015 update. Eur Urol. 2015;68(5):868–79.

17. Bertz S, Abee C, Schwarz-Furlan S, Alfer J, Hofstadter F, Stoehr R, Hartmann A, Gaumann AK. Increased angiogenesis and FGFR protein expression indicate a favourable prognosis in bladder cancer. Virchows Archiv. 2014;465(6):687–95.

18. di Martino E, Tomlinson DC, Williams SV, Knowles MA. A place for precision medicine in bladder cancer: targeting the FGFRs. Future Oncol (London, England). 2016;12(19):2243–63.

19. Green DA, Rink M, Xylinas E, Matin SF, Stenzl A, Roupret M, Karakiewicz PI, Scherr DS, Shariat SF. Urothelial carcinoma of the bladder and the upper tract: disparate twins. J Urol. 2013;189(4):1214–21.

20. Lee JY, Kim K, Sung HH, Jeon HG, Jeong BC, Seo SI, Jeon SS, Lee HM, Choi HY, Kwon GY, et al. Molecular characterization of urothelial carcinoma of the bladder and upper urinary tract. Transl Oncol. 2018;11(1):37–42.

21. Moss TJ, Qi Y, Xi L, Peng B, Kim TB, Ezzedine NE, Mosqueda ME, Guo CC, Czerniak BA, Ittmann M, et al. Comprehensive genomic characterization of upper tract urothelial carcinoma. Eur Urol. 2017;72(4):641–9.

22. Sfakianos JP, Cha EK, Iyer G, Scott SN, Zabor EC, Shah RH, Ren Q, Bagrodia A, Kim PH, Hakimi AA, et al. Genomic characterization of upper tract urothelial carcinoma. Eur Urol. 2015;68(6):970–7.

23. Neuzillet Y, Paoletti X, Ouerhani S, Mongiat-Artus P, Soliman H, de The H, Sibony M, Denoux Y, Molinie V, Herault A, et al. A meta-analysis of the relationship between FGFR3 and TP53 mutations in bladder cancer. PLoS One. 2012;7(12):e48993.

24. Jager W, Xue H, Hayashi T, Janssen C, Awrey S, Wyatt AW, Anderson S, Moskalev I, Haegert A, Alshalalfa M, et al. Patient-derived bladder cancer xenografts in the preclinical development of novel targeted therapies. Oncotarget. 2015;6(25):21522–32.

25. Sequist LV, Cassier P, Varga A, Tabernero J, Schellens JH, Delord J-P, LoRusso P, Camidge DR, Medina MH, Schuler M, et al. Abstract CT326: phase I study of BGJ398, a selective pan-FGFR inhibitor in genetically preselected advanced solid tumors. Cancer Res. 2014;74(19 Supplement):CT326.

26. Tabernero J, Bahleda R, Dienstmann R, Infante JR, Mita A, Italiano A, Calvo E, Moreno V, Adamo B, Gazzah A, et al. Phase I dose-escalation study of JNJ-42756493, an oral pan-fibroblast growth factor receptor inhibitor, in patients with advanced solid tumors. J Clin Oncol. 2015;33(30):3401–8.

27. Costa R, Carneiro BA, Taxter T, Tavora FA, Kalyan A, Pai SA, Chae YK, Giles FJ. FGFR3-TACC3 fusion in solid tumors: mini review. Oncotarget. 2016;7(34):55924–38.

28. Pal SK, Rosenberg JE, Hoffman-Censits JH, Berger R, Quinn DI, Galsky MD, Wolf J, Dittrich C, Keam B, Delord JP, et al. Efficacy of BGJ398, a fibroblast growth factor receptor 1-3 inhibitor, in patients with previously treated advanced urothelial carcinoma with FGFR3 alterations. Cancer Discov. 2018; 8(7):812–21.

29. Loriot Y, Necchi A, Park SH, García-Donas J, Huddart RA, Burgess EF, Fleming MT, Rezazadeh A, Mellado B, Varlamov S, et al. Erdafitinib (ERDA; JNJ-42756493), a pan-fibroblast growth factor receptor (FGFR) inhibitor, in patients (pts) with metastatic or unresectable urothelial carcinoma (mUC) and FGFR alterations (FGFRa): Phase 2 continuous versus intermittent dosing. J Clin Oncol. 2018;36(6_suppl):411.

30. Jiang YZ, Yu KD, Bao J, Peng WT, Shao ZM. Favorable prognostic impact in loss of TP53 and PIK3CA mutations after neoadjuvant chemotherapy in breast cancer. Cancer Res. 2014;74(13):3399–407.

31. Tan SH, Sapari NS, Miao H, Hartman M, Loh M, Chng WJ, Iau P, Buhari SA, Soong R, Lee SC. High-throughput mutation profiling changes before and 3 weeks after chemotherapy in newly diagnosed breast Cancer patients. PLoS One. 2015;10(12):e0142466.

29

Prognostic significance of the combination of preoperative hemoglobin and albumin levels and lymphocyte and platelet counts (HALP) in patients with renal cell carcinoma after nephrectomy

Ding Peng[1,2†] ⓘ, Cui-jian Zhang[1,2,3,4†], Qi Tang[1,2,3,4], Lei Zhang[1,2,3,4], Kai-wei Yang[1,2,3,4], Xiao-teng Yu[1,2,3,4], Yanqing Gong[1,2,3,4], Xue-song Li[1,2,3,4*], Zhi-song He[1,2,3,4] and Li-qun Zhou[1,2,3,4*]

Abstract

Background: To evaluate the prognostic significance of the novel index combining preoperative hemoglobin and albumin levels and lymphocyte and platelet counts (HALP) in renal cell carcinoma (RCC) patients.

Methods: We enrolled 1360 patients who underwent nephrectomy in our institution from 2001 to 2010. The cutoff values for HALP, neutrophil-to-lymphocyte ratio and platelet-to-lymphocyte ratio were defined by using X-tile software. Survival was analyzed by the Kaplan–Meier method, with differences analyzed by the log-rank test. Multivariate Cox proportional-hazards model was used to evaluate the prognostic significance of HALP for RCC.

Results: Low HALP was significantly associated with worse clinicopathologic features. Kaplan-Meier and log-rank tests revealed that HALP was strongly correlated with cancer specific survival ($P < 0.001$) and Cox multivariate analysis demonstrated that preoperative HALP was independent prognostic factor for cancer specific survival (HR = 1.838, 95%CI:1.260–2.681, $P = 0.002$). On predicting prognosis by nomogram, the risk model including TNM stage, Fuhrman grade and HALP score was more accurate than only use of TNM staging.

Conclusions: HALP was closely associated with clinicopathologic features and was an independent prognostic factor of cancer-specific survival for RCC patients undergoing nephrectomy. A nomogram based on HALP could accurately predict prognosis of RCC.

Keywords: Renal cell carcinoma, Prognosis, HALP, Nephrectomy

Background

Renal cancer accounts for 2% to 3% of all cancers, and the rate of renal cell carcinoma (RCC) has increased by 1.6% per year for the past 10 years [1]. Approximately 90% of renal cancer is RCC, and surgery is the only curative treatment. About 20% of RCC patients have advanced stage disease, and for those with localized RCC, nearly 30% show recurrence after tumor resection [2, 3]. Therefore, we need better prognostic models to improve prognosis.

The TNM stage, reflecting tumor invasion, lymph node metastasis and distant metastasis, is the most widely used system for predicting RCC prognosis [2]. However, because of heterogeneous prognoses, the outcomes of some patients with the same stage of cancer may be completely different. Therefore, we need useful biomarkers to increase the prognostic accuracy in RCC.

Increasing evidence supports that inflammation and nutrition are involved in the initiation and progression of various cancers, including RCC [4]. Hematologic parameters including albumin and hemoglobin levels and lymphocytes,

* Correspondence: pineneedle@sina.com; zhoulqmail@sina.com
†Equal contributors
[1]Department of Urology, Peking University First Hospital, No. 8, Xishiku Street, Xicheng District, Beijing 100034, China
Full list of author information is available at the end of the article

neutrophils and platelets counts are easily acquired laboratory data reflecting inflammation and nutrition status and
have been extensively studied. Numerous studies have reported the prognostic value of serum albumin and
hemoglobin levels and lymphocyte and platelet counts for
various cancers, including RCC [5–8]. However, the disad-
vantage of these indicators is that each reflects only one respect of inflammation or nutrition. Further studies found
that the combination of those factors in an index such as
the prognostic nutritional index (PNI), combining albumin
level and lymphocyte count, or the neutrophil-to-
lymphocyte ratio (NLR), lymphocyte-to-monocyte ratio
(LMR) or platelet-to-lymphocyte ratio (PLR) could more
accurately predict prognosis than a single index [9–12].

A novel index combining hemoglobin and albumin levels
and lymphocyte and platelet counts (HALP) has been
found significantly associated with outcomes in colorectal
and gastric cancer [13, 14]. In this study, we investigated
the clinical value of this index in RCC patients undergoing
nephrectomy.

Methods
Patients
We included 1360 patients with histologically confirmed
RCC. All patients were underwent nephrectomy in the
Department of Urology, Peking University First Hospital, between 2001 and 2010. Clinicopathologic characteristics and
laboratory data were collected. Follow-up care including abdominal ultrasonography or abdominal CT, chest X-ray, and
laboratory tests was performed at regular intervals (3-month
intervals in years 1 to 3, 6-month intervals in years 4 to 5,
and 12-month intervals in years 6 to 10 after diagnosis).

Statistical analysis
Data are presented as number (percentage) for categorical
variables and median (interquartile range [IQR]) for continuous variables. HALP was calculated as hemoglobin level
(g/L) × albumin level (g/L) × lymphocyte(/L)/platelet count
(/L), NLR as neutrophil-to-lymphocyte count and PLR as
platelet-to-lymphocyte count. The cut-off values for NLR,
PLR and HALP were determined by using X-tile v3.6.1
(Yale University) [15]. The X-tile software was able to compare the P values of different cut-off values for a continuous
variable and determine the best cut-off value with the most
significant P value. Chi-square test was used to analyze an
association of clinicopathologic data with HALP. The
Kaplan-Meier survival method was used to estimate
cancer-specific survival (CSS), with log-rank test used to
test significant differences. The significant variables in the
univariate analysis were included in the Cox proportional-
hazards regression multivariate survival analyses by Forward LR method. Statistical analyses involved use of SPSS
v22.0 (SPSS Inc., Chicago, IL, USA) and $P < 0.05$ was considered statistically significant.

Results
Patient characteristics
We included 1360 patients (952 men, median age
55 years [IQR 46–65]) (Table 1). The median follow-up
was 67 months (IQR 36–74) and 139 (10.2%) patients

Table 1 Basline clinicopathologic characteristics of 1360
patients with renal cell carcinoma (RCC) undergoing
nephrectomy

Characteristics	Total $n = 1360$
Age, years, median (IQR)	55 (46–65)
Female sex	408 (30%)
Histology subtype	
ccRCC	1228 (90.29%)
non-ccRCC	132 (9.71%)
Location	
left	626 (46.03%)
right	697 (51.25%)
bilateral	37 (2.72%)
Fuhrman grade	
1	374 (27.5%)
2	738 (54.26%)
3	237 (17.43%)
4	11 (0.81%)
T-stage	
1	1015 (74.63%)
2	113 (8.32%)
3	225 (16.54%)
4	7 (0.51%)
N status	
negative	1327 (97.57%)
positive	33 (2.43%)
ASA grade	
1	192 (14.12%)
2	1072 (78.82%)
3&4	96 (7.06%)
Sarcomatoid transformation	65 (4.78%)
Metastasis	61 (4.48%)
Lymphovascular invasion	100 (7.35%)
Necrosis	419 (3.08%)
Hypoalbuminemia	53 (3.9%)
Anemia	267 (19.6%)
NLR, median (IQR)	2.13 (1.60–2.85)
PLR, median (IQR)	124.07 (97.33–165.22)
HALP, median (IQR)	47.48 (33.21–63.45)

Data are n (%) unless indicated. *IQR* interquartile ratio, *ccRCC* clear-cell
renal cell carcinoma, *ASA* American Society of Anesthesiologists, *NLR*
neutrophil-to-lymphocyte ratio, *PLR* platelet-to-lymphocyte ratio, *HALP*
hemoglobin and albumin levels and lymphocyte and platelet counts

died due to RCC during follow-up. The 5-year estimated CSS was 89.4% for all patients.

Association of HALP and clinicopathologic features
We detected cut-off values for HALP, 31.2; NLR, 2.9; and PLR, 198.3 (Fig. 1 and Additional file 1: Figure S1) for dividing patients into low and high HALP, NLR and PLR groups. Decreased HALP level was associated with being female, older age, high Fuhrman grade and high T stage and N and M positive status, sarcomatoid transformation, tumor necrosis, lymphovascular invasion and low NLR or PLR (Table 2).

Association of HALP with patient outcomes
On univariate analysis, all included clinicopathologic features except for age ($P = 0.287$), gender ($P = 0.226$), histology subtype ($P = 0.385$) and American Society of Anesthesiologists grade ($P = 0.964$) were significantly related to survival outcomes (Table 3). Anemia and hypoalbuminemia, high PLR and low HALP were all significantly associated with worse survival (Fig. 2). On multivariate analyses, prognostic factors for CSS with RCC were Fuhrman grade (HR 1.767, 95% CI 1.177–2.652, $P = 0.006$), T stage (3.890, 2.510–6.030, $P < 0.001$), N stage (2.480, 1.526–4.032, $P < 0.001$), M stage (4.728, 3.090–7.233, $P < 0.001$) and HALP (1.838, 1.260–2.681, $P = 0.002$) (Table 3).

Nomogram of HALP-based risk model for RCC
We next used nomogram to predict 3- and 5-year CSS for individual patients. Independent prognostic factors in the multivariate analysis including Fuhrman grade, TNM status and HALP were included in the nomogram (Fig. 3). Similar to multivariate findings, with nomogram, high Fuhrman grade and advanced TNM status were associated with poor prognosis and high HALP with favorable prognosis.

The calibration curves of the nomogram showed that the predictive probability of 3- and 5-year survival was closely related to the actual 3- and 5-year survival (Fig. 4).

The C-index was 0.881 (95% CI: 0.853–0.909) by this nomogram compared with 0.846 (0.812–0.880) with the TNM staging system. Hence, the risk model including TNM stage, Fuhrman grade and HALP had better prognostic prediction accuracy than the only TNM system.

Discussion
In this study, we evaluated the prognostic significance of the novel index HALP combining hemoglobin and albumin levels and lymphocyte and platelet counts in RCC patients undergoing nephrectomy. HALP was closely associated with clinicopathologic features. Univariate and multivariate analyses demonstrated that HALP was an independent predictor of CSS for RCC patients undergoing nephrectomy. Furthermore, the nomogram based on HALP could predict prognosis more accurately than the TNM system.

There are several known predictive models of RCC such as TNM stage and the Stage, Size, Grading and Necrosis (SSIGN) model [16]. Inflammatory and nutritional indicators based on hematologic parameters such as albumin and hemoglobin levels and lymphocyte, neutrophil and platelet counts were also associated with outcomes with RCC. Moreover, several indicators combined with hematologic parameters, including NLR, LMR, and PLR, were more accurate predictors [6, 9, 10, 12]. Recently, indicators combining albumin level with LMR or NLR were found significantly associated with outcomes [17, 18], which suggests better prediction of outcomes by combining inflammatory and nutritional indicators.

Accumulating evidence suggests the important role of the inflammatory response and nutritional status in cancer progression and metastasis. Overall, 30% of cancer patients were found with cancer-related anemia (CRA) at the time of diagnosis and CRA was associated with more advanced cancer stage [19]. CRA is believed to be associated with chronic blood loss, iron deficiency, and vitamin B12 or folate nutritional deficiency. Meanwhile, imbalanced inflammation regulation, such as increased

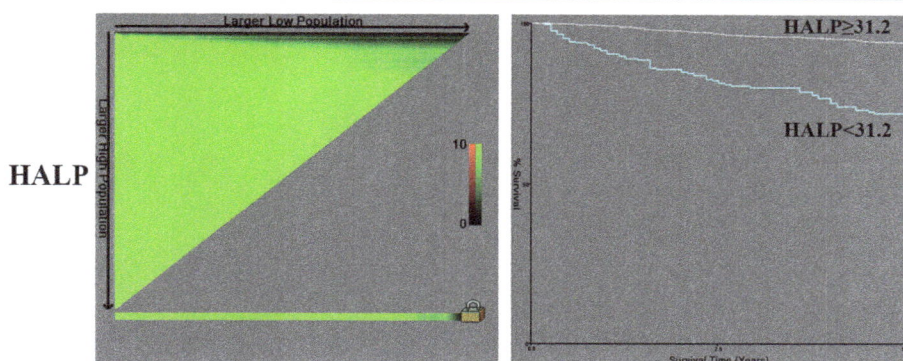

Fig. 1 Cut off value for hemoglobin and albumin levels and lymphocyte and platelet counts (HALP) by using X-tile

Table 2 Association of baseline clinicopathologic characteristics and HALP

Variable	n (%)	low (%)	HALP[a] high (%)	P value
All patients	1360	291 (21.40%)	1069 (78.60%)	
Gender				< 0.001
male	952 (70.00%)	162 (17.02%)	790 (82.98%)	
female	408 (30.00%)	129 (31.62%)	279 (68.38%)	
Age, years				< 0.001
≤ 65	997 (73.31%)	186 (18.66%)	811 (81.34%)	
>65	363 (26.69%)	105 (28.93%)	258 (71.07%)	
Histology subtype				0.695
ccRCC	1228 (90.29%)	261 (21.25%)	967 (78.75%)	
non-ccRCC	132 (9.71%)	30 (22.73%)	102 (77.27%)	
ASA grade				0.361
1 + 2	1264 (92.94%)	268 (21.20%)	996 (78.80%)	
3 + 4	96 (7.06%)	23 (23.96%)	68 (76.04%)	
Fuhrman grade				< 0.001
1 + 2	1112 (81.76%)	177 (15.92%)	935 (84.08%)	
3 + 4	248 (18.24%)	113 (45.56%)	130 (54.44%)	
T stage				< 0.001
1 + 2	1128 (82.94%)	173 (15.34%)	955 (84.66%)	
3 + 4	232 (17.06%)	118 (50.86%)	113 (49.14%)	
N status				< 0.001
negative	1327 (97.57%)	270 (20.35%)	1057 (79.65%)	
positive	33 (2.43%)	21 (63.64%)	12 (36.36%)	
Metastasis				< 0.001
negative	1299 (95.51%)	258 (19.86%)	1041 (80.14%)	
positive	61 (4.49%)	33 (54.10%)	28 (45.90%)	
Sarcomatoid transformation				< 0.001
absent	1295 (95.22%)	245 (18.92%)	1050 (81.08%)	
present	65 (4.78%)	46 (70.77%)	19 (29.23%)	
Tumor necrosis				< 0.001
absent	940 (69.12%)	158 (16.81%)	782 (83.19%)	
present	420 (30.88%)	133 (31.67%)	286 (68.33%)	
Lymphovascular invasion				< 0.001
absent	1260 (92.65%)	249 (19.76%)	1011 (80.24%)	
present	100 (7.35%)	42 (42%)	58 (58%)	
NLR				< 0.001
high	317 (23.3%)	166 (52.37%)	151 (47.63%)	
low	1043 (76.7%)	125 (11.98%)	918 (88.02%)	
PLR				< 0.001
high	195 (14.3%)	180 (92.31%)	15 (7.69%)	
low	1165 (85.7%)	111 (9.53%)	1054 (90.47%)	

[a]data are number of patients for those with HALP < and ≥ 31.2

Table 3 Univariate and multivariate analyses of factors associated with cancer-specific survival for RCC patients

Variable	Univariate analysis P	Multivariate analysis	
		HR (95% CI)	P
Age (>65 vs ≤65)	0.287		
Gender (female vs male)	0.226		
Histology subtype (non-ccRCC vs ccRCC)	0.385		
ASA grade (3 + 4 vs 1 + 2)	0.964		
Fuhrman grade (3 + 4 vs 1 + 2)	< 0.001	1.767 (1.177–2.652)	0.006
T stage (3 + 4 vs 1 + 2)	< 0.001	3.890 (2.510–6.030)	< 0.001
N status (positive/negative)	< 0.001	2.480 (1.526–4.032)	< 0.001
M status (positive vs negative)	< 0.001	4.728 (3.090–7.233)	< 0.001
Sarcomatous differentiation (present vs absent)	< 0.001		
Lymphovascular invasion (present vs absent)	< 0.001		
Necrosis (present vs absent)	< 0.001		
Hypoalbuminemia (present vs absent)	< 0.001		
Anemia (present vs absent)	< 0.001		
NLR (high vs low)	< 0.001		
PLR (high vs low)	< 0.001		
HALP (low vs high)	< 0.001	1.838 (1.260–2.681)	0.002

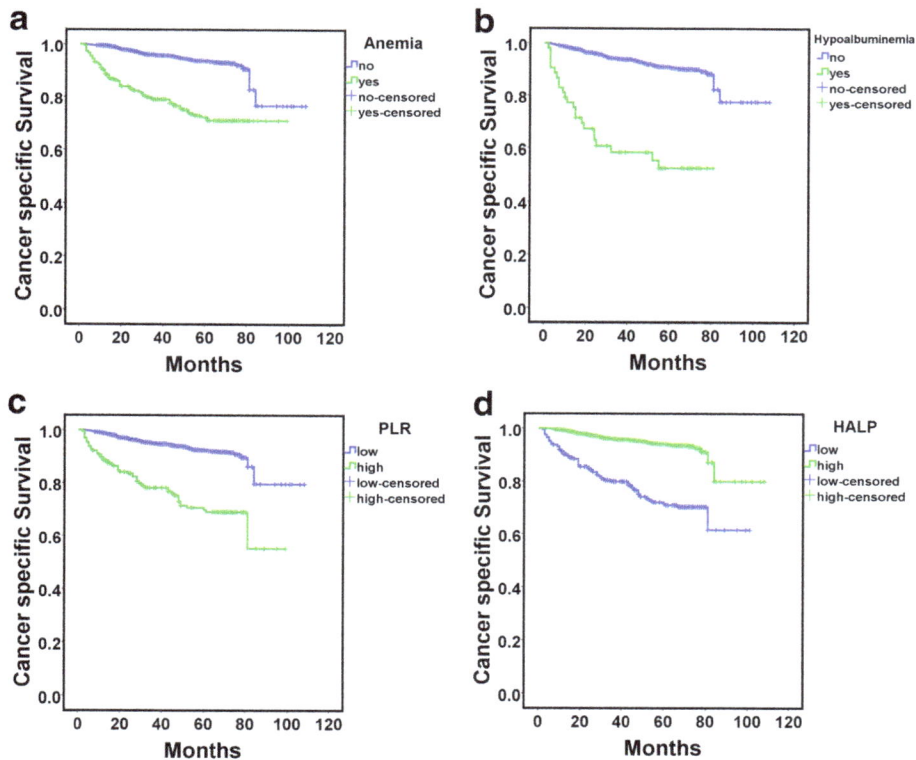

Fig. 2 Kaplan-Meier curves for cancer-specific survival in patients with RCC according to anemia (**a**), hypoalbuminemia (**b**), platelet-to-lymphocyte ratio (PLR)(**c**) and hemoglobin and albumin levels and lymphocyte and platelet counts (HALP) (**d**)

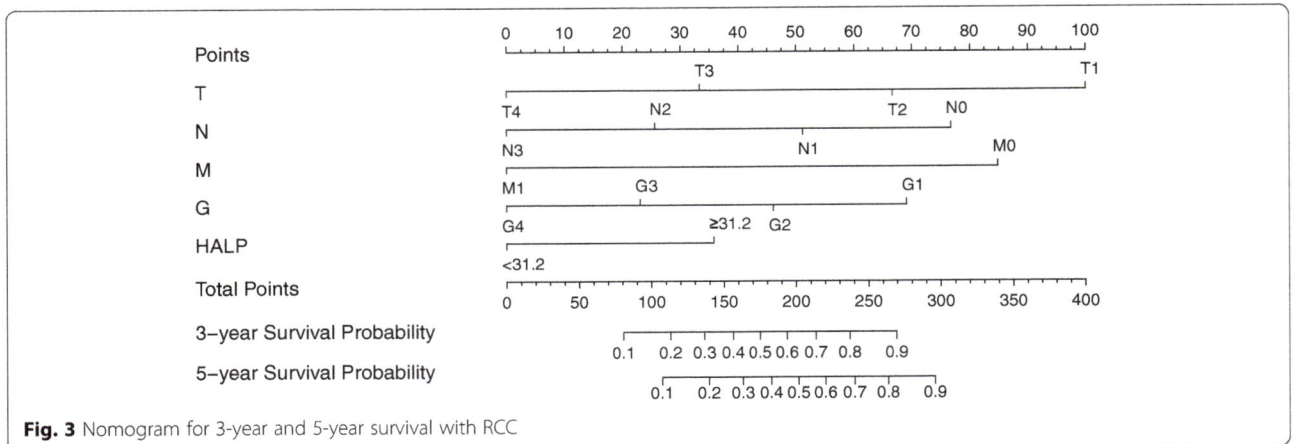

Fig. 3 Nomogram for 3-year and 5-year survival with RCC

hepcidin and reactive oxygen species stress, in cancer patients is also responsible for CRA [20]. Serum albumin is synthesized specially in the liver and known as a negative acute-phase protein. In addition, systemic factors such as inflammation and stress could affect serum albumin level. Therefore, decreased serum albumin level represents a malnutrition status and also a sustained systemic inflammation response. As important indicators of nutrition and inflammation, anemia and hypoalbuminemia are widely reported to be associated with worse outcomes in various cancers including RCC [7, 8]. Morgan et al. [21] reported that for locoregional RCC patients undergoing nephrectomy, 25% of patients have anemia and 5.1% have hypoalbuminemia. The authors also found hypoalbuminemia (< 35 g/L), unintentional preoperative weight loss $\geq 5\%$ and preoperative BMI $<$ 18.5 kg/m2 as reflecting nutritional deficiency (ND) and that anemia and ND were independent predictors of overall mortality and disease-specific mortality. Preoperative hypoalbuminemia and anemia were also found to predict transfusion during radical nephrectomy for RCC [5]. We observed 3.9% hypoalbuminemia and

19.6% anemia in our patients, which is consistent with previous study. On univariate analysis, both anemia and hypoalbuminemia were associated with worse survival.

Cancer-related inflammation is considered the seventh hallmark of cancer, playing a conflicting role in tumor initiation and progression in that both tumor-antagonizing and -promoting leukocytes can be found [22]. Elevated neutrophil count is associated with cytokine secretion and contributes to tumor angiogenesis, promotion and metastasis. CD4+ and CD8+ T lymphocytes can enhance cancer immune-surveillance to inhibit tumour cell proliferation, invasion and metastasis [23]. Increased neutrophil count and decreased lymphocyte count might be responsible for a weak and insufficient immune response to tumors and strongly associated with a poor survival in advanced cancer [24, 25].

Recent data implied that the activation of platelets is crucial for cancer progression by promoting angiogenesis, extracellular matrix degradation, and release of growth factors, which are essential components of tumor growth and metastatic [26]. In addition, platelets adhering to tumor cells could secrete vascular endothelial growth

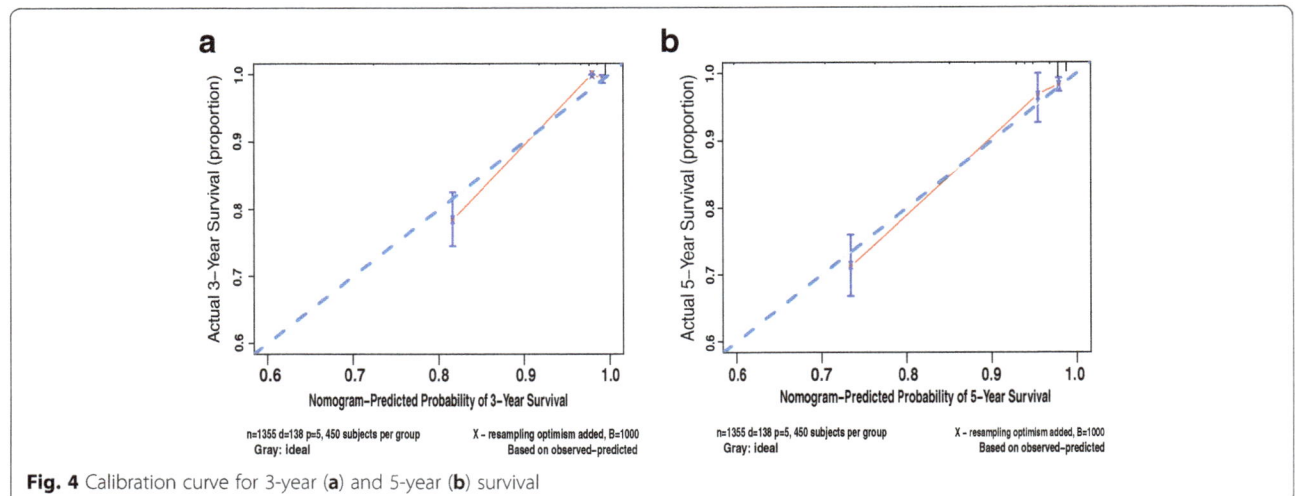

Fig. 4 Calibration curve for 3-year (**a**) and 5-year (**b**) survival

factor(VEGF), which induces microvessel permeability, promotes extravasation of cancer cells, and induces neoangiogenesis [27]. Platelet count was found a significant predictor of RCC-specific mortality [28]. Recently, tumor-educated blood platelets (TEPs) were implicated as central players in the systemic and local responses to tumor growth. As well, the RNA profile in TEPs could provide a valuable platform for liquid biopsy [29].

Systemic inflammation markers including NLR, LMR, and PLR have been found associated with survival in many solid tumors including RCC [6, 10, 30, 31]. Among those indicators, the finding of elevated NLR and PLR indicated increased neutrophil and platelet count and decreased lymphocyte count associated with worse outcomes. In our study, elevated NLR and PLR were associated with worse CSS on univariate analysis. However, on multivariate analyses, HALP rather than NLR and PLR remained an independent prognostic factor.

We used nomogram of independent prognostic factors found on multivariate analyses including HALP and evaluated their accuracy by calibration curves. The predictive accuracy was better with HALP than the TNM system. TNM stage may be an important factor in RCC, but other factors such as HALP could be included and improve the prediction of outcomes.

The major limitations of the present study are its retrospective nature and the single-center design. Additional large and prospective studies are needed to confirm these findings.

Conclusions

HALP was closely associated with clinicopathologic features of RCC patients undergoing nephrectomy and was an independent prognostic factor of CSS. A nomogram based on HALP could accurately predict prognosis with RCC. Preoperative HALP could be a novel indicator to evaluate the outcome for RCC patients after nephrectomy.

Abbreviations
CRA: cancer-related anemia; CSS: cancer-specific survival; LMR: lymphocyte-to-monocyte ratio; NLR: neutrophil-to-lymphocyte ratio; PLR: platelet-to-lymphocyte ratio; PNI: prognostic nutritional index; RCC: renal cell carcinoma

Acknowledgements
We sincerely thank the patients for their participation in this study.

Funding
This work was supported by the National Natural Science Foundation of China (Grant Number: 81372746 and 81672546).

Authors' contributions
DP: Project development, Data analysis, Manuscript writing. CZ: Project development, Data analysis, Manuscript writing. QT, LZ, KY, XY, YG, ZH: Data collection or management. XL & LZ: Project development. All authors read and approved the final manuscript.

Competing interests
The authors declare that they have no competing interests.

Author details
[1]Department of Urology, Peking University First Hospital, No. 8, Xishiku Street, Xicheng District, Beijing 100034, China. [2]Institute of Urology, Peking University, Beijing 100034, China. [3]National Urological Cancer Center, Beijing 100034, China. [4]Urogenital Diseases (male) Molecular Diagnosis and Treatment Center, Peking University, Beijing 100034, China.

References
1. Motzer RJ, Jonasch E, Agarwal N, Beard C, Bhayani S, Bolger GB, et al. Kidney cancer, version 3.2015. Journal of the National Comprehensive Cancer Network : JNCCN. 2015;13(2):151–9.
2. Ljungberg B, Bensalah K, Canfield S, Dabestani S, Hofmann F, Hora M, et al. EAU guidelines on renal cell carcinoma: 2014 update. Eur Urol. 2015;67(5):913–24.
3. Hsieh JJ, Purdue MP, Signoretti S, Swanton C, Albiges L, Schmidinger M, et al. Renal cell carcinoma. Nat Rev Dis Primers. 2017;3:17009–28.
4. Senbabaoglu Y, Gejman RS, Winer AG, Liu M, Van Allen EM, de Velasco G, et al. Tumor immune microenvironment characterization in clear cell renal cell carcinoma identifies prognostic and immunotherapeutically relevant messenger RNA signatures. Genome Biol. 2016;17(1):231–56.
5. Kim K, Seo H, Chin JH, Son HJ, Hwang JH, Kim YK. Preoperative hypoalbuminemia and anemia as predictors of transfusion in radical nephrectomy for renal cell carcinoma: a retrospective study. BMC Anesthesiol. 2015;15:103–10.
6. Chang Y, Fu Q, Xu L, Zhou L, Liu Z, Yang Y, et al. Prognostic value of preoperative lymphocyte to monocyte ratio in patients with nonmetastatic clear cell renal cell carcinoma. Tumour Biol. 2016;37(4):4613–20.
7. Corcoran AT, Kaffenberger SD, Clark PE, Walton J, Handorf E, Piotrowski Z, et al. Hypoalbuminaemia is associated with mortality in patients undergoing cytoreductive nephrectomy. BJU Int. 2015;116(3):351–7.
8. Stenman M, Laurell A, Lindskog M. Prognostic significance of serum albumin in patients with metastatic renal cell carcinoma. Med Oncol. 2014; 31(3):841–9.
9. Sun J, Ning H, Sun J, Qu X. Effect of hypertension on preoperative neutrophil-lymphocyte ratio evaluation of prognosis of renal cell carcinoma. Urol Oncol. 2016;34(5):239. e239-215
10. Gunduz S, Mutlu H, Tural D, Yildiz O, Uysal M, Coskun HS. Platelet to lymphocyte ratio as a new prognostic for patients with metastatic renal cell cancer. Asia-Pac J Clin Oncol. 2015;11(4):288–92.
11. Ohno Y, Nakashima J, Ohori M, Gondo T, Hatano T, Tachibana M. Followup of neutrophil-to-lymphocyte ratio and recurrence of clear cell renal cell carcinoma. J Urol. 2012;187(2):411–7.
12. Hofbauer SL, Pantuck AJ, de Martino M, Lucca I, Haitel A, Shariat SF, et al. The preoperative prognostic nutritional index is an independent predictor of survival in patients with renal cell carcinoma. Urol Oncol. 2015;33(2):68. e61-67
13. Chen XL, Xue L, Wang W, Chen HN, Zhang WH, Liu K, et al. Prognostic significance of the combination of preoperative hemoglobin, albumin, lymphocyte and platelet in patients with gastric carcinoma: a retrospective cohort study. Oncotarget. 2015;6(38):41370–82.
14. Jiang H, Li H, Li A, Tang E, Xu D, Chen Y, et al. Preoperative combined hemoglobin, albumin, lymphocyte and platelet levels predict survival in patients with locally advanced colorectal cancer. Oncotarget. 2016;7:72076–83.
15. Camp RL, Dolled-Filhart M, Rimm DL. X-tile: a new bio-informatics tool for biomarker assessment and outcome-based cut-point optimization. Clin Cancer Res. 2004;10(21):7252–9.
16. Frank I, Blute ML, Cheville JC, Lohse CM, Weaver AL, Zincke H. An outcome prediction model for patients with clear cell renal cell carcinoma treated with radical nephrectomy based on tumor stage, size, grade and necrosis: the SSIGN score. J Urol. 2002;168(6):2395–400.
17. Wang YQ, Jin C, Zheng HM, Zhou K, Shi BB, Zhang Q, et al. A novel prognostic inflammation score predicts outcomes in patients with ovarian cancer. Clin Chim Acta. 2016;456:163–9.
18. Chang Y, An H, Xu L, Zhu Y, Yang Y, Lin Z, et al. Systemic inflammation score predicts postoperative prognosis of patients with clear-cell renal cell carcinoma. Brit J Cancer. 2015;113(4):626–33.
19. Ludwig H, Van Belle S, Barrett-Lee P, Birgegard G, Bokemeyer C, Gascon P, et al. The European Cancer Anaemia survey (ECAS): a large, multinational, prospective survey defining the prevalence, incidence, and treatment of anaemia in cancer patients. Eur J Cancer. 2004;40(15):2293–306.

20. Maccio A, Madeddu C, Gramignano G, Mulas C, Tanca L, Cherchi MC, et al. The role of inflammation, iron, and nutritional status in cancer-related anemia: results of a large, prospective, observational study. Haematologica. 2015;100(1):124–32.

21. Morgan TM, Tang D, Stratton KL, Barocas DA, Anderson CB, Gregg JR, et al. Preoperative nutritional status is an important predictor of survival in patients undergoing surgery for renal cell carcinoma. Eur Urol. 2011;59(6):923–8.

22. Hanahan D, Weinberg RA. Hallmarks of cancer: the next generation. Cell. 2011;144(5):646–74.

23. Mantovani A, Allavena P, Sica A, Balkwill F. Cancer-related inflammation. Nature. 2008;454(7203):436–44.

24. Hoffmann TK, Dworacki G, Tsukihiro T, Meidenbauer N, Gooding W, Johnson JT, et al. Spontaneous apoptosis of circulating T lymphocytes in patients with head and neck cancer and its clinical importance. Clin Cancer Res. 2002;8(8):2553–62.

25. Bindea G, Mlecnik B, Fridman WH, Pages F, Galon J. Natural immunity to cancer in humans. Curr Opin Immunol. 2010;22(2):215–22.

26. Labelle M, Begum S, Hynes RO. Platelets guide the formation of early metastatic niches. P Natl Acad Sci USA. 2014;111(30):e3053–61.

27. Suzuki K, Aiura K, Ueda M, Kitajima M. The influence of platelets on the promotion of invasion by tumor cells and inhibition by antiplatelet agents. Pancreas. 2004;29(2):132–40.

28. Karakiewicz PI, Trinh QD, Lam JS, Tostain J, Pantuck AJ, Belldegrun AS, et al. Platelet count and preoperative haemoglobin do not significantly increase the performance of established predictors of renal cell carcinoma-specific mortality. Eur Urology. 2007;52(5):1428–36.

29. Best MG, Sol N, Kooi I, Tannous J, Westerman BA, Rustenburg F, et al. RNA-Seq of tumor-educated platelets enables blood-based pan-Cancer, multiclass, and molecular pathway Cancer diagnostics. Cancer Cell. 2015; 28(5):666–76.

30. Shin JS, Suh KW, Oh SY. Preoperative neutrophil to lymphocyte ratio predicts survival in patients with T1-2N0 colorectal cancer. J Surg Oncol. 2015;112(6):654–7.

31. Hsu JT, Liao CK, Le PH, Chen TH, Lin CJ, Chen JS, et al. Prognostic value of the preoperative neutrophil to lymphocyte ratio in Resectable gastric Cancer. Medicine. 2015;94(39):e1589–95.

Perineural invasion as an independent predictor of biochemical recurrence in prostate cancer following radical prostatectomy or radiotherapy

Li-jin Zhang[1*], Bin Wu[1], Zhen-lei Zha[1†], Wei Qu[2†], Hu Zhao[1†], Jun Yuan[1] and Ye-jun Feng[1]

Abstract

Background: Although numerous studies have shown that perineural invasion (PNI) is linked to prostate cancer (PCa) risk, the results have been inconsistent. This study aimed to explore the association between PNI and biochemical recurrence (BCR) in patients with PCa following radical prostatectomy (RP) or radiotherapy (RT).

Methods: According to the PRISMA statement, we searched the PubMed, EMBASE, Chinese National Knowledge Infrastructure (CNKI) and Wan Fang databases from inception to May 2017. Hazard ratios (HRs) and 95% confidence intervals (95% CIs) were extracted from eligible studies. Fixed or random effects model were used to calculate pooled HRs and 95% CIs according to heterogeneity. Publication bias was calculated by Begg's test.

Results: Ultimately, 19 cohort studies that met the eligibility criteria and that involved 13,412 patients (82-2,316 per study) were included in this meta-analysis. The results showed that PNI was associated with higher BCR rates in patients with PCa after RP (HR=1.23, 95% CI: 1.11, 1.36, $p<0.001$) or RT (HR=1.22, 95% CI: 1.12, 1.34, $p<0.001$). No potential publication bias was found among the included studies in the RP group (p-Begg = 0.124) or the RT group (p-Begg = 0.081).

Conclusions: This study suggests that the presence of PNI by histopathology is associated with higher risk of BCR in PCa following RP or RT, and could serve as an independent prognostic factor in patients with PCa.

Keywords: Perineural invasion, Prostate cancer, Radical prostatectomy, Radiotherapy, Biochemical recurrence, Meta-analysis

Background

Prostate cancer (PCa) is the most common newly diagnosed cancer in males, with 1.6 million new cases per year; PCa is the third most common cause of cancer-related death in men [1]. Despite the use of radical prostatectomy (RP) and radiotherapy (RT) as initial therapies for localized PCa, approximately 18 % of patients eventually experience biochemical recurrence (BCR) [2].

* Correspondence: stzlj913729553@163.com
†Equal contributors
[1]Departments of Urology, Affiliated Jiang-yin Hospital of the Southeast University Medical College, Jiang-yin 214400, China
Full list of author information is available at the end of the article

Therefore, it is crucial to identify the patients who are at an increased risk of BCR after RP or RT. Preoperative prostate-specific antigen (p-PSA) levels [3], Gleason score (GS) [4] and pathological stage [5] are widely used as traditional risk factors for BCR. However, there is a growing interest in the identification of a new prognostic marker to improve the evaluation of the likelihood of BCR in PCa patients after local treatment.

Perineural invasion (PNI), which is considered a major mechanism for the extraprostatic spread of PCa [6], has been increasingly recognized as a novel prognostic marker [7]. However, whether PNI might be a prognostic factor for BCR is still under debate [8]. Some authors suggest that the presence of PNI is associated with adverse oncological outcomes and a higher risk of BCR, whereas others argue that PNI is not an independent predictor of BCR.

Therefore, to further clarify the relationship between PNI and the risk of BCR in PCa, we performed this systematic review and meta-analysis to evaluate whether the presence of PNI has a prognostic impact on BCR in patients following RP or RT.

Methods
Search strategy
According to the PRISMA guidelines [9], a systematic literature search of the PubMed, EMBASE, Chinese National Knowledge Infrastructure (CNKI) and Wan Fang databases was performed (up to May 2017). The search strategy used the following: ("prostate cancer" or "prostate AND neoplasms") and ("radical prostatectomy" or "radiotherapy") and ("perineural invasion") and ("biochemical recurrence"). We also manually searched for potentially relevant studies from the references listed in the selected review articles. The language of the publications was limited to English and Chinese.

Inclusion and exclusion criteria
The inclusion criteria for the eligible studies were as follows: (1) all patients were diagnosed with histologically confirmed PCa, and PNI in RP specimens and biopsy specimens were assessed by pathologists; (2) all patients underwent RP or RT; (3) BCR after RP was defined as a detectable or rising PSA value after surgery that was ≥0.2 ng/ml with a second confirmation (American Urological Association [10]) ; BCR after RT was defined as a rise in PSA level of ≥2 ng/ml above the nadir (American Society for Radiation Oncology and Radiation Therapy Oncology Group in Phoenix [11]); (4) the risk of BCR was estimated as hazard ratios (HRs) with corresponding 95% confidence intervals (CIs) or the risk could be calculated from the original articles; (5) the study was of a prospective or retrospective cohort design; (6) the articles were published in English or Chinese. The exclusion criteria were as follows: (1) letters, reviews, case reports, editorials and author responses; (2) non-human studies; (3) studies that did not analyze the outcome after PNI and BCR; (4) duplicate articles; (5) articles contained elements that were inconsistent with the inclusion criteria.

Data extraction and Study Quality
The data of the eligible studies were extracted independently by two investigators (Zhen-lei Zha and Wei Qu). Any discrepancies were resolved by discussion with a third reviewer (Hu Zhao). The following data were extracted from the included studies: first author, year of publication, country, recruitment period, sample size,

patient's age, preoperative PSA level, Gleason score, pathological stage, positive percentage of PNI, definition of BCR, follow-up time and the HR(95%CI) of PNI for BCR. When the study provided the results of both the multivariate and univariate outcomes, we chose the multivariate model. The quality of the eligible studies was evaluated according to the Newcastle-Ottawa scale (NOS) [12], which include 3 domains with 8 items. Studies with scores of 7 or more stars were considered high-quality studies.

Statistical analyses
All statistical analyses in this meta-analysis were performed by Stata 12.0 software (Stat Corp, College Station, TX, USA).The association between PNI and BCR outcome was presented as summary relative risk estimates (SRREs) and 95% CIs. Heterogeneity between studies was assessed using Q and I^2 statistics. $P < 0.10$ or $I^2 > 50\%$ was considered significant heterogeneity. A random effects model was used when obvious heterogeneity was observed, but otherwise, a fixed-effects model was used. Sensitivity analysis was used to estimate the reliability of the pooled results via the sequential omission of each study. Subgroup analyses were performed to examine potential sources of heterogeneity according to the adjusted parameters. Publication bias was assessed by funnel plots and was statistically determined by Begg's tests; a p value < 0.05 was considered statistically significant.

Results
Search results
The search and selection process for eligible studies is shown in Fig. 1. In all, 222 articles were initially identified. Among them, 73 duplicates were excluded. After the abstracts were screened, 93 articles were excluded for the following reasons: non-human studies, letters, case reports, reviews, and other obvious irrelevant studies. A further 37 articles were excluded after full-text review because the results did not reported PNI on the BCR. Finally, 19 retrospective cohort studies met our inclusion criteria and were included in the meta-analysis. Of these, 13 studies with 10,807patients were analyzed to investigate whether PNI acts as a predictive biomarker of BCR in PCa following RP. Six studies with 2,605 patients were evaluated to determine the relationship between PNI and the risk of BCR in PCa following RT.

Characteristics of the included studies
The main characteristics of the included studies are shown in Tables 1 and 2. All articles included were published in English, except for one, which was published Chinese [13]. All studies were published between 2003

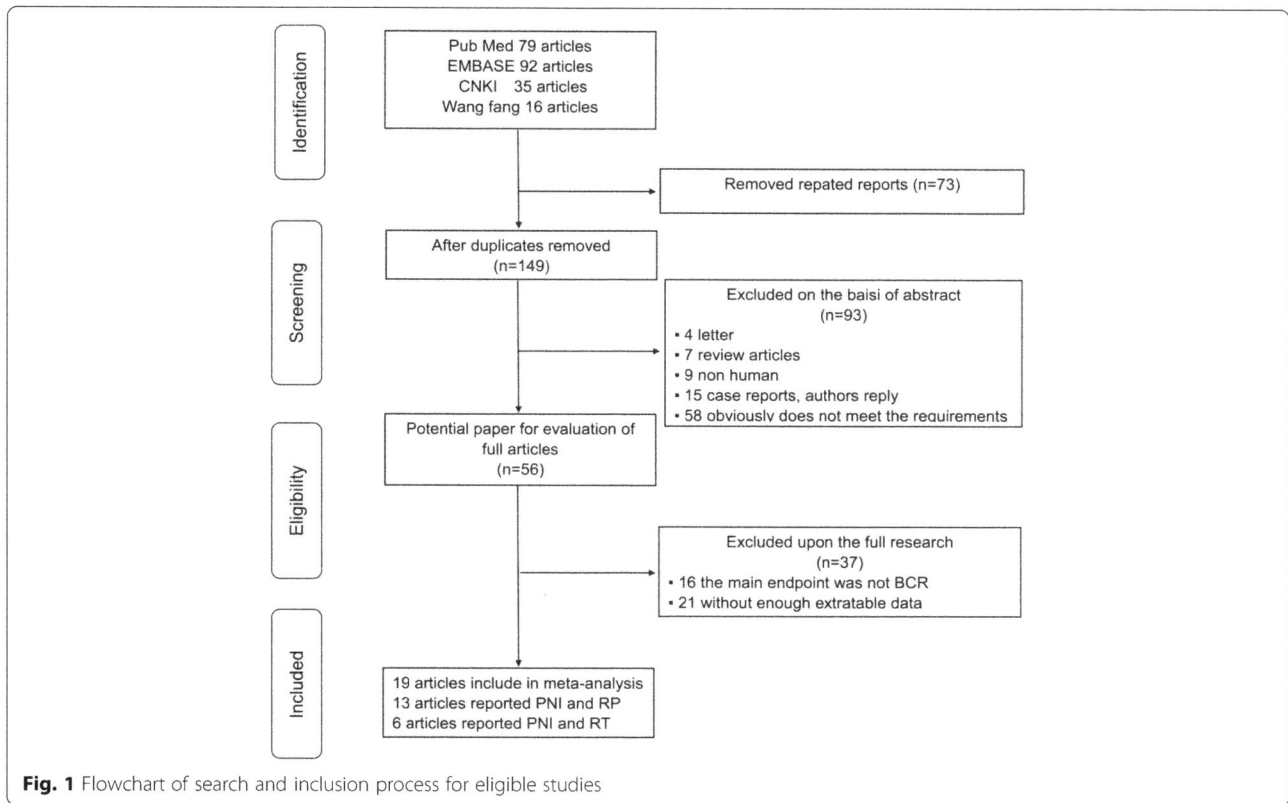

Fig. 1 Flowchart of search and inclusion process for eligible studies

and 2017, and the median duration of follow-up varied from 18.4 to 108 months. Patients in these studies were all diagnosed with PCa and received RP (13 studies) or RT (6 studies). Of the 19studies, 9 originated in Asia, and 10 were conducted in the other regions (USA, Australia, Belgium, Canada). This meta-analysis was based on a total sample size of 13,412 patients, of which 4,197 patients were reported to have PNI. Regarding the GS, 8,306 patients presented with a GS ≥7. For quality evaluated by the NOS, all the studies were found to be of high quality.

Relationship between PNI and BCR after RP
The forest plots of the meta-analyses are shown in Fig. 2. A random effects model was applied because the heterogeneity was evident among these studies (p= 0.025, I^2= 48.6%). The pooled HR indicated that the presence of PNI was associated with a higher risk of BCR in patients with PCa after RP (HR=1.23, 95% CI: 1.11, 1.36, p<0.001). According to the sensitivity analysis, the SRRE ranged from 1.18 (95% CI: 1.09, 1.29) to 1.26 (95% CI: 1.14, 1.38) (Fig. 4a). In the subgroup analyses, we found that the heterogeneity was decreased significantly in some models, such as those of geographical region ("other regions") and, age <65 years. It should also be noted that; the results of the subgroup analyses were consistent with

the primary findings (Table 3). Furthermore, no statistical evidence of publication bias was found as assessed by Begg's tests (p = 0.124) (Fig. 5a).

Association between PNI and BCR following RT
As shown in Fig. 3, the pooled HR from 6 studies indicated that PNI was an independent risk factor for BCA in PCa following RT (HR=1.22, 95% CI: 1.12, 1.34, p<0.001). Due to the lack of evidence of heterogeneity among the studies (p= 0.176, I^2 = 34.7%), a fixed effects model was applied. The SRRE for BCR ranged from1.20 (95% CI: 1.07, 1.34) to 1.27(95% CI: 1.15, 1.42) according to the sensitivity analysis (Fig. 4b). The results of the subgroup analysis showed that PNI in a sample size ≥ 500 cases was significantly associated with BCR (n=3, HR=1.20, 95% CI: 1.09, 1.31, p <0.001) (Table 3). Begg's tests (p = 0.081) provided no evidence of substantial publication bias in these studies (Fig. 5b).

Discussion
With the wide spread use of the serum PSA level in PCa screening, most patients with newly diagnosed PCa present with clinically localized or locally advanced disease [14]. RP and RT have become the standard local treatments for localized PCa. However, approximately 1/3 of patients will develop BCR after RP, and 25~33% will

Table 1 Characteristics of the included studies on PNI in patients with PCa following RP

Author	Year	Country	Recruitment period	sample size	Age (years)	p-PSA (ng/ml)	GS≥7 (n.%)	Pathological stage ≥ pT2 (n.%)	PNI (n.%)	Follow-up (months)	NOS (score)
Ito et al. [32]	2003	Japan	1989-1998	82	Mean 66.5	Mean 17.2	47 (57.3%)	50(61%)	64 (78%)	Mean 21.7	7
Jeon et al. [25]	2009	Korea	1995-2004	237	Mean 64.5	Mean 11.2	183 (77.2%)	237(100%)	100 (42.2%)	Median 21.6	8
Lee et al. [18]	2010	Korea	1999-2010	361	Mean 69	Mean 15.6	160 (44.3%)	361(100%)	188 (52.1%)	Mean 42.2	7
Loeb et al. [33]	2010	USA	2002-2007	1256	Mean 56.1	Mean 5.7	293 (23.3%)	297(23.6%)	188 (15%)	Mean 33.6	8
Muramaki et al. [34]	2010	Japan	2003-2007	174	Mean 67.5	Mean 9.5	150 (86.2%)	128(73.6%)	107 (83.6%)	Median 44.3	7
Jung et al. [35]	2011	Korea	2005-2009	407	Mean 63.2	Mean 10.3	247 (60.7%)	307(75.4%)	129 (31.7%)	Median 18.4	7
Lee et al. [36]	2015	Korea	2011-2012	752	Mean 66	Mean 9.3	605 (80.5%)	260(34.6%)	483 (64.2%)	Mean 28.3	7
Reeves et al. [27]	2015	Australia	2005-2012	1497	Median 62	NR	1306 (87.2%)	1173 (78%)	1173 (78.4%)	Median 14	7
Watkins et al. [37]	2015	USA	2003-2010	279	Median 62	Median 5.5	80 (28.7%)	279(100%)	193 (69%)	Median 52.7	8
Zhu et al. [13]	2016	China	2002-2014	502	Median 67	Median 12.9	248 (49.4%)	502(100%)	411 (81.9%)	Median 28.6	7
Kang et al. [24]	2016	Korea	2003-2014	2034	Median 67	Median 7.4	1726 (84.9%)	NR	252 (12.4%)	Median 48	7
Kim et al. [38]	2016	Korea	2005-2016	2316	Median 65	Median 7.4	1621 (69.9%)	2316(100%)	NR	Median 60	8
Aoun et al. [5]	2017	Belgium	1990-2013	910	Mean 64	Median 6.8	189 (20.8%)	910(100%)	305 (33.5%)	Median 108	7

GS: Gleason score; PNI: perineural invasion; NR: not reported;NOS: Newcastle–Ottawa Scale; p-PSA: preoperative PSA

Table 2 Characteristics of the included studies on PNI in patients with PCa following RT

Author	Year	Country	Recruitment period	sample size	Age (years)	p-PSA (ng/ml)	GS≥7 (n.%)	PNI (n.%)	Radiotherapy	Follow-up (months)	NOS (score)
Copp et al[39]	2005	USA	1997-2000	93	Median 69.1	Median 9.1	34(36.6%)	17(18.3%)	EBRT	Median 45	7
Yu et al[19]	2007	USA	1993-2002	657	Mean 68	NR	238(36.2%)	112 (19.1%)	EBRT	Median 68	7
Pina et al[40]	2010	Canada	1999-2008	339	Mean 61.9	Mean 5.7	45(13.3%)	89(26.3%)	BT	Median 32	8
Feng et al[41]	2011	USA	1998-2008	718	Median 69.4	Median 8.3	474(66%)	220(34%)	EBRT	Median 62.2	8
Ding et al[30]	2012	USA	1998-2003	185	Median 69	NR	47(25.4%)	10(5%)	BT/ EBRT	Median 80	7
Spratt et al[42]	2013	USA	1989-2011	613	Median 70	NR	613(100%)	156(25.4%)	EBRT	Median 72	7

GS: Gleason score; PNI: perineural invasion; EBRT: external beam radiotherapy; BT: brachytherapy; NR: not reported; NOS: Newcastle–Ottawa Scale; p-PSA: preoperative PSA

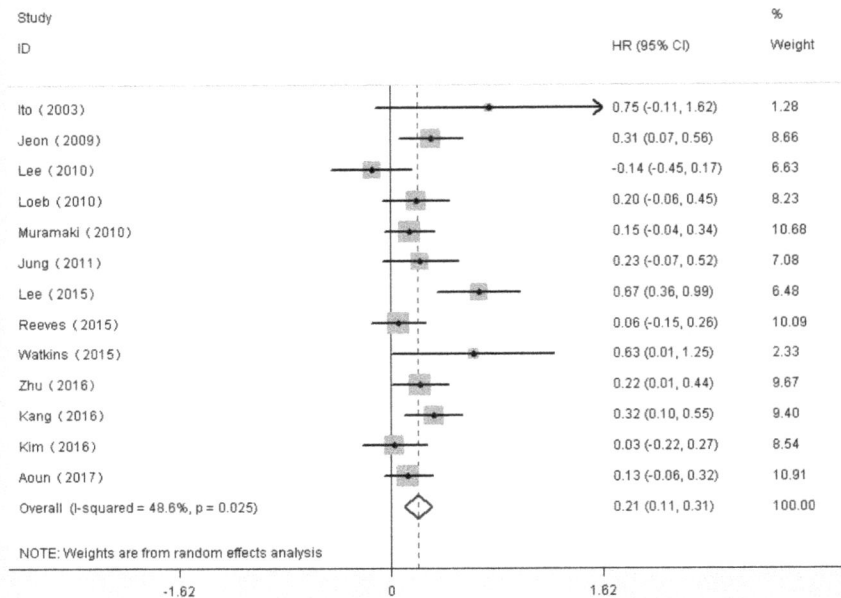

Study ID	HR (95% CI)	% Weight
Ito (2003)	0.75 (-0.11, 1.62)	1.28
Jeon (2009)	0.31 (0.07, 0.56)	8.66
Lee (2010)	-0.14 (-0.45, 0.17)	6.63
Loeb (2010)	0.20 (-0.06, 0.45)	8.23
Muramaki (2010)	0.15 (-0.04, 0.34)	10.68
Jung (2011)	0.23 (-0.07, 0.52)	7.08
Lee (2015)	0.67 (0.36, 0.99)	6.48
Reeves (2015)	0.06 (-0.15, 0.26)	10.09
Watkins (2015)	0.63 (0.01, 1.25)	2.33
Zhu (2016)	0.22 (0.01, 0.44)	9.67
Kang (2016)	0.32 (0.10, 0.55)	9.40
Kim (2016)	0.03 (-0.22, 0.27)	8.54
Aoun (2017)	0.13 (-0.06, 0.32)	10.91
Overall (I-squared = 48.6%, p = 0.025)	0.21 (0.11, 0.31)	100.00

NOTE: Weights are from random effects analysis

Fig. 2 Forest plots for PNI and outcomes of BCR in PCa patients following RP

experience BCR after RT [15]. Therefore, the characterization of the pathological features that may predict BCR is important for counseling patients and in directing the initial or adjuvant therapy. To date, seminal vesicle [16], surgical margins and extracapsular extension [17] are widely used as risk predictors of BCR in PCa. However, these are inferior and cannot accurately predict the risk of BCR in patients with PCa and complicated tumor backgrounds. Therefore, more sensitive and specific markers of risk are needed.

The phenomenon of peripheral nerve involvement has been overlooked for a long time, but it is now gaining recognition as a potential component of the cancer microenvironment [18]. PNI is defined as cancer cell tracking along or around a nerve within the perineural space [19]. It has been demonstrated that PNI may be a route of metastasis for many different cancers (pancreatic [20], bladder [21] and colorectal [22]). Patients with PNI have a higher risk of extraprostatic extension detected at the time of RP [23]; in other words, these patients have an increased risk of BCR.

However, the clinical significance of PNI in PCa following RP or RC is still controversial. Kang [24] and Jeon [25] showed that PNI is an adverse pathologic parameter and an independent predictor for BCR in PCa patients who undergo RP. Similarly, Yu [19] and Wong [26] considered that PNI is an independent

risk factor associated with an increased risk of BCR in patients who undergo external beam radiotherapy. On the contrary, Reeves [27] and Freedland [28] reported that PNI is not correlated with extracapsular extension and BCR in PCa after RP. Nevertheless, Weight [29] suggested that the presence of PNI is not a significant predictor of BCR in patients undergoing brachytherapy (BT) for PCa, and Ding[30] demonstrated a significant independent association between PNI and an increased risk of biochemical failure in 185 PCa patients who received BT.

The conflicting results from different studies prompted us to perform this meta-analysis. For this study, we analyzed 19 studies that included 13,412 patients with PCa, of which 4,197 (31.2%) had PNI. Our results demonstrate that PNI was associated with a higher risk of BCR in PCa patients who underwent RP (p <0.001) or RT (p <0.001). These findings are similar to those reported by Kang [24] and Yu [19]. Notably, the overall findings in the present meta-analysis were consistently independent of geographical region, age, p-PSA, sample size, publication year, and follow-up in the RP group; the findings were also independent of age and sample size in the RT series. In the sensitivity analysis, we sequentially excluded each study, and the reliability and robustness of the results were confirmed. Moreover, no evidence of significant publication bias was

Table 3 Summary and subgroup analyses of the eligible studies

Analysis specification	No. of studies	Study heterogeneity I²(%)	$P_{heterogeneity}$	Effects model	Pooled HR(95% CI)	P-Value
Radical prostatectomy						
Overall	13	48.6	0.025	Random	1.23 (1.11, 1.36)	<0.001
Geographical region						
Asia	9	57.8	0.013	Random	1.26 (1.10, 1.45)	0.001
Other regions	4	6	0.363	Fixed	1.23 (1.11, 1.36)	0.027
Age(years)						
≥65	7	67.2	0.006	Random	1.25 (1.04, 1.50)	0.015
<65	6	0	0.425	Fixed	1.20 (1.08, 1.32)	<0.001
p-PSA(ng/ml)						
≥10	4	44.4	0.126	Fixed	1.21 (1.01, 1.46)	0.037
<10	8	57.8	0.027	Random	1.28 (1.10, 1.49)	0.001
Sample size(cases)						
≥ 500	7	45.7	0.101	Fixed	1.23 (1.03, 1.47)	0.002
< 500	6	57.5	0.028	Random	1.24 (1.08, 1.41)	0.026
Median follow-up(months)						
≥ 30	7	34.9	0.162	Fixed	1.34 (1.12, 1.61)	0.001
< 30	6	57.9	0.036	Random	1.16 (1.11, 1.36)	0.014
Radiotherapy						
Overall	6	34.7	0.176	Fixed	1.22 (1.12, 1.34)	<0.001
Age(years)						
≥65	4	44.8	0.143	Fixed	1.21 (1.11, 1.33)	<0.001
<65	2	38.8	0.201	Fixed	1.45 (0.93, 2.24)	0.097
Sample size(cases)						
≥ 500	3	0	0.495	Fixed	1.20 (1.09, 1.31)	<0.001
< 500	3	31.0	0.235	Fixed	1.68 (1.18, 2.39)	0.004

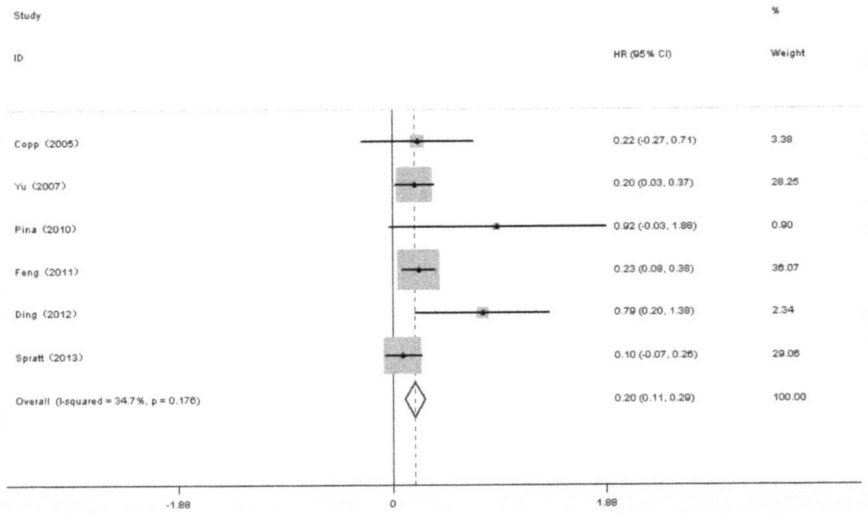

Fig. 3 Forest plots for PNI and outcomes of BCR in PCa patients following RT

found in this analysis according to Funnel plots and Begg's tests. Although subgroup analyses were conducted in the RP and RT groups, significant heterogeneity still existed in some subgroups. The relevant results indicated that these factors were not potential sources of high heterogeneity.

Several potential limitations of our meta-analysis need to be addressed. First, all the included studies were retrospective cohort studies, and data extracted from those studies may have led to inherent potential bias as an unmeasured and uncontrolled confounder. Second, only papers in English and Chinese were selected, and thus some studies that were published in other languages may have otherwise been eligible. Therefore, both selection and publication bias are possible. Third, the pathological diagnosis of PCa and the detection method of PNI varied throughout the eligible studies. Collectively, these factors may promote significant heterogeneity. Fourth, substantial heterogeneity was identified across the studies, and although subgroup analyses were conducted to explore the source of the heterogeneity, heterogeneity still existed in certain categories of analysis. Thus, our results should be interpreted with caution.

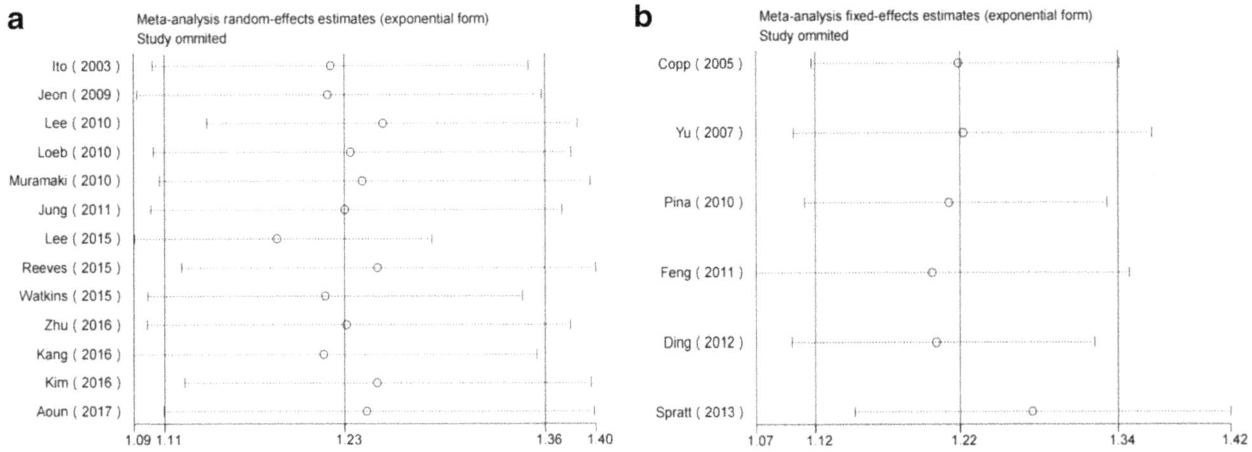

Fig. 4 a: Sensitivity analysis for PNI and BCR in PCa following RP; **b**: Sensitivity analysis for PNI and BCR in PCa following RT

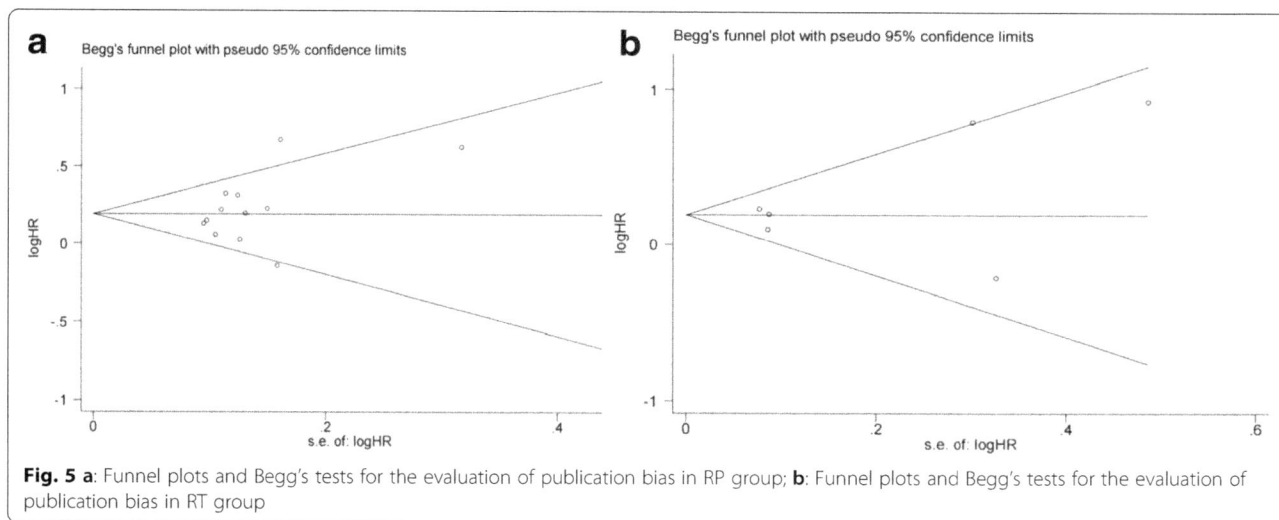

Fig. 5 a: Funnel plots and Begg's tests for the evaluation of publication bias in RP group; **b**: Funnel plots and Begg's tests for the evaluation of publication bias in RT group

Conclusions

To conclude, despite the limitations listed above, this meta-analysis suggested the prognostic and clinicopathological importance of PNI in PCa. The results demonstrated that the presence of PNI is associated with a high risk of BCR whether the patient undergoes RP or RT. Since BCR has been reported to lead to distant metastasis and cancer death [31], we suggested that some patients with PCa and PNI may benefit from adjuvant local or systemic therapy. However, more randomized controlled trials with standardized methods and long-term follow-up are needed to verify our results.

Abbreviations

BCR: Biochemical recurrence; CIs: Confidence intervals; HRs: Hazard ratios; NOS: Newcastle–Ottawa Scale; PCa: Prostate cancer; PNI: Perineural invasion; PSA: Prostate-specific antigen; RP: Radical prostatectomy; RT: Radiotherapy

Acknowledgements
Not applicable.

Funding
No funding was supposed in our study

Authors' contributions
LJZ and BW designed the research; ZLZ, WQ and HZ performed the literature search; JY and YJF analyzed the data and interpreted the results, LJZ wrote the paper. All authors approved the final manuscript.

Competing interests
The authors declare they have no competing interests.

Author details
[1]Departments of Urology, Affiliated Jiang-yin Hospital of the Southeast University Medical College, Jiang-yin 214400, China. [2]Departments of Pharmacy, Affiliated Jiang-yin Hospital of the Southeast University Medical College, Jiang-yin 214400, China.

References
1. Siegel RL, Miller KD, Jemal A. Cancer Statistics, 2017. CA: a cancer journal for clinicians. 2017;67(1):7–30.
2. Fossati N, Karnes RJ, Cozzarini C, Fiorino C, Gandaglia G, Joniau S, Boorjian SA, Goldner G, Hinkelbein W, Haustermans K, et al. Assessing the Optimal Timing for Early Salvage Radiation Therapy in Patients with Prostate-specific Antigen Rise After Radical Prostatectomy. European urology. 2016;69(4):728–33.
3. Qi P, Tsivian M, Abern MR, Banez LL, Tang P, Moul JW, Polascik TJ. Long-term oncological outcomes of men undergoing radical prostatectomy with preoperative prostate-specific antigen <2.5 ng/ml and 2.5-4 ng/ml. Urologic oncology. 2013;31(8):1527–32.
4. Kir G, Seneldir H, Gumus E. Outcomes of Gleason score 3 + 4 = 7 prostate cancer with minimal amounts (<6%) vs >/=6% of Gleason pattern 4 tissue in needle biopsy specimens. Annals of diagnostic pathology. 2016;20:48–51.
5. Aoun F, Albisinni S, Henriet B, Tombal B, Van Velthoven R, Roumeguere T. Predictive factors associated with biochemical recurrence following radical prostatectomy for pathological T2 prostate cancer with negative surgical margins. Scandinavian journal of urology. 2017;51(1):20–6.
6. Ayala GE, Dai H, Ittmann M, Li R, Powell M, Frolov A, Wheeler TM, Thompson TC, Rowley D. Growth and survival mechanisms associated with perineural invasion in prostate cancer. Cancer research. 2004;64(17):6082–90.
7. Cohn JA, Dangle PP, Wang CE, Brendler CB, Novakovic KR, McGuire MS, Helfand BT. The prognostic significance of perineural invasion and race in men considering active surveillance. BJU international. 2014;114(1):75–80.
8. Haki Yuksel O, Urkmez A, Verit A: Can perineural invasion detected in prostate needle biopsy specimens predict surgical margin positivity in D'Amico low risk patients? Archivio italiano di urologia, andrologia : organo ufficiale [di] Societa italiana di ecografia urologica e nefrologica 2016, 88(2):89-92.
9. Liberati A, Altman DG, Tetzlaff J, Mulrow C, Gotzsche PC, Ioannidis JP, Clarke M, Devereaux PJ, Kleijnen J, Moher D. The PRISMA statement for reporting systematic reviews and meta-analyses of studies that evaluate health care interventions: explanation and elaboration. Journal of clinical epidemiology. 2009;62(10):e1–34.
10. Thompson IM, Valicenti RK, Albertsen P, Davis BJ, Goldenberg SL, Hahn C, Klein E, Michalski J, Roach M, Sartor O, et al. Adjuvant and salvage radiotherapy after prostatectomy: AUA/ASTRO Guideline. The Journal of urology. 2013;190(2):441–9.
11. Roach M 3rd, Hanks G, Thames H Jr, Schellhammer P, Shipley WU, Sokol GH, Sandler H. Defining biochemical failure following radiotherapy with or without hormonal therapy in men with clinically localized prostate cancer: recommendations of the RTOG-ASTRO Phoenix Consensus Conference. International journal of radiation oncology, biology, physics. 2006;65(4):965–74.
12. Stang A. Critical evaluation of the Newcastle-Ottawa scale for the assessment of the quality of nonrandomized studies in meta-analyses. European journal of epidemiology. 2010;25(9):603–5.

13. Zhu YJ, Wang YQ, Pan JH, Dong BJ, Xu F, Sha JJ, Xue W. Huang YR: [Value of perineural invasion in prostatectomy specimen in the assessment on tumor progression and prognosis]. Zhonghua wai ke za zhi [Chinese journal of surgery]. 2016;54(3):217–21.

14. Lee DJ, Mallin K, Graves AJ, Chang SS, Penson DF, Resnick MJ, Barocas DA. Recent Changes in Prostate Cancer Screening Practices and Epidemiology. J Urol. 2017;198(6):1230–40.

15. Fakhrejahani F, Madan RA, Dahut WL. Management Options for Biochemically Recurrent Prostate Cancer. Current treatment options in oncology. 2017;18(5):26.

16. Porcaro AB, de Luyk N, Corsi P, Sebben M, Tafuri A, Tamanini I, Processali T, Cerruto MA, Migliorini F, Brunelli M, et al. Bilateral lymph node micrometastases and seminal vesicle invasion associated with same clinical predictors in localized prostate cancer. Tumori. 2017; 103(3):299–306.

17. Psutka SP, Feldman AS, Rodin D, Olumi AF, Wu CL, McDougal WS. Men with organ-confined prostate cancer and positive surgical margins develop biochemical failure at a similar rate to men with extracapsular extension. Urology. 2011;78(1):121–5.

18. Lee JT, Lee S, Yun CJ, Jeon BJ, Kim JM, Ha HK, Lee W, Chung MK. Prediction of perineural invasion and its prognostic value in patients with prostate cancer. Korean journal of urology. 2010;51(11):745–51.

19. Yu HH, Song DY, Tsai YY, Thompson T, Frassica DA, DeWeese TL. Perineural invasion affects biochemical recurrence-free survival in patients with prostate cancer treated with definitive external beam radiotherapy. Urology. 2007;70(1):111–6.

20. Liang D, Shi S, Xu J, Zhang B, Qin Y, Ji S, Xu W, Liu J, Liu L, Liu C, et al. New insights into perineural invasion of pancreatic cancer: More than pain. Biochimica et biophysica acta. 2016;1865(2):111–22.

21. Muppa P, Gupta S, Frank I, Boorjian SA, Karnes RJ, Thompson RH, Thapa P, Tarrell RF, Herrera Hernandez LP, Jimenez RE, et al. Prognostic significance of lymphatic, vascular and perineural invasion for bladder cancer patients treated by radical cystectomy. Pathology. 2017;49(3): 259–66.

22. Zhou Y, Wang H, Gong H, Cao M, Zhang G, Wang Y. Clinical significance of perineural invasion in stages II and III colorectal cancer. Pathology, research and practice. 2015;211(11):839–44.

23. DeLancey JO, Wood DP, Jr., He C, Montgomery JS, Weizer AZ, Miller DC, Jacobs BL, Montie JE, Hollenbeck BK, Skolarus TA: Evidence of perineural invasion on prostate biopsy specimen and survival after radical prostatectomy. Urology 2013, 81(2):354-357.

24. Kang M, Oh JJ, Lee S, Hong SK, Lee SE, Byun SS. Perineural Invasion and Lymphovascular Invasion are Associated with Increased Risk of Biochemical Recurrence in Patients Undergoing Radical Prostatectomy. Annals of surgical oncology. 2016;23(8):2699–706.

25. Jeon HG, Bae J, Yi JS, Hwang IS, Lee SE, Lee E. Perineural invasion is a prognostic factor for biochemical failure after radical prostatectomy. International journal of urology : official journal of the Japanese Urological Association. 2009;16(8):682–6.

26. Wong WW, Schild SE, Vora SA, Halyard MY. Association of percent positive prostate biopsies and perineural invasion with biochemical outcome after external beam radiotherapy for localized prostate cancer. International journal of radiation oncology, biology, physics. 2004;60(1):24–9.

27. Reeves F, Hovens CM, Harewood L, Battye S, Peters JS, Costello AJ, Corcoran NM. Does perineural invasion in a radical prostatectomy specimen predict biochemical recurrence in men with prostate cancer? Canadian Urological Association journal = Journal de l'Association des urologues du Canada. 2015;9(5-6):E252–5.

28. Freedland SJ, Csathy GS, Dorey F, Aronson WJ. Percent prostate needle biopsy tissue with cancer is more predictive of biochemical failure or adverse pathology after radical prostatectomy than prostate specific antigen or Gleason score. The Journal of urology. 2002;167(2 Pt 1): 516–20.

29. Weight CJ, Ciezki JP, Reddy CA, Zhou M, Klein EA. Perineural invasion on prostate needle biopsy does not predict biochemical failure following brachytherapy for prostate cancer. International journal of radiation oncology, biology, physics. 2006;65(2):347–50.

30. Ding W, Lee J, Chamberlain D, Cunningham J, Yang L, Tay J. Twelve-month prostate-specific antigen values and perineural invasion as strong independent prognostic variables of long-term biochemical outcome after prostate seed brachytherapy. International journal of radiation oncology, biology, physics. 2012;84(4):962–7.

31. Pagano MJ, Whalen MJ, Paulucci DJ, Reddy BN, Matulay JT, Rothberg M, Scarberry K, Patel T, Shapiro EY, RoyChoudhury A, et al. Predictors of biochemical recurrence in pT3b prostate cancer after radical prostatectomy without adjuvant radiotherapy. Prostate. 2016;76(2):226–34.

32. Ito K, Nakashima J, Mukai M, Asakura H, Ohigashi T, Saito S, Tachibana M, Hata J, Murai M. Prognostic implication of microvascular invasion in biochemical failure in patients treated with radical prostatectomy. Urologia internationalis. 2003;70(4):297–302.

33. Loeb S, Epstein JI, Humphreys EB, Walsh PC. Does perineural invasion on prostate biopsy predict adverse prostatectomy outcomes? BJU international. 2010;105(11):1510–3.

34. Muramaki M, Miyake H, Kurahashi T, Takenaka A, Fujisawa M. Characterization of the anatomical extension pattern of localized prostate cancer arising in the peripheral zone. BJU international. 2010;105(11):1514–8.

35. Jung JH, Lee JW, Arkoncel FR, Cho NH, Yusoff NA, Kim KJ, Song JM, Kim SJ, Rha KH. Significance of perineural invasion, lymphovascular invasion, and high-grade prostatic intraepithelial neoplasia in robot-assisted laparoscopic radical prostatectomy. Annals of surgical oncology. 2011;18(13):3828–32.

36. Lee D, Lee C, Kwon T, You D, Jeong IG, Hong JH, Ahn H, Kim CS. Clinical features and prognosis of prostate cancer with high-grade prostatic intraepithelial neoplasia. Korean journal of urology. 2015;56(8):565–71.

37. Watkins JM, Laszewski M, Watkins PL, Dufan TA, Adducci C. Margin involvement at prostatectomy for clinically localized prostate cancer: does a low-risk group exist? Practical radiation oncology. 2015;5(1):e31–6.

38. Kim DK, Koo KC, Abdel Raheem A, Kim KH, Chung BH, Choi YD, Rha KH. Single Positive Lymph Node Prostate Cancer Can Be Treated Surgically without Recurrence. PLoS One. 2016;11(3):e0152391.

39. Copp H, Bissonette EA, Theodorescu D. Tumor control outcomes of patients treated with trimodality therapy for locally advanced prostate cancer. Urology. 2005;65(6):1146–51.

40. Pina AG, Crook JM, Kwan P, Borg J, Ma C. The impact of perineural invasion on biochemical outcome after permanent prostate iodine-125 brachytherapy. Brachytherapy. 2010;9(3):213–8.

41. Feng FY, Qian Y, Stenmark MH, Halverson S, Blas K, Vance S, Sandler HM, Hamstra DA. Perineural invasion predicts increased recurrence, metastasis, and death from prostate cancer following treatment with dose-escalated radiation therapy. International journal of radiation oncology, biology, physics. 2011;81(4):e361–7.

42. Spratt DE, Zumsteg Z, Ghadjar P, Pangasa M, Pei X, Fine SW, Yamada Y, Kollmeier M, Zelefsky MJ. Prognostic importance of Gleason 7 disease among patients treated with external beam radiation therapy for prostate cancer: results of a detailed biopsy core analysis. International journal of radiation oncology, biology, physics. 2013;85(5):1254–61.

Decolonization potential of 0.02%polyhexanide irrigation solution in urethral catheters under practice-like in vitro conditions

Florian H. H. Brill[1]*, Henrik Gabriel[1], Holger Brill[1], Jan-Hendrik Klock[1], Joerg Steinmann[2,3] and Andreas Arndt[4]

Abstract

Background: Long-term use of indwelling urethral catheters is associated with high risk of urinary tract infection (UTI) and blockage, which may in turn cause significant morbidity and reduce the life of the catheter. A 0.02% polyhexanide irrigation solution has been developed for routine mechanical rinsing together with bacterial decolonization of suprapubic and indwelling urethral catheters.

Methods: Using a practice-like in vitro assay and standard silicon catheters, artificially contaminated with clinically relevant bacteria, experiments were carried out to evaluate the bacterial decolonization potential of polyhexanide vs. 1) no intervention (standard approach) and 2) irrigation with a saline (NaCl 0.9%) solution. Swabbing and irrigation was used to extract the bacteria.

Results: Irrigation with polyhexanide reduced the microbial population vs. the control catheters by a factor of $1.64 \log_{10}$ (swab extraction) and by a factor of $2.56 \log_{10}$ (membrane filtration). The difference in mean microbial counts between the two groups (0.90) was statistically significant in favor of polyhexanide when the liquid extraction method was used ($p = 0.034$). The difference between the two groups using the swab extraction method did not reach statistical significance.

Conclusions: The saline and polyhexanide solutions are able to reduce bacterial load of catheters, which shows a combined mechanical and antimicrobial effect. Further research is required to evaluate the long-term tolerability and efficacy of polyhexanide in clinical practice.

Keywords: Bacterial decolonization, Biofilm, Polyhexanide, Urinary catheter, Urinary tract infection

Background

The long-term use of indwelling urethral and suprapubic catheters to manage intractable urinary incontinence and retention is commonplace in both hospital and especially community healthcare settings [1–9]. Surveys of nursing homes across Europe and the US have shown that between 8 to 10% of residents have indwelling urinary catheters [3, 4]. The long-term catheterization patient population is a heterogeneous group, many of which are elderly people who have chronic disabilities [10, 11]. Long-term catheterization can lead to significant patient morbidity and mortality caused by associated complications [10]. The most common complications that occur are urinary tract infection (UTI) and catheter blockage, which can affect up to 70% of catheterized patients [9–11]. Enteric pathogens (e.g. *Escherichia coli*) are most commonly responsible; however, *Pseudomonas* species, *Enterococcus* species, *Staphylococcus aureus*, coagulase-negative staphylococci, *Enterobacter* species and yeasts are also known to cause infection [12]. Bacteria gain access to the urinary tract either extra- or intraluminally and form biofilm colonies, which may adhere to the catheter surface and drainage bag [12–15]. As well as providing a source of infection, biofilm

* Correspondence: florian.b@brillhygiene.com
[1]Dr. Brill + Partner GmbH Institute for Hygiene and Microbiology, Stiegstück 34, 22339 Hamburg, Germany
Full list of author information is available at the end of the article

formation is also implicated in encrustation and blockage of catheters [14].

Bacteria within biofilms are morphologically and physiologically different from planktonic bacterial cells and are often resistant to systemic antibiotic treatment, making them difficult to eradicate [13]. However, there is evidence suggesting that physical removal, i.e. mechanical rinsing, is the best method of biofilm elimination, and regular cleansing is required to prevent regrowth of the bacteria [16]. Nevertheless, current guidance does not recommend an active approach for catheter management [17, 18]. The standard clinical approach is not to intervene and therefore removal of the catheter may be the only option [3].

Broad-spectrum antimicrobial agents such as polyhexanide that kill microorganisms have shown to be appropriate agents to use for mechanical rinsing and removal of biofilm across a range of applications [16, 19]. The aim of this study was to investigate whether taking an active approach with a mechanical irrigation with normal saline solution and a combined approach with a polyhexanide solution is efficient for decolonizing urethral catheters. The bactericidal activity of the polyhexanide solution was tested in vitro using a suspension assay. In addition, the bacterial decolonization potential was tested using a practice-like in vitro assay with standard catheters, which were artificially contaminated. The polyhexanide solution and irrigation with a normal saline solution were compared to no intervention (standard approach).

Methods

The decolonization activity of a polyhexanide solution (Uro-Tainer® 0.02% Polyhexanide, B. Braun Medical Ltd., Sempach, Switzerland) and normal saline solution was assessed in the presented study. For the time being polyhexanide is used in wound antiseptics with 0.02% and 0.04% concentration [20]. The 0.02% concentration is recommended for clean wounds. As in the application for transurethral catheter decolonization in most cases clean conditions without blood are expected, the lower concentration has been selected to reduce the risk for irritation in patients.

Bactericidal activity in suspension assay

The suspension tests were performed according to EN 13727 [21] against the following six bacteria strains: *Staphylococcus aureus* (ATCC 6538), *Enterococcus hirae* (ATCC 10541), *Escherichia coli K12* (ATCC 11229, *Proteus mirabilis* (ATCC 14153), *Pseudomonas aeruginosa* (ATCC 15442), *Klebsiella pneumoniae* (ATCC 16609). The bacteria were incubated for 48 h at 36 ± 1 °C. They were exposed to the polyhexanide solution at 50 and 80% v/v for 5, 15, 30 and 60 min under clean conditions

(0.3 g/L bovine serum albumin). A combination of 80 g/L polysorbate 80, 60 g/L saponin, 6 g/L lecithin, 20 g/L sodium dodecyl sulphate in A. dest. was validated and used as neutralizing solution.

Catheter decolonization assay

The test bacteria were *Escherichia coli* (ATCC 11229), *Proteus mirabilis* (ATCC 14153) and methicillin-resistant *Staphylococcus aureus* (MRSA) (ATCC 33592). The devices used in all experiments were 41 cm long transurethral silicon balloon catheters with a nelaton-top, size ch. 18 (B. Braun Melsungen Ltd., Germany).

The experimental set up of the in-vitro decolonization assay was as follows:

- The catheters were contaminated with 5 ml of a mixed suspension of the test organisms (10^8 to 10^9 colony forming units [cfu] per ml simulating worst-case conditions) in caseinpepton-soy bean pepton-bouillon daily for 3 days (Fig. 1).
- The contaminated catheters were incubated for a total of 72 h at 36 °C ± 1 °C.
- All catheters were irrigated twice daily with a flow of 400 ml of the synthetic urine (composition according to EN 1616: 25 g/L urea, 9 g/L NaCl, 2.5 g/L Potassium hydrogenorthophosphate, dipotassium hydrogenorthophosphate, 3 g/L ammonium chloride 2 g/L kreatinin, 3 g/L sodium sulphite in A. dest. + 3 g/L % bovine serum albumin [22]) during the incubation period.
- After incubation and the treatment of the catheter with normal saline or polihexanide or no treatment respectively the catheters were irrigated with 100 ml of neutralizer solution (1 g/L polysorbate 80, 1 g/L

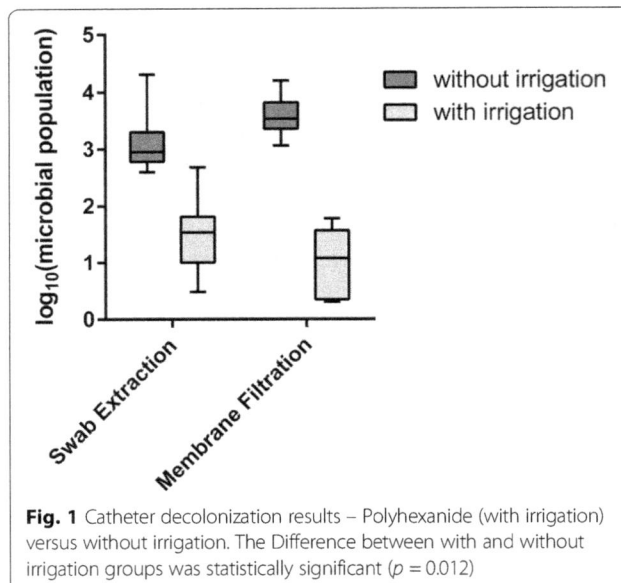

Fig. 1 Catheter decolonization results – Polyhexanide (with irrigation) versus without irrigation. The Difference between with and without irrigation groups was statistically significant ($p = 0.012$)

lecithine, 1 g/L histidine, 2 g/L Sodium dodecyl sulphate) and the microbial count in the solution was determined by membrane filtration of 50 ml and with serial dilution tests (liquid extraction method).

- In addition, all catheters were cut with a sterile scalpel and the content of the inner lumen of the catheters was extracted with a sterile cotton swab. The swab was suspended in normal saline solution and the microbial count was determined with a serial dilution assay (swab extraction method).
- The endpoint, i.e. $\log_{10}$ reduction factor (RF) in microbial count, was calculated for the treatment groups vs. the control no treatment group.
- The statistical difference between the groups was evaluated by the one-sided unpaired Wilcoxon rank sum test [23].

In the first experiment according to above described methodology a total of 20 contaminated catheters were included. Ten were used as growth control in the no treatment group and 10 were treated with polyhexanide solution by connecting the device to the catheter as described in the instructions for use. After the exposure time of 5 min the microbial count was determined.

The second catheter decolonization experiment was similar to the first experiment. A total of 30 catheters were included. Ten catheters were treated with 100 ml 0.9% NaCl solution with an exposure time of 5 min. Additional 10 catheter were treated with 100 ml of the polihexanide solution with an exposure time of 5 min. The remaining 10 catheters were used as growth control and not treated.

Results

In the suspension test assay according to EN 13727 the polyhexanide solution was shown to have bactericidal activity in vitro against *Staphylococcus aureus, Enterococcus hirae, Pseudomonas aeruginosa, Escherichia coli, Proteus mirabilis* and *Klebsiella pneumonia* under clean conditions (Table 1).

The results of the first catheter decolonization assay are summarized in Fig. 1. The control catheters (standard approach i.e. no intervention) had a mean microbial population of 3.12 $\log_{10}$ (range 2.60–4.31 $\log_{10}$) when measured using the swab extraction method and 3.57 $\log_{10}$ (range 3.06–4.20 $\log_{10}$) when the membrane filtration method was used. The catheters irrigated with the polyhexanide solution had a mean microbial population of 1.47 $\log_{10}$ (range 0.48–2.68 $\log_{10}$) when measured using the swab extraction method and 1.01 $\log_{10}$ (0.30–1.60 $\log_{10}$) when the membrane filtration method was used. The difference in the mean microbial count between the two groups was statistically significant in favor of the polyhexanide solution for both methods of analysis ($p = 0.012$).

Irrigation of the catheters with the polyhexanide solution reduced the microbial population compared to that of the control catheters by a factor of 1.64 $\log_{10}$ (1.12–2.30 $\log_{10}$) when measured using the swab extraction method and by a factor of 2.56 $\log_{10}$ (1.46–3.20 $\log_{10}$) using the membrane filtration method.

The results of the second catheter decolonization assay are summarized in Table 2. The catheters irrigated with NaCl 0.9% had a mean microbial population of 2.37 $\log_{10}$ (± 0.196) when measured using the swab extraction method and 1.70 $\log_{10}$ (± 0.458) when the membrane filtration method was used. The catheters irrigated with the polyhexanide solution had a mean microbial

Table 1 Bactericidal activity of polyhexanide 0.02% solution against different reference strains

Test Sample/ Test Organism Microbial Count Control NO	lg-reduction factor after minutes				
	Conc. in %	5	15	30	60
Staphylococcus aureus (ATCC 6538), NO = 7.62	50.00	≥ 7.62	≥ 7.62	≥ 7.62	≥ 7.62
	80.00	≥ 7.62	≥ 7.62	≥ 7.62	≥ 7.62
Enterococcus hirae (ATCC 10541), NO = 7.42	50.00	≥ 7.42	≥ 7.42	≥ 7.42	≥ 7.42
	80.00	≥ 7.42	≥ 7.42	≥ 7.42	≥ 7.42
Escherichia coli K12 (ATCC 11229), NO = 7.26	50.00	n.c.	≥ 6.56	≥ 7.26	≥ 7.26
	80.00	3.93	≥ 7.26	≥ 7.26	≥ 7.26
Proteus mirabilis (ATCC 14153), NO = 7.76	50.00	≥ 7.76	≥ 7.76	≥ 7.76	≥ 7.76
	80.00	≥ 7.76	≥ 7.76	≥ 7.76	≥ 7.76
Pseudomonas aeruginosa (ATCC 15442), NO = 7.35	50.00	n.c.	5.58	≥ 7.43	≥ 7.43
	80.00	≥ 7.35	≥ 7.43	≥ 7.43	≥ 7.43
Klebsiella pneumonia (ATCC 16609), NO = 7.66	50.00	5.18	≥ 7.66	≥ 7.66	6.96
	80.00	≥ 7.66	≥ 7.66	≥ 7.66	6.96

n.c. not calculable

Table 2 Catheter decolonization results – polyhexanide 0.02% versus NaCl 0.9%

Catheter	Swab Extraction Method			Membrane Filtration Method		
	log with NaCl	log with polyhexanide	Difference NaCl – polyhexanide	log with NaCl	log with polyhexanide	Difference NaCl – polyhexanide
1	2.34	2.48	−0.13	1.00	1.00	0.00
2	2.48	1.48	1.00	1.00	1.00	0.00
3	2.48	1.30	1.18	2.00	0.00	2.00
4	2.48	1.48	1.00	2.00	0.00	2.00
5	2.48	1.48	1.00	2.00	2.00	0.00
6	2.48	2.48	0.00	2.00	2.00	0.00
7	2.48	2.48	0.00	1.00	1.00	0.00
8	2.48	2.48	0.00	2.00	1.00	1.00
9	2.08	2.48	−0.40	2.00	0.00	2.00
10	1.90	2.48	−0.57	2.00	0.00	2.00
Mean	2.37	2.06	0.31[a]	1.70	0.80	0.90[b]
Standard deviation	0.196	0.514	0.628	0.458	0.748	0.943
No of catheters		10			10	

[a]The difference between the polyhexanide and NaCl groups is not statistically significant ($p = 0.173$) for the swab extraction method
[b]The difference between the polyhexanide and NaCl groups is statistically significant ($p = 0.034$) for the liquid extraction method

population of 2.06 $\log_{10}$ (± 0.514) when measured using the swab extraction method and 0.80 $\log_{10}$ (± 0.748) when the membrane filtration method was used. The difference in mean microbial count between the two groups (0.90) was statistically significant in favor of the polyhexanide solution when the liquid extraction method was used ($p = 0.034$). However, the difference between the two groups using the swab extraction method was not statistically significant ($p = 0.173$).

Discussion

This study has demonstrated that the polyhexanide solution has bactericidal activity in vitro against microorganisms which have been commonly associated with development of UTI in catheterized patients [12, 15]. Furthermore, this is the first in vitro study to demonstrate the potential role of polyhexanide for bacterial decolonization of urinary catheters.

The current literature on bacterial decolonization of urethral catheters is largely restricted to treatment with a range of systemic antibiotic regimens [24]. In a study by Jones et al. it has been shown that MRSA was able to colonize a silastic rubber surface even in the presence of prophylactic vancomycin or rifampicin [25]. Furthermore, other studies have shown that the lowest concentration required to eradicate bacterial biofilm for many antibiotics may exceed the maximum therapeutic dose level [26–29].

As an alternative to systemic antibiotic treatment efforts have been made to develop catheters coated with hydrophilic gels or antibacterial agents (such as silver) to prevent bacterial adhesion [30] .However, none of these

developments have been shown to resist biofilm formation, especially in patients with *Proteus mirabilis* UTI [30]. One explanation for this lack of success is that this approach does not involve mechanical rinsing or irrigation.

In comparison to antibiotics and use of coated catheters it is suggested that polyhexanide might provide an effective, non-systemic approach to bacterial decolonization of urinary catheters. Polyhexanide has been successfully used for bacterial decolonization and prevention of biofilm formation in wound management [19, 31–35]. In an in vitro study rinsing with polyhexanide solution significantly reduced MRSA biofilm at 48 and 72 h compared to two saline solutions ($p < 0.05$) [32]. In addition to its bactericidal properties, polyhexanide has also been shown to have anti-adhesive properties due to its chemical nature (i.e. cationic), which may have the potential to help prevent biofilm formation [31].

The present study has shown that mechanical rinsing with 0.9% NaCl solution and a 0.02% solution of polyhexanide was shown to be significantly and consistently more effective at reducing the bacterial colonization of the catheters compared to no intervention (standard approach). However, there was no significant difference seen in microbial count between the polihexanide compared to the control groups when the swab extraction method was used.

The results of this study were achieved in experiments that were designed to replicate practice-like conditions as closely as possible. Silicone catheters used routinely in practice were contaminated with a combination of clinically relevant bacteria (e.g. *Proteus mirabilis* and MRSA) and a solution of synthetic urine and incubated for several days at body temperature. The polyhexanide solution and the saline solution were used according to the manufacturer's instructions to rinse the catheters for 5 min as used in clinical practice. However, the study has some limitations: the experiments were performed with only one type of catheter. The inoculation with mixed bacterial strains was not standardized in terms of growth of the included species. The microbial counts of the three test bacteria were not determined separately. Therefore, it is possible that the effect of the treatments is not balanced against all bacteria. Also it is possible that some bacteria turned into viable, but not culturable (VBNC) status especially after antimicrobial treatment. As we used standard test bacteria under laboratory conditions on solid media, it is unlikely but possible that this has influenced the results. In addition, practice-like in vitro conditions cannot replace in vivo studies and therefore the results may not directly translate into the clinical setting. Further research is required to demonstrate the efficacy of the polyhexanide as well as 0.9% NaCl solution across a range of catheter types and materials available in clinical practice. Research is also required in patients to evaluate the tolerability and clinical effectiveness of the polyhexanide solution when used for routine catheter maintenance in the short- and long-term.

In summary, the results of this study have shown that a 0.02% polihexanide and 0.9% NaCl solution is able to significantly reduce bacterial load of catheters, which shows a combined mechanical and antimicrobial effect. Further research is required to demonstrate the tolerability and efficacy of the polyhexanide solution in daily clinical practice.

Abbreviations
MRSA: Methicillin-resistant *Staphylococcus aureus*; RF: Reduction factor; UTI: Urinary tract infection

Authors' contributions
FHHB, HG, HB, J-HK and AA were involved in the development of the method, the planning of the laboratory tests. HG and J-HK were responsible for data analysis. FHHB, JS and AA prepared the manuscript for important intellectual content and also approved the final version for journal submission. All authors read and approved the final manuscript.

Competing interest
The study was partially financially supported by B. Braun Medical Ltd. FHHB was an employee for B. Braun Medical Ltd. between 2006 and 2010. AA is an employee of B. Braun Medical Ltd.

Author details
[1]Dr. Brill + Partner GmbH Institute for Hygiene and Microbiology, Stiegstück 34, 22339 Hamburg, Germany. [2]Institute of Medical Microbiology, University Hospital Essen, Essen, Germany. [3]Institute of Clinical Hygiene, Medical Microbiology and Infectiology, Paracelsus Medical University, Klinikum Nürnberg, Nuremberg, Germany. [4]Department of Research and Development, B. Braun Medical Ltd., Sempach, Switzerland.

References
1. Greene T, Kiyoshi-Teo H, Reichert H, Krein S, Saint S. Urinary catheter indications in the United States: results from a national survey of acute care hospitals. Infect Control Hosp Epidemiol. 2014;35:96–8.
2. Gokula RR, Hickner JA, Smith MA. Inappropriate use of urinary catheters in elderly patients at a midwestern community teaching hospital. Am J Infect Control. 2004;32:196–9.
3. Wilde MH, Getliffe K. Urinary catheter care for older adults. Ann Long Term Care. 2006;14: article 6051. Available at http://www.annalsoflongtermcare.com/article/6051 Last accessed July 2016
4. McNulty C, Freeman E, Smith G, et al. Prevalence of urinary catheterization in UK nursing homes. J Hosp Infect. 2003;55:119–23.
5. Milligan F. Male sexuality and urethral catheterisation: a review of the literature. Nurs Stand. 1999;13:43–7.
6. Henry M. Catheter confusion. Nurs Times. 1992;88:65–72.
7. Crow R, Mulhall A, Chapman RB. Indwelling catheterization and related nursing practice. J Adv Nurs. 1988;13:489–95.
8. Crow R, Chapman RG, Roe BH, Wilson JA. A study of patients with an indwelling urethral catheter and related nursing practice. In: University of Surrey 1986: nursing practice research unit.
9. Roe BH, Brocklehurst JC. Study of patients with indwelling catheters. J Adv Nurs. 1987;12:713–8.
10. Wilde MH, McDonald MV, Brasch J, et al. Long-term urinary catheter users self-care practices and problems. J Clin Nurs. 2013;22:356–67.
11. Khan AA, Mathur S, Feneley R, Timoney AG. Developing a strategy to reduce the high morbidity of patients with long-term urinary catheters: the BioMed catheter research clinic. BJU Int. 2007;100:1298–301.
12. Brusch JL. Catheter-related urinary tract infection: Transmission and pathogens. Available at http://emedicine.medscape.com/article/2040035-overview. Last accessed July 2016.
13. Costerton JW, Lewandowski Z, Caldwell DE, Korber DR, Lappin-Scott HM. Microbial biofilms. Annu Rev Microbiol. 1995;49:711–45.
14. Pratt RJ, Pellowe CM, Wilson JA, et al. epic2: national evidence-based guidelines for preventing healthcare-associated infections in NHS hospitals in England. J Hosp Infect. 2007;65(Suppl 1):S1–64.
15. Goldsworthy MJH. Gene expression of *Pseudomonas aeruginosa* and MRSA with a catheter-associated urinary tract infection biofilm model. Biosci Horiz. 2008;1:28–37.
16. Gilliver S. PHMB a well-tolerated antiseptic with no reported toxic effects. J Wound Care/ Activa Healthcare Supplement 2009;S9–14. http://lohmann-rauscher.co.uk/downloads/clinical-evidence/SXP025-SGilliver-PHMB-a-well-tolerated-antiseptic-with-.pdf.
17. Robert Koch Institut. Infection prevention in the home. Recommendations of the Commission for Hospital Hygiene and Infection Production of the Robert Koch institute (RKI). Bundesgesundheitsblatt Gesundheitsforschung Gesundheitsschutz. 2005;48:1061–80.
18. Conway LJ, Larson EL. Guidelines to prevent catheter-associated urinary tract infection: 1980 to 2010. Heart Lung. 2012;41:271–83.
19. Bradbury S, Fletcher J. Prontosan® made easy. 2011;2:1–6. http://www.woundsinternational.com/media/issues/418/files/content_9864.pdf.
20. Egli-Gany D, Brill FHH, Hintzpeter M, Andreé S, Pavel FHH. Evaluation of the antiseptic efficacy and local tolerability of a Polihexanide-based antiseptic on resident skin Flora. Adv Skin Wound Care. 2012;25(9):404–8.
21. DIN EN 13727: Chemical disinfectants and antiseptics - quantitative suspension test for the evaluation of bactericidal activity in the medical area - test method and requirements (phase 2, step 1); German version EN 13727:2012+A2:2015.
22. EN 1616: Sterile uretheral catheters for single use (includes amendment A1: 1999); German version EN 1616:1997 + A1:1999.
23. European Committee for Standardization. Chemical disinfectants and antiseptics. In: Hygienic handrub. Test method and requirements (phase 2/step 2); German version EN 1500; 1997.

24. Buehlmann M, Bruderer T, Frei R, Widmer AF. Effectiveness of a new decolonisation regimen for eradication of extended-spectrum β-lactamase-producing Enterobacteriaceae. J Hosp Infect. 2011;77:113–7.
25. Jones SM, Morgan M, Humphrey TJ, Lappin-Scott H. Effect of vancomycin and rifampicin on meticillin-resistant *Staphylococcus aureus* biofilms. Lancet. 2001;357:40–1.
26. Koseoglu H, Aslan G, Esen N, Sen BH, Coban H. Ultrastructural stages of biofilm development of *Escherichia coli* on urethral catheters and effects of antibiotics on biofilm formation. Urology. 2006;68:942–6.
27. Olson ME, Ceri H, Morck DW, Buret AG, Read RR. Biofilm bacteria: formation and comparative susceptibility to antibiotics. Can J Vet Res. 2002;66:86–92.
28. Conley J, Olson ME, Cook LS, Ceri H, Phan V, Davies HD. Biofilm formation by group a streptococci: is there a relationship with treatment failure? J Clin Microbiol. 2003;41:4043–8.
29. Phillips L, Wolcott RD, Fletcher J, Schultz GS. Biofilms made easy. 2010;1:1–6. http://www.woundsinternational.com/media/issues/288/files/content_8851.pdf.
30. Stickler DJ. Bacterial biofilms and the encrustation of urethral catheters. Biofouling. 1996;9:293–305.
31. Afinogenova AG, Grabovskaya KB, Kuleshevich EV, Suvorov AN, Afinogenova AG. Effects of biguanides on the formation of streptococcal biofilms using a human embryo skin fibroblast cell culture. Infect in Surg. 2011;1:5–13.
32. Perez R, Davies SC, Kaehn K. Effect of different wound rinsing solutions on MRSA biofilm in a porcine wound model. Wund Manage. 2010;4(2):44–8.
33. Romanelli M, Dini V, Barbanera S, Bertone MS. Evaluation of the efficacy and tolerability of a solution containing propyl betaine and polyhexanide for wound irrigation. Skin Pharmacol Physiol. 2010;23(Suppl 1):41–4.
34. Moller A, Nolte A, Kaehn K. Experiences with the use of PHMB-containing wound products in the management of chronic wounds — results of a methodical and retrospective analysis of 953 patients. Wund Manage. 2008; 3:112–7.
35. Andriessen AE, Eberlein T. Assessment of a wound cleansing solution in the treatment of problem wounds. Wounds. 2008;20(6):171–5.

Permissions

Contributors

Andrew Stickley
The Stockholm Center for Health and Social Change (SCOHOST), Södertörn University, Huddinge 141 89, Sweden

Ziggi Ivan Santini
The Danish National Institute of Public Health, University of Southern Denmark, Oester Farimagsgade 5A, 1353 Copenhagen, Denmark

Ai Koyanagi
Parc Sanitari Sant Joan de Déu, Universitat de Barcelona, Fundació Sant Joan de Déu/ CIBERSAM, Barcelona, Spain

Yunjin Bai, Yin Tang, Lan Deng, Xiaoming Wang, Yubo Yang, Jia Wang and Ping Han
Department of Urology, Institute of Urology, West China Hospital, Sichuan University, Guoxue Xiang#37, Chengdu, Sichuan 610041, China

A. Waldmann
Institute for Social Medicine and Epidemiology, University Luebeck, Ratzeburger Allee 160 (Hs 50), 23562 Luebeck, Germany

A. Schmick
Institute for Social Medicine and Epidemiology, University Luebeck, Ratzeburger Allee 160 (Hs 50), 23562 Luebeck, Germany
Department of Emergency Medicine, Klinik Hirslanden, Witellikerstrasse 40, 8032 Zurich, Switzerland

M. Juergensen
Institute for Social Medicine and Epidemiology, University Luebeck, Ratzeburger Allee 160 (Hs 50), 23562 Luebeck, Germany

Institute for History of Medicine and Science Studies, University Luebeck, Koenigstr. 42, 23552 Luebeck, Germany

A. Katalinic
Institute for Social Medicine and Epidemiology, University Luebeck, Ratzeburger Allee 160 (Hs 50), 23562 Luebeck, Germany
Institute for Cancer Epidemiology, University Luebeck, Ratzeburger Allee 160 (Hs 50), 23562 Luebeck, Germany

V. Rohde
Medical Practice of Urology, Auguststr. 4, 23611 Bad Schwartau, Germany

Hongyan Ren
Department of Urology, The First Affiliated Hospital of Chongqing Medical University, No. 1 Youyi Road, Yuzhong District, Chongqing 400016, China

Ping Tang
Department of Cardiology, The First Affiliated Hospital of Chongqing Medical University, No. 1 Youyi Road, Yuzhong District, Chongqing 400016, China

Qinghua Zhao
Department of Nursing, The First Affiliated Hospital of Chongqing Medical University, No. 1 Youyi Road, Yuzhong District, Chongqing 400016, China

Guosheng Ren
Molecular Oncology and Epigenetics Laboratory, The First Affiliated Hospital of Chongqing Medical University, No. 1 Youyi Road, Yuzhong District, Chongqing 400016, China

Yoshiyuki Miyazawa, Yoshitaka Sekine, Takahiro Syuto, Masashi Nomura, Hidekazu Koike, Hiroshi Matsui, Yasuhiro Shibata, Kazuto Ito and Kazuhiro Suzuki
Department of Urology, Gunma University Graduate School of Medicine, 3-9-22 Showa-machi, Maebashi, Gunma 371-8511, Japan

Long-sheng Wang, Shao-jun Chen, Jun-feng Zhang, Meng-nan Liu, Jun-hua Zheng and Xu-dong Yao
Department of Urology, Shanghai Tenth People's Hospital, Tongji University, School of Medicine, Shanghai 200072, China

Brenda Sirovich, Douglas J. Robertson and Philip P. Goodney
White River Junction VA Medical Center, 215 N Main Street, White River Junction, VT 05009, USA
The Dartmouth Institute for Health Policy and Clinical Practice, Geisel School of Medicine at Dartmouth College, Hanover, NH, USA

Florian R. Schroeck
White River Junction VA Medical Center, 215 N Main Street, White River Junction, VT 05009, USA
Section of Urology, Dartmouth Hitchcock Medical Center, Lebanon, NH, USA
Norris Cotton Cancer Center, Dartmouth Hitchcock Medical Center, Lebanon, NH, USA
The Dartmouth Institute for Health Policy and Clinical Practice, Geisel School of Medicine at Dartmouth College, Hanover, NH, USA

John D. Seigne
Section of Urology, Dartmouth Hitchcock Medical Center, Lebanon, NH, USA
Norris Cotton Cancer Center, Dartmouth Hitchcock Medical Center, Lebanon, NH, USA
The Dartmouth Institute for Health Policy and Clinical Practice, Geisel School of Medicine at Dartmouth College, Hanover, NH, USA

Saori Yonekubo, Satoshi Tatemichi, Kazuyasu Maruyama and Mamoru Kobayashi
Central Research Laboratories, Kissei Pharmaceutical Co., Ltd, 4365-1 Kashiwabara, Hotaka, Azumino-City, Nagano-Pref 399-8304, Japan

Yoko Saitoh-Maeda1, Takashi Kawahara, Yasuhide Miyoshi1, Sohgo Tsutsumi1, Daiji Takamoto1, Kota Shimokihara, Yuutaro Hayashi, Taku Mochizuki, Mari Ohtaka, Manami Nakamura, Yusuke Hattori, Jun-ichi Teranishi, Yasushi Yumura and Hiroji Uemura
Departments of Urology and Renal Transplantation, Yokohama City University Medical Center, 4-57 Urafune-cho, Minami-ku, Yokohama, Kanagawa 2320024, Japan

Kimito Osaka, Hiroki Ito, Kazuhide Makiyama, Noboru Nakaigawa and Masahiro Yao
Department of Urology, Yokohama City University Graduate School of Medicine, Yokohama, Japan

Taku Mochizuki, Daiji Takamoto, Yusuke Hattori, Jun-ichi Teranishi, Yasuhide Miyoshi, Yasushi Yumura and Hiroji Uemura
Departments of Urology and Renal Transplantation, Yokohama City University Medical Center, 4-57 Urafune-cho, Minami-ku, Yokohama, Kanagawa, 2320024, Japan

Takashi Kawahara
Departments of Urology and Renal Transplantation, Yokohama City University Medical Center, 4-57 Urafune-cho, Minami-ku, Yokohama, Kanagawa, 2320024, Japan
Department of Urology, Yokohama City University, Graduate School of Medicine, Yokohama, Japan

Kazuhide Makiyama and Masahiro Yao
Department of Urology, Yokohama City University, Graduate School of Medicine, Yokohama, Japan

Marloes J. Tijnagel, Jeroen R. Scheepe and Bertil F. M. Blok
Department of Urology, Erasmus University Medical Center, P.O. Box 2040 3000 CA Rotterdam, The Netherlands

Lujia Zou, Shanhua Mao, Shenghua Liu, Limin Zhang, Tian Yang, Yun Hu, Qiang Ding and Haowen Jiang
Department of Urology, Huashan Hospital, Fudan University, No.12 Wulumuqi Middle Road, Shanghai 200040, People's Republic of China

Daniel N. Cagney and Pierre Thirion
Department of Radiation Oncology, St. Luke's Radiation Oncology Network, Highfield Road Rathgar, Dublin, Ireland

Mary Dunne, Carmel O'Shea, Marie Finn, Emma Noone, Martina Sheehan, Lesley McDonagh, Lydia O'Sullivan and John Armstrong
Department of Radiation Oncology, St. Luke's Radiation Oncology Network, Highfield Road Rathgar, Dublin, Ireland
Clinical Trials Unit, St. Luke's Radiation Oncology Network, Dublin, Ireland

Jae-Yoon Kim, Seok-Ho Kang, Jun Cheon, Jeong-Gu Lee, Je-Jong Kim and Sung-Gu Kang
Department of Urology, Korea University College of Medicine, 73 Inchon-Ro, Sungbuk-gu, Seoul 136-705, Republic of Korea

Takuma Narita, Shingo Hatakeyama, Takuya Koie, Shogo Hosogoe, Teppei Matsumoto, Osamu Soma, Hayato Yamamoto, Yuki Tobisawa and Takahiro Yoneyama
Department of Urology, Hirosaki University Graduate School of Medicine, 5 Zaifu-cho, Hirosaki 036-8562, Japan

Chikara Ohyama
Department of Urology, Hirosaki University Graduate School of Medicine, 5 Zaifu-cho, Hirosaki 036-8562, Japan
Department of Advanced Transplant and Regenerative Medicine, Hirosaki University Graduate School of Medicine, Hirosaki, Japan

Tohru Yoneyama and Yasuhiro Hashimoto
Department of Advanced Transplant and Regenerative Medicine, Hirosaki University Graduate School of Medicine, Hirosaki, Japan

Ran Cheng, Meng Zhao and Kefang Wang
School of Nursing, Shandong University, No.44, Wenhua Xi Road, Jinan, Shandong 250012, China

Dongjuan Xu
School of Nursing, Shandong University, No.44, Wenhua Xi Road, Jinan, Shandong 250012, China
School of Nursing, Purdue University, West Lafayette, Indiana 47907, USA

Aixia Ma
Department of endocrinology, Qilu Hospital of Shandong University, Jinan, Shandong 250012, China

Zhongyu Jian, Shijian Feng, Yuntian Chen, Xin Wei, Deyi Luo, Hong Li and Kunjie Wang
Department of Urology, Institute of Urology (Laboratory of Reconstructive Urology), West China Hospital, Sichuan University, No. 37 Guo Xue Xiang, Chengdu, Sichuan 610041, People's Republic of China

Ronald Wagner Pereira Coelho, Janise Silva Moreno and Leudivan Ribeiro Nogueira
Aldenora Bello Cancer Hospital, Seroa da Mota Street, Apeadouro, São Luís 65031-630, Brazil

Jaqueline Diniz Pinho
Federal University of Pará, Brazil, Gov. José Malcher Avenue, Belém 66055-260, Brazil

Dimitrius Vidal e Oliveira Garbis, Athiene Maniva Teixeira do Nascimento and Laisson de Moura Feitoza
Federal University of Maranhão, São Luís, Brazil, dos Portugueses Avenue, Bacanga, São Luís 65080-805, Brazil

José Ribamar Rodrigues Calixto
Federal University of Maranhão, São Luís, Brazil, dos Portugueses Avenue, Bacanga, São Luís 65080-805, Brazil
University Hospital of Federal University of Maranhão, Barão de Itapari Street, Centro, São Luís, Brazil

Joyce Santos Larges
University Hospital of Federal University of Maranhão, Barão de Itapari Street, Centro, São Luís, Brazil

Gyl Eanes Barros Silva
University Hospital of Federal University of Maranhão, Barão de Itapari Street, Centro, São Luís, Brazil
Department of Radiology and Pathology, Ribeirão Preto Medical School of University of São Paulo, Bandeirantes Avenue, Monte Alegre, Ribeirão Preto 14049-900, Brazil
Ribeirão Preto Medical School - USP, Av. Bandeirantes, 3900, Ribeirão Preto, SP 14048-900, Brazil

Leandra Naira Zambelli Ramalho
Department of Radiology and Pathology, Ribeirão Preto Medical School of University of São Paulo, Bandeirantes Avenue, Monte Alegre, Ribeirão Preto 14049-900, Brazil

Antônio Augusto Moura da Silva
Public Heath Department, Federal University of Maranhão, São Luís, Brazil, dos Portugueses Avenue, Bacanga, São Luís 65080-805, Brazil

Dingyi Liu, Qi Tang, Haidong Wang, Jian Wang, Yanfeng Zhou, Jiashun Yu and Wenmin Li
Department of Urology, Department of Radiology, Shanghai Punan Hospital, Shanghai, People's Republic of China

Mingwei Wang, Wenlong Zhou and Boke Liu
Department of Urology, Shanghai Jiao Tong University Medical School Affiliated Ruijin Hospital, 197 Ruijin Er Road, Shanghai 200025, People's Republic of China

Yuan Shao
Department of Urology, Shanghai Jiao Tong University Medical School Affiliated Ruijin Hospital, 197 Ruijin Er Road, Shanghai 200025, People's Republic of China
Department of Urology, Shanghai Jiao Tong University Medical School Affiliated Ruijin Hospital North, 999 Xiwang Road, Shanghai 201801, People's Republic of China

Weimu Xia
Department of Urology, Chinese People's Liberation Army Hospital 184, Yingtan, People's Republic of China

Sang Hu
Department of Urology, Shanghai Post and Telecommunication Hospital, 666 Changle Road, Shanghai 200040, People's Republic of China

Karthik Rao
Johns Hopkins University School of Medicine, Baltimore, MD, USA

Stella Liang and Michael Cardamone
Financial Analysis Unit, Johns Hopkins Health System, Baltimore, MD, USA

Nrupen Bhavsar
Department of Epidemiology, Johns Hopkins Bloomberg School of Public Health, Baltimore, MD, USA

Corinne E. Joshu
Department of Epidemiology, Johns Hopkins Bloomberg School of Public Health, Baltimore, MD, USA
Sidney Kimmel Comprehensive Cancer Center at Johns Hopkins, Baltimore, MD, USA

Elizabeth A. Platz
Department of Epidemiology, Johns Hopkins Bloomberg School of Public Health, Baltimore, MD, USA
Sidney Kimmel Comprehensive Cancer Center at Johns Hopkins, Baltimore, MD, USA
Department of Urology and the James Buchanan Brady Urological Institute, Johns Hopkins University School of Medicine, Baltimore, MD, USA

William G. Nelson
Sidney Kimmel Comprehensive Cancer Center at Johns Hopkins, Baltimore, MD, USA
Department of Urology and the James Buchanan Brady Urological Institute, Johns Hopkins University School of Medicine, Baltimore, MD, USA
Department of Environmental Health Sciences, Johns Hopkins Bloomberg School of Public Health, Baltimore, MD, USA

Kyle Marmen
Johns Hopkins Health Care, Glen Burnie, Baltimore, MD, USA

H. Ballentine Carter
Department of Urology and the James Buchanan Brady Urological Institute, Johns Hopkins University School of Medicine, Baltimore, MD, USA

Michael C. Albert
Johns Hopkins Community Physicians, Johns Hopkins Medical Institutions, Baltimore, MD, USA

Craig E. Pollack
Department of Medicine, Johns Hopkins University School of Medicine, 2024 E. Monument Street, Suite 2-519, Baltimore, MD 21287, USA

Yan-Fei Jia and Qian Feng
Lanzhou University Second Hospital, Lanzhou 730020, People's Republic of China

Zheng-Yan Ge
Xiyuan Hospital, China Academy of Traditional Chinese Medicine, Beijing 100091, People's Republic of China

Ying Guo, Fang Zhou, Kai-Shu Zhang and Yi-Qun Gu
Graduate School of Peking Union Medical College, No. 9 Dongdansantiao, Dongcheng District, Beijing 100730, People's Republic of China
National Health and Family Planning Key Laboratory of Male Reproductive Health, Department of Male Clinical Research, National Research Institute for Family Planning, Beijing 100081, People's Republic of China

Wei Wang, Wen-Hong Lu and Xiao-Wei Liang
National Health and Family Planning Key Laboratory of Male Reproductive Health, Department of Male Clinical Research, National Research Institute for Family Planning, Beijing 100081, People's Republic of China

Liang Cao, Cheng-ming Jia, Lei-tao Wu, Ying-qi Li, Wen Wang and Jing Ma
Department of Traditional Chinese Medicine, Xijing Hospital, Fourth Military Medical University, Xi'an 710032, People's Republic of China

Sha Zhang, Wei He and Zhe Li
Shanxi University of Chinese Medicine, Xian yang 712046, People's Republic of China

Atif Ali hashmi, Zubaida Fida Hussain, Muhammad Irfan, Erum Yousuf Khan, Naveen Faridi and Hanna Naqvi
Liaquat National Hospital and Medical College, Karachi, Pakistan

Muhammad Muzzammil Edhi
Brown University, Providence, RI, USA

Amir Khan
Kandahar University, Kandahar, Afghanistan

Jie Yang, Pei Lu, Ke-liang Chen and Wei Zhang
Department of Urology, First Affiliated Hospital of Nanjing Medical University, Nanjing 210029, Jiangsu, China

Rong-zhen Tao
Department of Urology, First Affiliated Hospital of Nanjing Medical University, Nanjing 210029, Jiangsu, China

Department of Urology, The Affiliated Jiangning Hospital with Nanjing Medical University, Nanjing, Jiangsu, China

Ying-heng Huang, Xiao-rong He, Li-di Wan, Jing Wang, Xin Tang and Meng-xing Chen
First Clinical Medical College, Nanjing Medical University, Nanjing, Jiangsu, China

Xin-kun Huang
Department of Urology, The Affiliated Jiangning Hospital with Nanjing Medical University, Nanjing, Jiangsu, China

F. Dimitriadis, J. Giannakis, S. Skouros and N. Sofikitis
Department of Urology, School of Medicine, Ioannina University, Ioannina, Greece

A. Zachariou
Department of Urology, School of Medicine, Ioannina University, Ioannina, Greece
3 Spyridi Street, 38221 Volos, Greece

C. Mamoulakis
Department of Urology, University General Hospital of Heraklion, University of Crete, Medical School, Heraklion, Greece

M. Filiponi
Department of Urology, ELPIS Hospital, Volos, Greece

P. Tsounapi and A. Takenaka
Department of Urology, School of Medicine, Tottori University, Yonago, Japan

Patrick Betschart, Dominik Abt and Hans-Peter Schmid
Department of Urology, Cantonal Hospital St. Gallen, St. Gallen, Switzerland

Valentin Zumstein
Department of Urology, Cantonal Hospital St. Gallen, St. Gallen, Switzerland
Department of Urology, University Medical Center Hamburg-Eppendorf, Hamburg, Germany

Cedric Michael Panje
Department of Radiation Oncology, Cantonal Hospital St. Gallen, St. Gallen, Switzerland

Paul Martin Putora
Department of Radiation Oncology, Cantonal Hospital St. Gallen, St. Gallen, Switzerland
Department of Radiation Oncology, Inselspital, Bern University Hospital, Bern, Switzerland

Yong-tong Zhu, Rui Hua, Song Quan and Qing-jun Chu
Reproductive Medicine Center, Department of Obstetrics and Gynecology, Nanfang Hospital/ The First School of Clinical Medicine, Southern Medical University, Guangzhou, China

Chun-yan Wang
Department of Neurology, Integrated Hospital of Traditional Chinese Medicine, Southern Medical University, Guangzhou, China

Wan-long Tan
Department of Urology, Nanfang Hospital, Southern Medical University, Guangzhou, China

Young Saing Kim
Division of Medical Oncology, Department of Internal Medicine, Gil Medical Center, Gachon University College of Medicine, Incheon, South Korea

Kyung Kim, Su Jin Lee and Se Hoon Park
Division of Hematology-Oncology, Department of Medicine, Sungkyunkwan University Samsung Medical Center, Sungkyunkwan University School of Medicine, 81 Irwon-ro, Gangnam-gu, Seoul 06351, South Korea

Ghee-Young Kwon
Department of Pathology and Translational Genomics, Sungkyunkwan University Samsung Medical Center, Seoul, South Korea

Ding Peng
Department of Urology, Peking University First Hospital, No. 8, Xishiku Street, Xicheng District, Beijing 100034, China
Institute of Urology, Peking University, Beijing 100034, China

Cui-jian Zhang, Qi Tang, Lei Zhang, Kai-wei Yang, Xiao-teng Yu, Yanqing Gong, Xue-song Li, Zhi-song He and Li-qun Zhou
Department of Urology, Peking University First Hospital, No. 8, Xishiku Street, Xicheng District, Beijing 100034, China
Institute of Urology, Peking University, Beijing 100034, China
National Urological Cancer Center, Beijing 100034, China
Urogenital Diseases (male) Molecular Diagnosis and Treatment Center, Peking University, Beijing 100034, China

Li-jin Zhang, Bin Wu, Zhen-lei Zha, Hu Zhao, Jun Yuan and Ye-jun Feng
Departments of Urology, Affiliated Jiang-yin Hospital of the Southeast University Medical College, Jiang-yin 214400, China

Wei Qu
Departments of Pharmacy, Affiliated Jiang-yin Hospital of the Southeast University Medical College, Jiang-yin 214400, China

Myong Kim, Cheryn Song and Hanjong Ahn
Department of Urology, Asan Medical Center, University of Ulsan College of Medicine, 88 Olympic-Ro 43 Gil Songpa-Gu, Seoul 05505, Republic of Korea

Se Un Jeong and Yong Mee Cho
Department of Pathology, Asan Medical Center, University of Ulsan College of Medicine, Seoul 05505, Republic of Korea

Jae Yoon Ro
Department of Pathology and Genomic Medicine, Houston Methodist Hospital, Weill Medical College of Cornell University, Houston, TX 10065, USA

Aram Kim
Department of Urology, Konkuk University Medical Center, Konkuk University School of Medicine, Seoul 05030, Republic of Korea

Michael Froehner, Ulrike Heberling, Vladimir Novotny, Stefan Zastrow and Manfred P. Wirth
Department of Urology, University Hospital Carl Gustav Carus, Technische Universität Dresden, Fetscherstrasse 74, D-01307 Dresden, Germany

Rainer Koch
Department of Medical Statistics and Biometry, University Hospital Carl Gustav Carus, Technische Universität Dresden, Fetscherstrasse 74, D-01307 Dresden, Germany

Matthias Hübler
Department of Anesthesiology, University Hospital Carl Gustav Carus, Technische Universität Dresden, Fetscherstrasse 74, D-01307 Dresden, Germany

Oliver W. Hakenberg
Department of Urology, University of Rostock, Ernst-Heydemann-Strasse 6, D-18055 Rostock, Germany

Takashi Kawahara, Yukari Ishiguro, Shinji Ohtake, Yusuke Ito, Hiroki Ito, Kazuhide Makiyama, Keiichi Kondo, Yasuhide Miyoshi, Yasushi Yumura1, Narihiko Hayashi, Hisashi Hasumi, Kimito Osaka, Kentaro Muraoka, Koji Izumi, Jun-ichi Teranishi, Masahiro Yao and Noboru Nakaigawa
Department of Urology, Yokohama City University Graduate School of Medicine, 3-9 Fukuura, Kanazawa-ku, Yokohama, Kanagawa 2360004, Japan

Hiroji Uemura
Department of Urology, Yokohama City University Graduate School of Medicine, 3-9 Fukuura, Kanazawa-ku, Yokohama, Kanagawa 2360004, Japan
Department of Urology and Renal Transplantation, Yokohama City University Medical Center, Yokohama, Japan

Ikuma Kato
Department of Pathology, Yokohama City University Hospital, Yokohama, Japan

Itamar Getzler, Zaher Bahouth, Ofer Nativ and Sarel Halachmi
Department of Urology, Bnai Zion Medical Center, Faculty of Medicine, Technion - Israel Institute of Technology, Golomb 47, 31048 Haifa, Israel

Jacob Rubinstein
Department of Mathematics, Technion - Israel Institute of Technology, Haifa, Israel

Florian H. H. Brill, Henrik Gabriel, Holger Brill and Jan-Hendrik Klock
Dr. Brill + Partner GmbH Institute for Hygiene and Microbiology, Stiegstück 34, 22339 Hamburg, Germany

Joerg Steinmann
Institute of Medical Microbiology, University Hospital Essen, Essen, Germany
Institute of Clinical Hygiene, Medical Microbiology and Infectiology, Paracelsus Medical University, Klinikum Nürnberg, Nuremberg, Germany

Andreas Arndt
Department of Research and Development, B. Braun Medical Ltd., Sempach, Switzerland

Index

A

Active Surveillance, 134-136, 138-140, 219

Adrenocortical Carcinoma, 71-74

Androgen Deprivation Therapy, 85, 89-90, 92, 135

Angiogenesis, 199, 202, 208

Antihypertensive Drug, 149-150, 161-162

B

Biochemical Recurrence, 211, 219-220

Bladder Cancer, 30-31, 35-36, 51-57, 66-67, 69-70, 99, 106, 163-164, 166-168, 202

Bladder Outlet Obstruction, 58, 65, 113

C

Calcium Channel Blocker, 162

Castration-resistant Prostate Cancer, 37, 41, 92

Chi-square Test, 11, 46, 76, 115, 165, 204

Chyluria, 128-132

Computed Tomography, 66, 73, 94, 101, 105, 128, 131-132, 170, 174

Cryotherapy, 135, 138

Cystectomy, 30, 35-36, 54, 66-67, 69-70, 99-101, 103-106, 163-165, 167-168, 196-200, 220

Cystometrogram, 58-59, 65

Cystoscopy, 51-53, 55, 93-97, 128-131

D

Dehydroepiandrosterone, 37-39, 41

Dihydrotestosterone, 37-39, 41

E

Electronic Health Record, 51-53, 55-56

Epidemiologic, 3, 8-9, 121, 126-127, 153, 162, 199

Epidermal Growth Factor Receptor, 49, 163, 167-168

Erectile Dysfunction, 27, 138, 183, 194-195

External Beam Radiotherapy, 92, 215-216, 220

F

Female Sexual Dysfunction, 176-177, 182-183

Flexible Ureteroscopy, 93, 169, 174-175

Flow Cytometry, 43, 46

G

Gene Expression, 62, 197, 225

Gleason Score, 85, 87, 135-136, 212, 214-215, 219-220

Glomerular Filtration Rate, 106

H

Holmium Laser Lithotripsy, 169-170, 173-175

Hydronephrosis, 81-83, 94-96, 98-106, 169-170, 172-174

I

Ileal Neobladder Construction, 99-101, 103-106

Immunohistochemistry, 40, 60, 163-164

Intracytoplasmic Sperm Injection, 192, 195

L

Laparoscopic Pyelolithotomy, 10-15, 18

Laparoscopic Ureterolithotomy, 93, 97-98

Laparoscopy, 16, 93, 98, 129

M

Magnetic Resonance Imaging, 73, 128, 132

Medication Adherence, 75, 78

Mirabegron, 176-183

N

Nephrectomy, 49, 203-205, 208-209

Nephrolithiasis, 18, 169, 172

Neurogenic Bladder, 65, 78

Neutrophil-to-lymphocyte Ratio (NLR), 71

Non-vascularized Bladder Graft, 79-80, 83

O

Overactive Bladder, 8, 58, 65, 75, 77-78, 107-113, 176, 181-183

Oxidative Stress, 141, 143, 146-148

P

Penile Cancer, 121-123, 126-127

Percutaneous Nephrolithotomy, 10, 12-15, 17-18, 172-174, 191

Perineural Invasion, 122, 125-126, 211-212, 214-215, 219-220

Phosphodiesterase-5 Inhibitor, 192

Polyhexanide, 221-226

Polymerase Chain Reaction, 197, 201

Progression-free Survival, 73, 92

Prostate Biopsy, 134, 139, 220

Prostate-specific Antigen, 92, 133, 139-140, 211, 219-220, 233

Psoas Muscle Index (PMI), 66

Pyelonephritis, 100, 105

R

Radical Cystectomy, 30, 35-36, 66-67, 69-70, 99-101, 103-106, 163, 165, 167, 196-197, 199-200, 220

Radiotherapy, 38, 85-86, 89-92, 105, 121-123, 125, 127, 135-136, 138, 163, 185, 191, 211-212, 215-217, 219-220

Randomized Controlled Trial, 11-12, 17-18, 29, 78, 92, 174

Renal Cell Carcinoma, 43-44, 48-50, 71, 74, 185, 191, 203-204, 209-210

Robot-assisted Radical Prostatectomy, 114, 120, 233

Robotic Surgery, 16

S

Sarcopenia, 66-70

Scrotal Hemorrhage, 192-195

Self-help Position Therapy (SHPT), 169, 171

Sex Hormone-binding Globulin, 141-142, 145, 147

Spinal Cord Injury, 76

Squamous Cell Carcinoma, 121, 126-127

Stone-free Rate, 10, 17, 174

Suprapubic Catheter, 114, 119-120

T

Testicular Sperm Aspiration, 192-193, 195

U

Ultrasonography, 12, 100, 195, 204

Unilateral Pedal Lymphangiography, 128, 132

Ureteral Stent, 54, 80, 93-94

Ureteroscopic Lithotripsy, 93, 95-98

Urethral Catheterization, 114, 117, 119

Urinary Diversion, 30, 32-33, 35-36, 83, 99, 104-106, 120

Urinary Incontinence, 1, 4-9, 75, 77-78, 107, 113, 117-118, 138, 176-177, 179-180, 182-183, 221

Urinary Tract Infection, 17, 78-79, 108-110, 112, 221, 225

Urolithiasis, 18, 98, 174-175, 184-185, 188, 190-191

Urothelial Carcinoma, 70, 106, 163-165, 196, 198, 200-202

www.ingramcontent.com/pod-product-compliance
Lightning Source LLC
Chambersburg PA
CBHW061255190326

41458CB00011B/3678